ESSENTIAL IMMUNOLOGY

Essential Immunology

IVAN M. ROITT
MA, DSc(Oxon), FRCPath
Professor and Head of Department of Immunology, Middlesex Hospital Medical School, London W1

FOURTH EDITION

BLACKWELL SCIENTIFIC PUBLICATIONS
OXFORD LONDON EDINBURGH
BOSTON MELBOURNE

Editorial offices:
Osney Mead, Oxford, OX2 OEL
8 John Street, London, WC1N 2ES
9 Forrest Road, Edinburgh, EH1 2QH
52 Beacon Street, Boston
Massachusetts 02108, USA
214 Berkeley Street, Carlton
Victoria 3053, Australia

First published 1971
Reprinted 1972 (twice), 1973 (twice)
Second edition 1974
Reprinted 1975
Third edition 1977
Reprinted 1978, 1979
Fourth edition 1980

Spanish editions 1972, 1975
Italian editions 1973, 1975
Portuguese edition 1973
French edition 1975
Dutch edition 1975
Japanese edition 1976
German edition 1977
Polish edition 1977

Set by Santype International Ltd
Salisbury, Wiltshire
Printed and bound in Great Britain by
Butler & Tanner Ltd
Frome, Somerset

DISTRIBUTORS

USA
Blackwell Mosby Book Distributors
11830 Westline Industrial Drive
St Louis, Missouri 63141

Canada
Blackwell Mosby Book Distributors
120 Melford Drive, Scarborough
Ontario, M1B 2X4

Australia
Blackwell Scientific Book Distributors
214 Berkeley Street, Carlton
Victoria 3053

British Library
Cataloguing in Publication Data

Roitt, Ivan Maurice
Essential immunology—4th ed.
1. Immunology
I. Title
616.07'9 QR181

ISBN 0 632 00739 7

TO MY FAMILY

Contents

Preface

The 3rd edition has undergone some very painful surgery and I hope the new model does justice to the exciting developments which continue to make immunology such a delight.

New sections have been introduced dealing with idiotypic networks, monoclonal antibodies, lymphoid malignancies and blood groups, while particular attention has been drawn to the subjects of amyloid, lymphocyte ontogeny, dendritic macrophages and granuloma formation. At the technical level, the fluorescence-activated cell sorter, laser nephelometry and immunochemical analysis of membrane components are introduced.

Sections on cell-mediated immune responses, the genetic basis of antibody variability and control, the biological significance of the major histocompatibility complex and the nature of the T-cell receptor, immune complex hypersensitivity and the aetiology and treatment of autoimmune disease, have all been radically revised.

I have stressed the role of the acute inflammatory reaction in the defence against infection and given fuller accounts of microbial killing mechanisms and the efficacy of communal vaccination programmes. In addition, the importance of seeing hypersensitivity reactions as an exaggeration of normal defence processes is underlined.

Many diagrams are new or have been revised and the quality of many of the photographs upgraded. In particular, the introduction of colour plates illustrating light microscopy of cells involved in the immune response and the appearance of certain dermal hypersensitivity reactions should be an improvement.

I am indebted for their invaluable knowledge and wisdom to my colleagues, Franco Bottazzo, Jonathan Brostoff, Anne Cooke, Deborah Doniach, Frank Hay, Peter Lydyard, Ian McConnell, Philip Penfold and John Playfair. As ever, my gratitude is due to Christine Meats for her help with secretarial and administrative matters.

Acknowledgements

First edition

While not wishing to saddle my colleagues with responsibility for some of the wilder views expressed in this book it would be ungrateful of me not to acknowledge with pleasure the helpful discussions I have had with Jonathan Brostoff, George Dick, Deborah Doniach, Frank Hay, Leslie Hudson, Gerald Jones and John Playfair. I would like to express my appreciation to my secretary, Gladys Stead, who helped to prepare and assemble the manuscript with her usual impeccable expertise and who always encouraged me when my authorship seemed to be faltering. I also wish to acknowledge my debt to Valerie Petts for her excellent help with the photographs. My thanks also to the many people who supplied material for the illustrations; they are acknowledged at the appropriate place in the text. In particular, Bill Weigle kindly let me have unpublished information. Finally let me say that the pain of converting blank paper to written manuscript at home was made bearable by the loving support and understanding of my wife and family.

Second edition

The necessity for a second edition has been dictated by the breakneck increase in immunological knowledge since this book was first written—clearly the subject has too many adherents! My colleagues will know how much I have appreciated their invaluable discussions; particularly I must mention Ita Askonas, Jonathan Brostoff, Deborah Doniach, Arnold Greenberg, Hilliard Festenstein, Frank Hay, M. Hobart, Leslie Hudson, D. L. Brown, John Playfair and Mac Turner. Once again I would have been lost without the admirable help of my secretary, Gladys Stead. Even the publishers have been nice!

Third edition

The indecent speed at which we lurch forward has necessitated radical revision of many sections in this new edition.

The anatomical basis of the immune response, immunity to infection and the biological significance of the major histocompatibility complex have all been given fuller treatment. A summary has been added to the end of each chapter which should be a help to those poor souls for whom circumstances make revision essential. The index has received serious attention and I hope it will be of greater value. I am most grateful to the many colleagues whom wisdom I have sought: Franco Bottazzo, Jonathan Brostoff, Peter Campbell, Deborah Doniach, Hilliard Festenstein, Peter Gould, Frank Hay, Peter Lachman, Ian McConnell, John Playfair and Martin Raff. Finally, my thanks are due to Miss Christine Meats for her most able and cheerful secretarial assistance.

1 Introduction

The essential function of the immune system is defence against infection. Babies born with a defect in a critical part of this system suffer continued infections and in many cases may die if recourse to advanced medical technology is not available. Lower animal forms possess so-called *innate* or *non-specific* immune mechanisms such as phagocytosis of bacteria by specialized cells, which afford them protection against infecting organisms. Additionally, higher animals have evolved an *adaptive* or *acquired immune response* which provides a flexible, *specific* and more effective reaction to different infections.

At the heart of the adaptive immune response lie three important features, memory, specificity and the recognition of 'non-self'. Our experience of the subsequent protection (*immunity*) afforded by exposure to many infectious illnesses can in fact lead us to this view.

We rarely suffer twice from such diseases as measles, mumps, chicken-pox, whooping cough and so forth. The first contact with an infectious organism clearly imprints some information, imparts some *memory*, so that the body is effectively prepared to repel any later invasion by that organism. This protection is provided by the adaptive immune response evoked as a reaction to the infectious agent behaving as an antigen (figure 1.1). One of the agents of the immune response is antibody which combines with antigen to cause its elimination.

By following the production of antibody on the first and second contacts with antigen we can see the basis for the development of immunity. For example, when we inject a bacterial product such as staphylococcal toxoid into a rabbit, several days elapse before antibodies can be detected in the blood; these reach a peak and then fall (figure 1.2). If we now allow the animal to rest and then give a second injection of toxoid, the course of events is dramatically altered. Within two to three days the antibody level in the blood rises steeply to reach much higher values than were observed in the *primary response*. This *secondary*

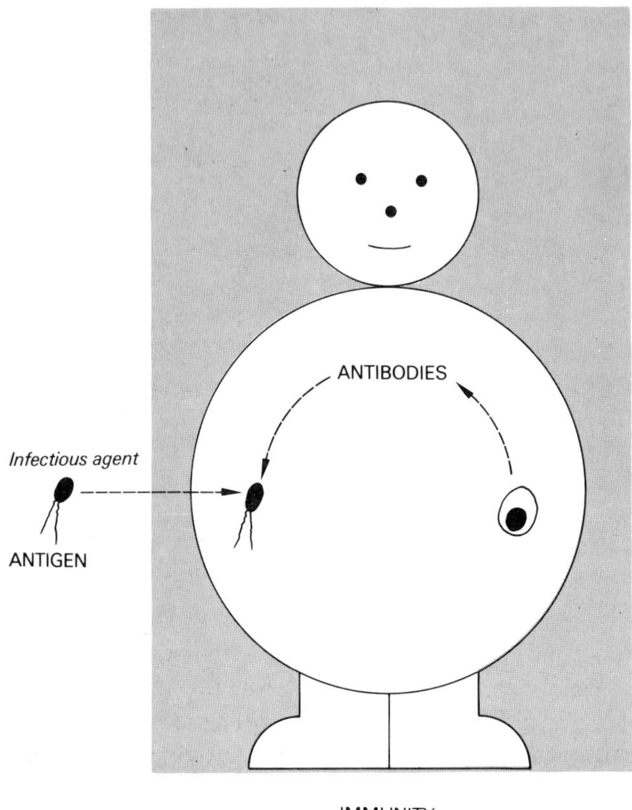

FIGURE 1.1. Antibodies (*anti*-foreign *bodies*) are produced by host white cells on contact with the invading micro-organism which is acting as an antigen (i.e. *gen*erates *anti*bodies). The individual may then be immune to further attacks.

response then is characterized by a more rapid and more abundant production of antibody resulting from the 'tuning up' or priming of the antibody-forming system to provide a population of memory cells after first exposure to antigen.

Vaccination utilizes this principle by employing a relatively harmless form of the antigen (e.g. a killed virus) as the primary stimulus to imprint 'memory'. The body's defences are thereby alerted and any subsequent contact with the virulent form of the organism will lead to a secondary response with an early and explosive production of antibody which will usually prevent the infection from taking hold.

Specificity was mentioned earlier as a fundamental feature of the adaptive immunological response. The establishment of memory or immunity by one organism does not confer

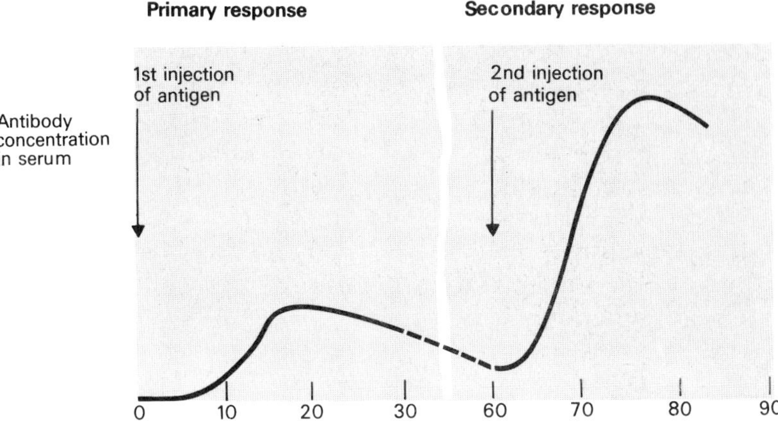

FIGURE 1.2. *Primary and secondary response.* A rabbit is injected on two separate occasions with staphylococcal toxoid. The antibody response on the second contact with antigen is more rapid and more intense.

protection against another unrelated organism. After an attack of measles we are immune to further infection but are susceptible to other agents such as the polio or mumps viruses. The body can, in fact, differentiate specifically between the two organisms.

This ability to recognize one antigen and distinguish it from another goes even further. The individual must also recognize what is foreign, i.e. what is '*non-self*'. The failure to discriminate between 'self' and 'non-self' could lead to the synthesis of antibodies directed against components of the subject's own body (*autoantibodies*) which in principle could prove to be highly embarrassing. On purely theoretical grounds it seemed to Burnet and Fenner that the body must develop some mechanism whereby 'self' and 'non-self' could be distinguished, and they postulated that those circulating body components which were able to reach the developing lymphoid system in the perinatal period could in some way be 'learnt' as 'self'. A permanent unresponsiveness or tolerance would then be created so that as immunological maturity were reached there would normally be an inability to respond to 'self' components. As we shall see later, these predictions have been amply verified.

The non-specific immunity mechanisms, such as the uptake of bacteria by phagocytic cells which we mentioned earlier, are not heightened by subsequent infections and in this respect differ fundamentally from the adaptive immune response. Clearly this has evolved to provide more effective defence in that the small fraction of immunological cells which are capable of recognizing the particular agents infecting the body at any one time increase in number and synthesize antibodies which greatly speed up the disposal of these organisms by facilitating their adherence to phagocytic cells (see chapter 7). In other words the specific adaptive immune response operates to a considerable extent by increasing the efficiency of the non-specific immunity systems.

Some historical perspectives

Space does not allow more than a cursory survey of some of the outstanding contributions to the early development of immunology.

India and China (ancient times)—Practice of 'variolation' in which protection against smallpox was obtained by inoculating live organisms from disease pustules (dangerous!).

Jenner (1798)—Protective effect of vaccination with non-virulent cowpox against smallpox infection (noting the pretty pox-free skin of the milkmaids).

Pasteur (1881)—Vaccine for anthrax using attenuated organisms.

Metchnikoff (1883)—Role of phagocytes in immunity.

Von Behring (1890)—Recognized antibodies in serum to diphtheria toxin.

Denys & Leclef (1895)—Phagocytosis greatly enhanced by immunization—innate response amplified by adaptive.

Ehrlich (1897)—Side-chain receptor theory of antibody synthesis.

Bordet (1899)—Lysis of cells by antibody requires co-operation of serum factors now collectively termed complement.

Landsteiner (1900)—Human ABO groups and natural isohaemagglutinins.

Richet & Portier (1902)—Anaphylaxis (opposite of prophylaxis).

Wright (1903)—Relation of opsonic activity to phagocytosis. (Basis for Sir Colenso Ridgeon's assertion in Shaw's 'The Doctor's Dilemma' that vaccines stimulate antibodies (opsonins) which 'butter' the germs for ingestion by phagocytes, in contrast with 'B.B.'s' resonant belief that any anti-toxin would non-specifically 'stimulate the phagocytes'.)

von Pirquet & Schick (1905)—Description of serum sickness following injection of foreign serum.

von Pirquet (1906)—Relation of immunity and hypersensitivity.

Fleming (1922)—Lysozyme

Zinsser (1925)—Contrast between immediate and delayed-type hypersensitivity.

Heidelberger & Kendall (1930–35)—Quantitative precipitin studies on antigen–antibody interactions.

Let us examine the work of Heidelberger and Kendall and its implications in more detail and with some benefit.

The classical precipitin reaction

When an antigen solution is mixed in correct proportions with a potent antiserum, a precipitate is formed. Quantitative analysis of this interaction by the method shown in figure 1.3 gives both the antibody content of the immune serum and also an indication of the valency of the antigen, i.e. the effective number of combining sites. This can vary enormously depending on the antigen, its size, and the species making the antibody. With rabbit antisera, ovalbumin may have a valency of 10 and human thyroglobulin as many as 40 combining sites on its surface. By splitting antigens into large fragments with proteolytic enzymes it has become clear that the separate combining areas on the surface of a given protein (called antigenic *determinants* or *epitopes*) are by no means identical.

It will be noted from the precipitin curve in figure 1.3 that as more and more antigen is added, an optimum is reached after which consistently less precipitate is formed. At this stage the supernatant can be shown to contain soluble complexes of antigen (Ag) and antibody (Ab), many of composition Ag_4Ab_3, Ag_3Ab_2 and Ag_2Ab. In extreme antigen excess (AgXS, figure 1.3) ultracentrifugal analysis reveals the complexes to be mainly of the form Ag_2Ab, suggesting that the rabbit antibodies studied are bivalent (figure 1.4; see also figures 2.5 and 2.6). Between these extremes the cross-linking of antigen and antibody will generally give rise to three-dimensional lattice structures, as suggested by Marrack, which coalesce to form large precipitating aggregates.

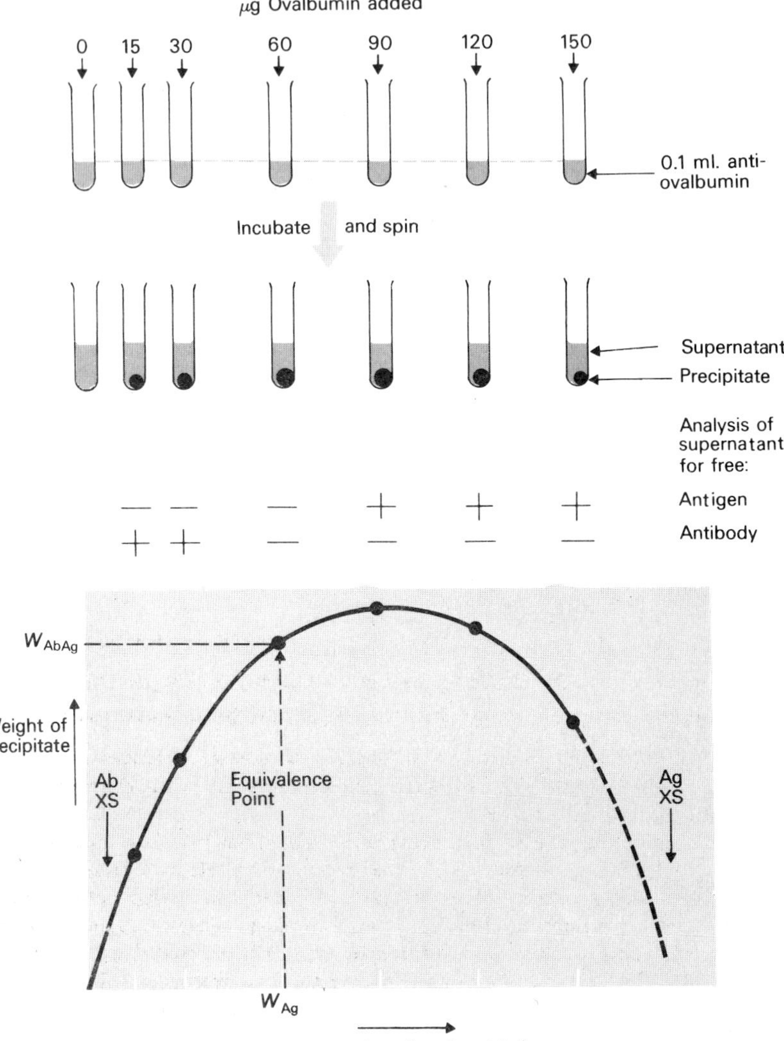

FIGURE 1.3. Quantitative precipitin reaction between rabbit anti-ovalbumin and ovalbumin (after Heidelberger & Kendall). Increasing amounts of ovalbumin are added to a constant volume of the antiserum placed in a number of tubes. After incubation the precipitates formed are spun down and weighed. Each supernatant is split into two halves: by adding antigen to one and antibody to the other, the presence of reactive antibody or antigen respectively can be demonstrated. The antibody content of the serum can be calculated from the equivalence point where no antigen or antibody is present in the supernatant. All the antigen added is therefore complexed in the precipitate with all the antibody available and the antibody content in 0·1 ml of serum would therefore be given by (W_{AgAb}–W_{Ag}). Analysis of the precipitate formed in antibody excess (AbXS), where the antigen-combining sites are largely saturated, gives a measure of the molar ratio of antibody to antigen in the complex and hence an estimate of the antigen valency.

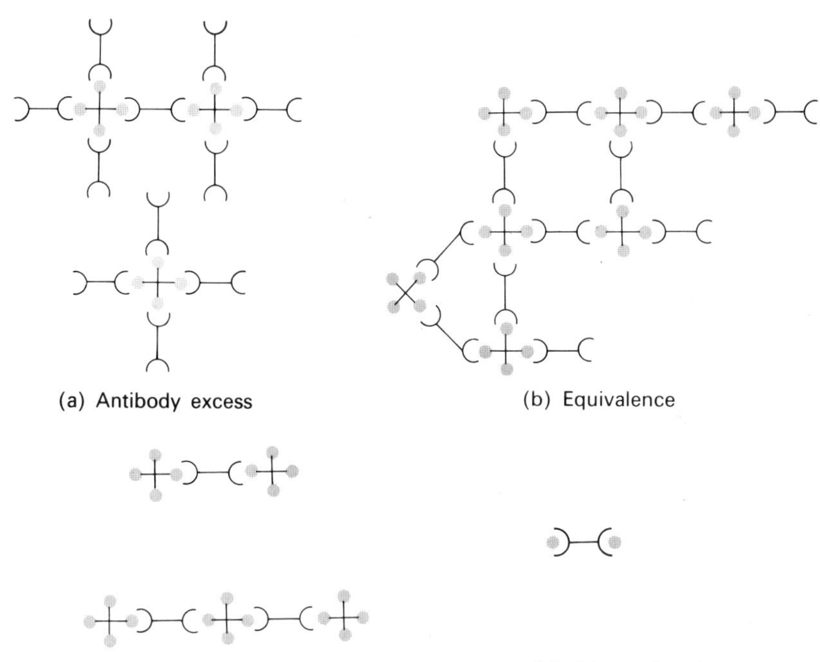

(d) Monovalent hapten

FIGURE 1.4. Diagrammatic representation of complexes formed between a hypothetical tetravalent antigen ( ) and bivalent antibody ( ) mixed in different proportions. In practice, the antigen valencies are unlikely to lie in the same plane or to be formed by identical determinants as suggested in the figure.

(a) In extreme antibody excess, the antigen valencies are saturated and the molar ratio Ab : Ag approximates to the valency of the antigen.

(b) At equivalence, large lattices are formed which aggregate to form a typical immune precipitate. This secondary aggregation, and hence precipitation tends to be inhibited by high salt concentration.

(c) In extreme antigen excess where the two valencies of each antibody molecule become rapidly saturated, the complex Ag_2Ab tends to predominate.

(d) A monovalent hapten binds but is unable to cross-link antibody molecules.

The basis of specificity

Much of our understanding of the factors governing antigen specificity has come from the studies of Landsteiner and of Pauling and their colleagues on the interaction of antibody with small chemically defined groupings termed *haptens*, a typical example being *m*-aminobenzene sulphonate (figure 1.5). Whereas an antigen will both evoke antibody formation and combine with the resulting antibody, *a hapten is defined as a small molecule which by itself cannot stimulate antibody synthesis but will combine with antibody once formed.*

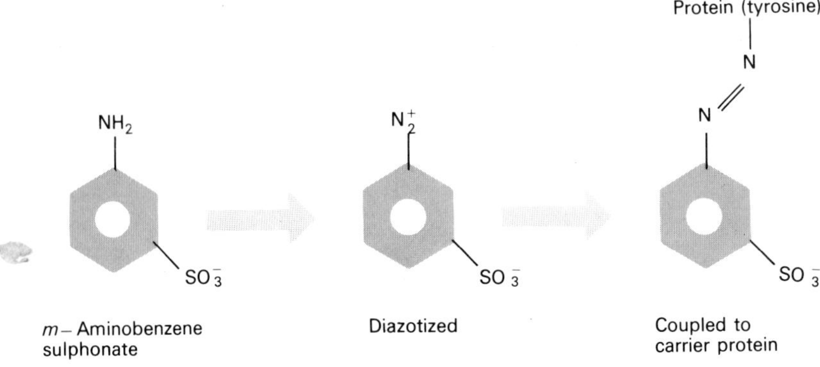

FIGURE 1.5. Coupling of hapten to carrier protein by diazotization.

The problem of how to produce these antibodies was solved by injecting the haptens coupled to proteins which acted as 'carriers'. It then became possible to relate variations in the chemical structure of a hapten to its ability to bind to a given antibody. In one experiment, antibodies raised to *m*-aminobenzene sulphonate were tested for their ability to combine with *ortho*, *meta* and *para* isomers of the hapten and related molecules in which the sulphonate group was substituted by arsonate or carboxylate (figure 1.6). The results are summarized in table 1.1. The hapten with the sulphonate group in the *ortho* position combines somewhat less well with the antibody than the original *meta* isomer, but the *para*-substituted compound (chemically similar to the *ortho*) shows very poor reactivity. The substitution of arsonate for sulphonate leads to weaker combination with the antibody; both groups are negatively charged and have a tetrahedral structure but the arsonate group is larger in size and has an extra H atom (figure 1.6). The aminobenzoates in which the sulphonate is substituted by the nega-

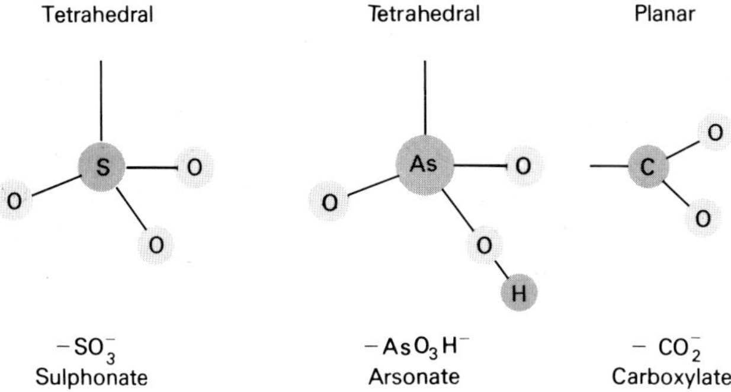

FIGURE 1.6. Configurations of the sulphonate, arsonate and carboxylate groups.

TABLE 1.1. Effect of variations in hapten structure on strength of binding to *m*-aminobenzene sulphonate antibodies

	NH_2 (R ortho)	NH_2 (R meta)	NH_2 (R para)
	ortho	*meta*	*para* isomers
R = sulphonate	+ +	+ + +	±
R = arsonate	−	+	−
R = carboxylate	−	±	−

Strength of binding is directly graded from negative (−) to very strong (+ + +). Since free haptens can only combine with one antibody-combining site and cannot therefore cross-link, they form only soluble complexes; their binding strength was assessed through their ability to inhibit precipitation by antibody of a new carrier protein substituted with several of the original hapten (*m*-aminobenzene sulphonate) groups per molecule (from Landsteiner K. & van der Scheer J. *J.exp.Med.* 1936, **63**, 325).

tively charged but planar carboxylate group show even less affinity for the antibody. It would appear that the overall *configuration* of the hapten is even more important than its *chemical* nature, i.e. the hapten is recognized by the overall three-dimensional shape of its outer electron cloud as distinct from its chemical reactivity. The production of antibodies against such strange moieties as benzene sulphonate and arsonate becomes more comprehensible if they are thought to be directed against a particular electron-cloud shape rather than a specific chemical structure. This view is consistent with the nature of antigen–antibody binding which is known not to involve covalent linkages.

THE FORCES BINDING ANTIGEN TO ANTIBODY

It should be stressed immediately that the forces which hold antigen and antibody together are in essence no different from the so-called 'non-specific' protein–protein interactions which occur between any two unrelated proteins (or other macromolecules) as, for example, human serum albumin and human transferrin. These intermolecular forces may be classified under four headings:

(a) *Electrostatic*

These are due to the attraction between oppositely charged ionic groups on the two protein side chains as, for example,

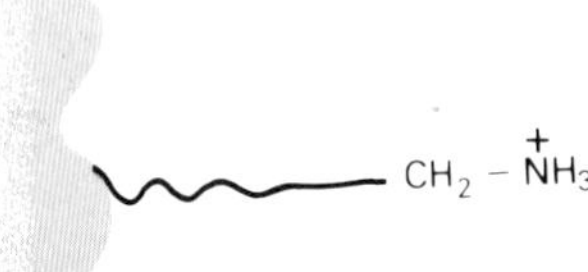
CH2 – NH3
OCO – CH2
Lysine side – chain
Aspartate side – chain

(a)

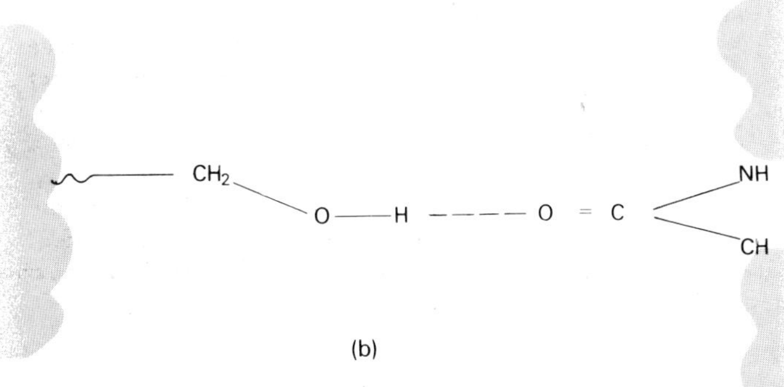
CH2
O — H – – – – O = C
NH
CH

(b)

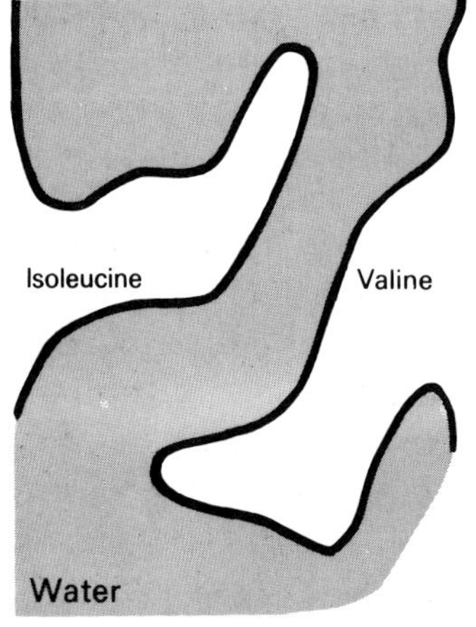
Isoleucine
Valine
Water

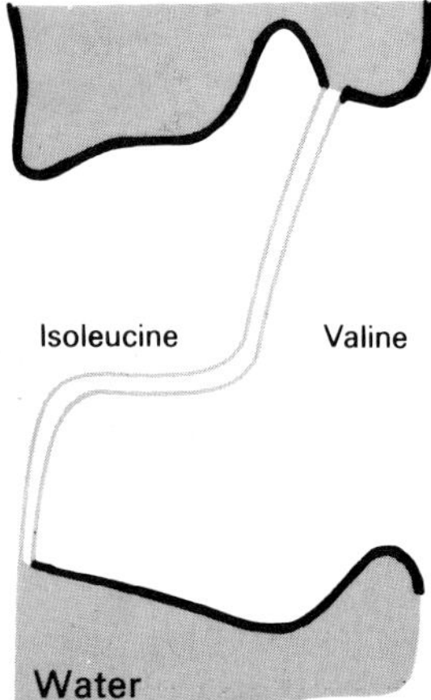
Isoleucine
Valine
Water

(c)

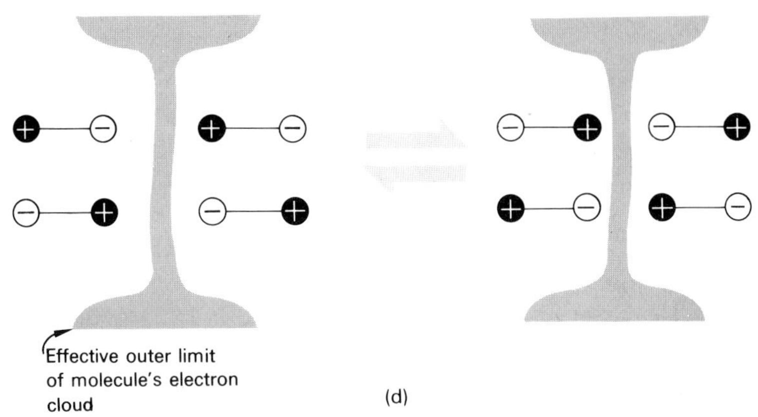

FIGURE 1.7. Protein–protein interactions.

(a) Coulombic attraction between oppositely charged ionic groupings.

(b) Hydrogen bonding between two proteins: the example shows an H-bond between a serine or threonine side-chain on one protein and a peptide carbonyl group on the other.

(c) Hydrophobic bonding: the region in which the water molecules are in contact with the hydrophobic groups (indicated by the thickened line) is considerably reduced when the hydrophobic groups on two proteins are in contact with each other and the lower free-energy of this system makes this a more probable state than separation of the hydrophobic groups.

(d) Van der Waals forces: the interaction between the electrons in the external orbitals of two different macromolecules may be envisaged (for simplicity!) as the attraction between induced oscillating dipoles in the two electron clouds.

an ionized amino group (NH_3^+) on a lysine of one protein and an ionized carboxyl group ($—COO^-$) of, say, aspartate on the other (figure 1.7a). The force of attraction (F) is inversely proportional to the square of the distance (d) between the charges, i.e.

$$F \propto 1/d^2$$

Thus as the charges come closer together, the attractive force increases considerably: if we halve the distance apart, we quadruple the attraction. Dipoles on antigen and antibody can also attract each other. In addition, electrostatic forces may be generated by charge transfer reactions between antibody and antigen; for example an electron-donating protein residue such as tryptophan could part with an electron to a group such as dinitrophenyl which is electron-accepting thereby creating an effective $+1$ charge on the antibody and -1 on the antigen.

(b) *Hydrogen bonding*

The formation of the relatively weak and reversible hydrogen bridges between hydrophilic groups such as .OH, $.NH_2$ and .COOH depends very much upon the close approach of the two molecules carrying these groups (figure 1.7b).

(c) *Hydrophobic*

In the same way that oil droplets in water merge to form a single large drop, so non-polar, hydrophobic groups such as the side chains of valine, leucine and phenylalanine, tend to associate in an aqueous environment. The driving force for this hydrophobic bonding derives from the fact that water in contact with hydrophobic molecules with which it cannot H-bond, will associate with other water molecules but the number of configurations which allow H-bonds to form will not be as great as that occurring when they are surrounded completely by other water molecules, i.e. the entropy is lower. The greater the area of contact between water and hydrophobic surfaces, the lower the entropy and the higher the energy state. Thus if hydrophobic groups on two proteins come together so as to exclude water molecules between them, the net surface in contact with water is reduced (figure 1.7c) and the proteins take up a lower energy state than when they are separated (in other words, there is a force of attraction between them). It has been estimated that hydrophobic forces may contribute up to 50% of the total strength of the antigen–antibody bond.

(d) *Van der Waals*

These are the forces between molecules which depend upon interaction between the external 'electron clouds'. The deviation of gaseous molecules of say nitrogen or hydrogen from 'ideal' behaviour according to the kinetic theory is attributable to the Van der Waals attractions between them. The nature of this interaction is difficult to describe in non-mathematical terms but it has been likened to a temporary perturbation of electrons in one molecule effectively forming a dipole which induces a dipolar perturbation in the other molecule, the two dipoles then having a force of attraction between them; as the displaced electrons swing back through the equilibrium position and beyond, the dipoles oscillate (figure 1.7d). The force of attraction is inversely proportional to the seventh power of the distance, i.e.

$$F \propto 1/d^7$$

and as a result this rises very rapidly as the interacting molecules come closer together.

This last point underlines one essential feature common to all four types of force—they depend upon the close approach of both molecules before the forces become of significant magnitude. And this is at the heart of the combination of antigen and antibody. By having *complementary* electron-cloud shapes on the combining site of the antibody and the surface determinant of the antigen, the two molecules can fit snugly together like a lock and key (figure 1.9a). The intermolecular distance becomes very small and the 'non-specific protein interaction forces' are considerably increased; the greater the areas of antigen and antibody which fit together, the greater the force of attraction, particularly if there is apposition of opposite charges and hydrophobic groupings.

ANTIBODY AFFINITY

The combination of antibody with the surface determinant of an antigen or a monovalent hapten molecule (cf. figure 1.4d) is reversible and the complex may readily dissociate, depending upon the strength of binding. This can be defined through the equilibrium constant (K) of the reaction:

$$\mathrm{Ab} + \mathrm{Hp} \rightleftharpoons \mathrm{AbHp}$$

(⊃—⊂)　(•)　(⊃—⊂•)

given by the mass action equation,

$$K = \frac{[\mathrm{AbHp}]}{[\mathrm{Ab}][\mathrm{Hp}]}$$

where [Ab] is the concentration of free antibody combining sites and [Hp] the concentration of free hapten. If the antibody and hapten fit together very closely, the equilibrium will lie well over to the right; we refer to such antibodies which bind strongly to the hapten as *high affinity antibodies*. At a certain *free* hapten concentration $[\mathrm{Hp_c}]$ where half of the antibody sites are bound, $[\mathrm{AbHp}] = [\mathrm{Ab}]$ and $K = 1/[\mathrm{Hp_c}]$, i.e. K is equal to the reciprocal of the concentration of free hapten at the equilibrium point where half the antibody sites are in the bound form. In other words, when an antibody has a high affinity constant and binds

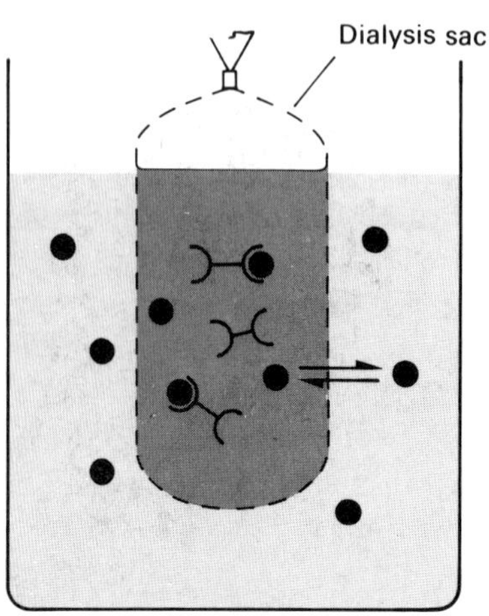

FIGURE 1.8. Antibody affinity determined by studying the equilibrium between antibody (⤙⤚) and hapten (●). Within the dialysis sac the hapten is partly in the free form and partly bound to antibody according to the affinity of the antibody. Only hapten can diffuse through the dialysis membrane and the external concentration then will equal the concentration of unbound hapten within the sac. Measurement of total hapten in the dialysis sac then enables the amount bound to antibody to be calculated. By repeating this at different concentrations of hapten, one can calculate the average affinity constant (K) as described in the text. Constant renewal of the external buffer will lead to total dissociation and loss of hapten from inside the dialysis sac showing the reversible nature of the antigen–antibody bond.

hapten strongly, it only needs a low hapten concentration to half-saturate the antibody. Affinity constants, which can be determined by methods such as that shown in figure 1.8, may reach values as high as 10^{11} litres/mole.

Analysis of the binding at different hapten concentrations generally shows a heterogeneity which indicates that most antisera, even those raised against antigens with a simple structure, contain a variety of different antibodies with a range of binding affinities which depend upon the area of contact between the antibody and the antigenic determinant, the closeness of fit (figure 1.9) and the distribution of charged and hydrophobic groups. If we bear in mind that antigen determinants are not two-dimensional as represented in the figures, but have a three-dimensional electron-cloud shape, one can realize that antibodies are confronted with very many different configurations even in a single determinant, depending upon the direction from which the antibody molecule approaches.

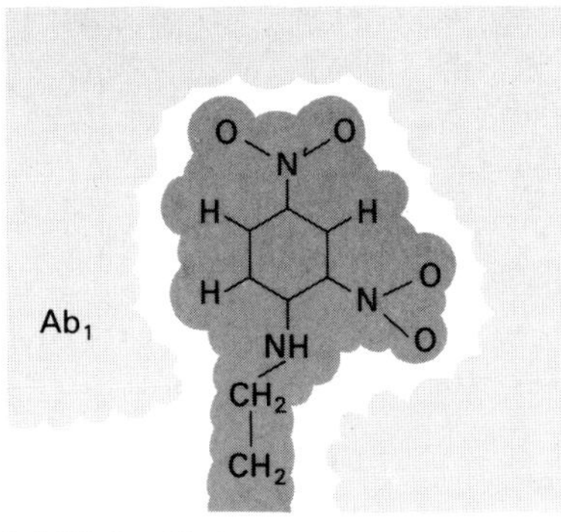

(a) High affinity

Ab_2

(b) Moderate affinity

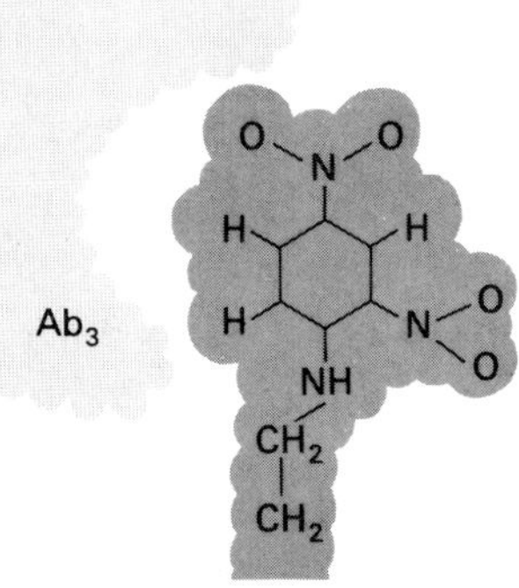

(c) Low affinity

FIGURE 1.9. Binding of antibodies present in the same antiserum with different affinities to the same hapten (dinitrobenzene linked to the amino group of lysine). (a) $Antibody_1$ fits with nearly the whole of the hapten and is thus of high affinity. (b) $Antibody_2$ fits with less of the molecule and not so closely, and has a moderate binding affinity while (c) the low affinity $antibody_3$ is complementary in shape to so little of the hapten surface that its binding energy is very little above that occurring between completely unrelated proteins. Only a portion of the antibody combining site is shown.

AVIDITY AND THE BONUS EFFECT OF MULTIVALENT BINDING

The strength of the interaction of antibody with a monovalent hapten or a single antigen determinant we have labelled antibody affinity. In most practical situations we are concerned with the interaction of an antiserum with a multivalent antigen molecule and the term employed to express this binding,

$$n\mathrm{Ab} + m\mathrm{Ag} \rightleftharpoons \mathrm{Ab}_n\mathrm{Ag}_m$$

is *avidity*. The factors which contribute to avidity are complicated. Not only must we contend with the heterogeneity of antibodies in a given serum which are directed against each determinant on the antigen, but we must also recognize that the differing amino acid sequences on different parts of a protein surface, for example, lead to the formation of a number of antigenic patches or determinants on a single molecule, each with its distinct shape and specificity.

The multivalence of most antigens leads to an interesting 'bonus' effect in which the binding of two antigen molecules by antibody is always greater than the arithmetic sum of the individual antibody links. This is illustrated in figure 1.10. The mechanism of this effect may be interpreted by considering an analogy. Let us fabricate an unheard of disease in which we cannot stop our hands opening and closing continuously. If we now try to hold an object in *one* hand it will fall the moment we open that hand. However, if we use *both* hands to hold the object, provided we open and close our hands at different times, there is much less chance of the object falling. The reversible combination of antigen and antibody is like the opening and closing of the hand; the more valencies holding the antigen the less likely it is to be lost when the complex dissociates at any one binding site (figure 1.11).

SPECIFICITY AND CROSS-REACTIONS

An antiserum raised against a given antigen can cross-react with a partially related antigen which bears one or more identical or similar determinants. In figure 1.12 it can be seen that an antiserum to antigen$_1$ will react less strongly with antigen$_2$ which bears just one identical determinant

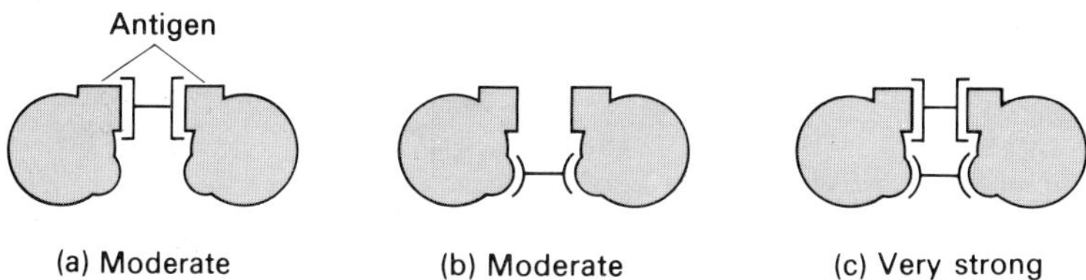

FIGURE 1.10. The 'bonus' effect of multivalent attachment on binding strength. The force binding the two antigen molecules in (c) with two antibody bridges is often at least 10 times greater than (a+b) where only single antibody molecules provide the link. The effect varies with *K* values; the weaker the affinity the more the bonus.

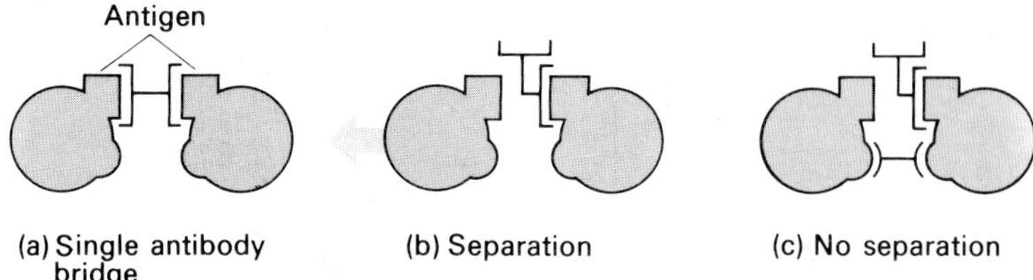

FIGURE 1.11. The mechanism of the bonus effect. Each antigen–antibody bond is reversible and with a single antibody bridge between two antigen molecules (a), dissociation of either bond could enable an antigen molecule to 'escape' as in (b). If there are two antibody bridges, even when one dissociates the other prevents the antigen molecule from escaping and holds it in position ready to reform the broken bond.

because only certain of the antibodies in the serum can bind. Antigen$_3$ which possesses a similar but not identical determinant will not fit as well with the antibody and the binding is even weaker. Antigen$_4$ which has no structural similarity at all will not react significantly with the antibody.* Thus, based upon stereochemical considerations, we can see why the avidity of the antiserum for antigens $_{2+3}$ is less than for the homologous antigen, while for the unrelated antigen$_4$ it is negligible. It is in this way that the *specificity* of an antiserum is expressed.

THE ANTIBODY SITE AND ANTIGEN DETERMINANTS

The forces which bind antigen to antibody are largely similar to those binding enzyme to substrate. The elucidation of

* If the antigenic determinant is appreciably smaller than the antibody site, there could be a cross-reaction with an unrelated antigen which bound fortuitously to the remainder of the site.

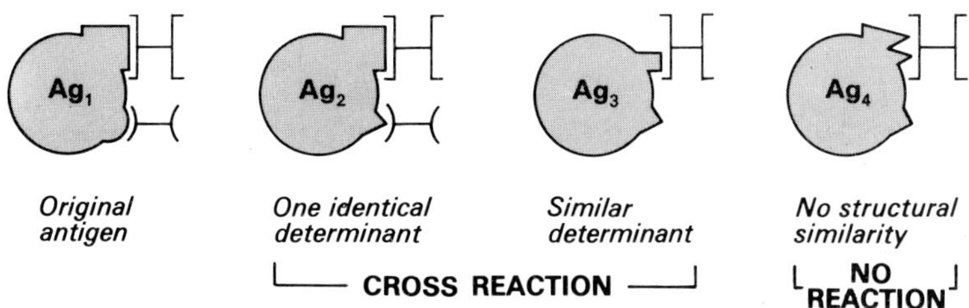

FIGURE 1.12. Specificity and cross-reaction. The avidity of the serum (antibodies ⊢[,)⊣( ) for $Ag_1 > Ag_2 > Ag_3 \gg Ag_4$ so that the serum shows specificity.

the three-dimensional structures of certain enzymes such as lysozyme by X-ray crystallography has shown that the substrate lies within a long cleft in the surface of the molecule. Similar studies on homogeneous antibody preparations indicate that the combining site is approximately 1.5–2.0 nm long, 1.5 nm wide and 0.5–1.2 nm deep (Poljak and colleagues).

These dimensions are consistent with studies using *linear* haptens formed from repeating units of sugar molecules (Kabat) or amino acids (Sela) which have indicated that the site probably accommodates roughly six such units. Of these units, the terminal one usually shows the highest binding energy to the antibody and may be termed the 'immunodominant' group; successive units contribute progressively less to the overall binding. Investigations by Benjamini into tobacco mosaic virus (TMV) protein and its antibodies have shown firstly that the C-terminal decapeptide has strong antibody-binding activity (figure 1.13a) and surprisingly, the antibody has a comparable affinity for the C-terminal tripeptide coupled with an octanoyl (hydrophobic) group at the N-terminal end (figure 1.13b). It would appear that the major contribution to specificity is made by the configuration of the three terminal amino acid residues, and that a further significant factor in the binding energy is derived from non-specific interaction with hydrophobic groupings further back in the antibody site. It will be of importance to know whether these results hold true for other antigens.

So far we have discussed the interaction of linear antigens with the antibody combining site. A different situation arises with globular proteins. Studies with synthetic antigens have shown that antibodies are formed against determinants accessible on the surface and not against residues buried within the molecule. This is so with globular proteins such as myoglobulin and staphylococcal nuclease, where the main antigenic determinants are located on those portions of the surface polypeptide chain which protrude as angular bends

(a) H_2N—Thr.Thr.Ala.Glu.Thr.Leu.Asp.Ala.Thr.Arg.COOH

(b) $CH_3(CH_2)_6CO$—Ala.Thr.Arg.COOH

FIGURE 1.13. The C-terminal decapeptide of TMV protein (a) and the octanoyl derivative of the C-terminal tripeptide (b) which have comparable antibody-binding activities.

capable of lying within an antibody cleft. The linear *sequence* of amino acids in the peptide chain is clearly important for specificity but the overall *conformation* of the peptide makes a very significant contribution to the energy of binding with antibody. Lysozyme provides a case in point: this protein has an intrachain-disulphide bond which forms a loop in the peptide chain. As Arnon has shown, certain antibodies reacting with lysozyme can be inhibited by prior addition of the isolated loop peptide. However, reduction of the disulphide bond destroys this inhibitory activity even though the linear chain so formed has an unchanged primary amino acid sequence.

It is worth emphasizing that our analysis has been concerned with the interaction of an antigenic determinant or a hapten with antibody but several further factors govern the ability of a given substance to act as an *antigen*, i.e. to stimulate the antigen-reactive cells in the host animal to produce antibody. These include the content of polymeric repeating structures, the rate of catabolism, the size, the degree of 'foreigness'—i.e. dissimilarity from self—and the ability of the body to recognize the substance (see chapter 3, p. 71).

Summary

The purpose of the immune response is to defend the host against infection. 'Non-specific' immune mechanisms (e.g. phagocytosis) are enhanced by the development of *adaptive* immunity characterized by memory, specificity and the recognition of non-self. The more rapid and intense antibody response which occurs on the second contact with antigen explains the protection afforded by a primary infection against subsequent disease and provides the rationale for the immunological education of the body by vaccination.

Antigens bind to antibodies reversibly by non-covalent molecular interactions including electrostatic, hydrogen-bonding, hydrophobic and Van der Waals forces which become significant when complementarity of shape between antigen and antibody allows them to approach each other closely ('lock and key' fit like enzyme and substrate).

The binding strength of an antibody for a single determinant or hapten is measured by *affinity*. The term *avidity* describes the binding of an antiserum for the whole antigen molecule, this being influenced relative to affinity, by the bonus effect of multivalency. Antibodies discriminate between two antigens, i.e. show *specificity*, by their greater avidity for one rather than the other. Where some determinants (epitopes) on two antigens are identical or similar, they will give cross-reactions directly dependent upon their relative binding strengths to the antibodies.

The antigenic determinant must be capable of lying within the groove forming the antibody combining site. With linear antigens, primary structure is crucially important for the formation of a determinant but in the case of globular molecules, tertiary conformation is usually of even greater significance.

Further reading

Cunningham A.J. (1978) *Understanding Immunology*. Academic Press, New York.

Davis B.D., Dulbecco R., Eisen H.N., Ginsberg H.S. & Wood W.B. (1973) *Microbiology* (Including Immunology) 2nd Edition. Harper International Edition.

Fongerean M. & Dansset J. (eds) (1980) *Progress in Immunology IV*. Academic Press, London. (Papers from the 4th Int. Congress of Immunology.)

Fudenberg H.H., Stites D.P., Caldwell J.L. & Wells J.V. (1978) *Basic and Clinical Immunology*, 2nd Edition. Lange Medical Publications, Los Altos, California.

Glynn L.E. & Steward M.W. (eds) (1977) *Immunochemistry: an Advanced Textbook*, Wiley, Chichester.

Hobart M.J. & McConnell I. (1980) *The Immune System: a course on the molecular and cellular basis of immunity*, 2nd edition. Blackwell Scientific Publications, Oxford.

Humphrey J.H. & White R.G. (1970) *Immunology for Students of Medicine*, 3rd Edition. Blackwell Scientific Publications, Oxford (Dated but scholarly.)

Kabat E.A. (1976) *Structural Concepts in Immunology and Immunochemistry*. Holt, Rinehart & Winston Inc, New York.

Richards F.F., Konigsberg W.H. & Rosenstein R.W. (1975) On the specificity of antibodies: Biochemical and biophysical evidence indicates the existence of polyfunctional antibody combining regions. *Science* **187**, 130.

Sela M. (ed) (1974) *The Antigens*. Academic Press, New York.

Thaler M.S., Klausner R.D. & Cohen H.J. (1977) *Medical Immunology*. Lippincot, Philadelphia.

Historical

Landsteiner K. (1946) *The Specificity of Serological Reactions*. Harvard University Press (reprinted 1962 by Dover Publications, New York).

Metchnikoff E. (1893) *Comparative Pathology of Inflammation*. Transl. F.A. and E.H. Starling. Kegan Paul, Trench, Trübner & Co., London.

Parish H.J. (1968) *Victory with Vaccines*. Livingstone, Edinburgh.

Series for the advanced student

* *Advances in Immunology* (Annual). Academic Press, London.
Progress in Allergy. S.Karger, Basle.
Modern Trends in Immunology. Butterworths, London.
* *Immunological Reviews* (ed. G. Moller). Munksgaard, Copenhagen.
Essays in Fundamental Immunology. Blackwell Scientific Publications, Oxford.
Contemporary Topics in Molecular Immunology. Plenum Press, N.Y.
Contemporary Topics in Immunobiology. Plenum Press, N.Y.
Protides of the Biological Fluids. Pergamon Press, Oxford.

* In depth treatment

Current information

Current Titles in Immunology, Transplantation & Allergy. MSK Books London.

Major journals

Nature, Lancet, Science, J.exp.Med., Immunology, J.Immunology, Clin.exp. Immunology, Mol. Immunol., Immunopharmacology, Infect & Immunity, Int.Arch.Allergy, Cell.Immunology, European J.Immunology, Scand.J.Immunol., Clin.Immunol. & Immunopath., J.Immunogenetics, J.Immunol.Methods, J.Reticuloendoth.Soc., Tissue Antigens, Immunogenetics, Transplantation, Ann.d'Immunologie, Cancer Immunol.Immunotherapy, J.Allergy Clin.Immunol., Clin.Allergy, Ann.Allergy, J.Clin.Lab.Immunology, Parasitic Immunol.

2 The immunoglobulins

The association of antibody activity with the classical γ-globulin fraction of serum was shown many years ago by Tiselius and Kabat. They hyperimmunized rabbits with pneumococcal polysaccharide to produce a high concentration of circulating antibody and then examined the effect of absorbing the serum with antigen on the electrophoretic profile. Only the γ-globulin fraction was significantly reduced after removal of antibody (figure 2.1). With the recognition of heterogeneity in the types of molecules which can function as antibodies, it has now become customary to use the general term 'immunoglobulin'. In each species, the immunoglobulin molecules can be subdivided into different classes on the basis of the structure of their 'backbone' (rather than on their specificity for given antigens). Thus, in the human for example, five major structural types or classes can be distinguished: immunoglobulin G (abbreviated to IgG), IgM, IgA, IgD and IgE.

The basic structure of the immunoglobulins

The antibody fraction of serum consists predominantly of one group of proteins with molecular weight around 150,000 (sedimentation coefficient $7S$)

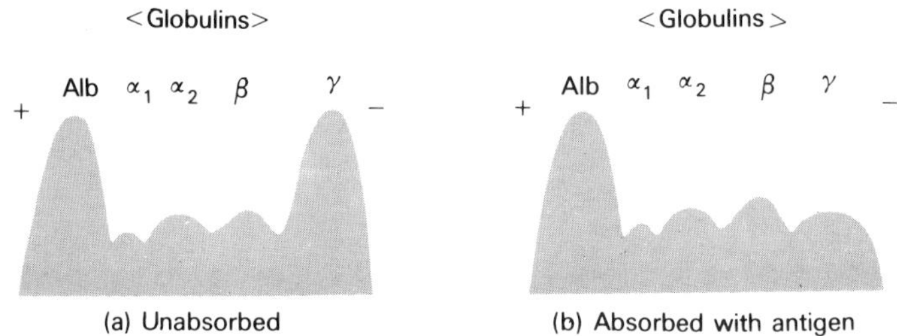

FIGURE 2.1. Association of antibody activity with γ-globulin serum fraction. Hyperimmune serum is separated into major fractions by electrophoresis before (a) and after (b) absorption with antigen. Only the γ-globulin fraction is reduced.

of which the major component is IgG, and another of molecular weight 900,000 (19*S* IgM). The IgG antibodies can be split by papain into three fragments (R.R. Porter). Two of these are identical and are able to combine with antigen to form a soluble complex which will not precipitate; these are therefore univalent antibody fragments and are given the nomenclature Fab ('fragment antigen binding'). The third fragment has no power to combine with antigen and is termed Fc ('fragment crystallizable' obtainable in crystalline form). Another proteolytic enzyme, pepsin, cleaves the Fc part from the remainder of the antibody molecule, leaving a large fragment (5*S*) which can still precipitate with antigen and is formulated as $F(ab')_2$ since it is clearly still divalent.

Antibodies can also be broken down into their constituent peptide chains. First the disulphide bonds linking different chains must be broken by reduction with *excess* of a sulphydryl reagent. The reduced molecule still has a sedimentation coefficient of 7*S* because the chains are held together by non-covalent forces but they can be separated by lowering the pH into two sizes of peptide chain termed *light* and *heavy chains* (G. Edelman).

On the basis of these findings Porter put forward a symmetrical four-peptide model for antibody consisting of two heavy and two light chains linked together by interchain disulphide bonds (figure 2.2). The formation of the various

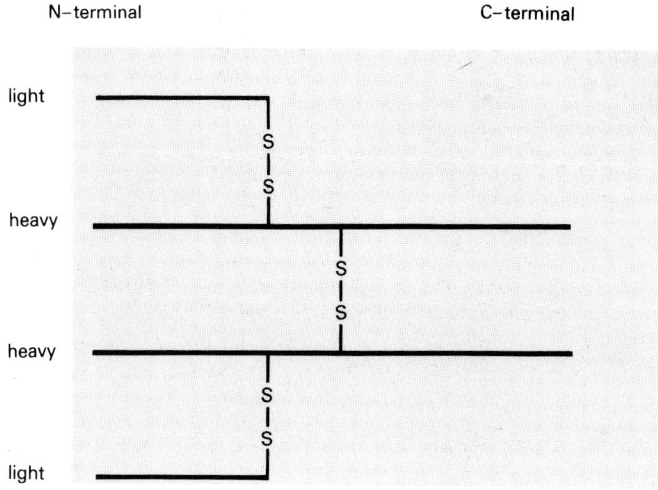

FIGURE 2.2. Antibody model proposed by R.R. Porter with two heavy and two light polypeptide chains held by interchain disulphide bonds. In the diagram the amino-terminal residue is on the left for each chain.

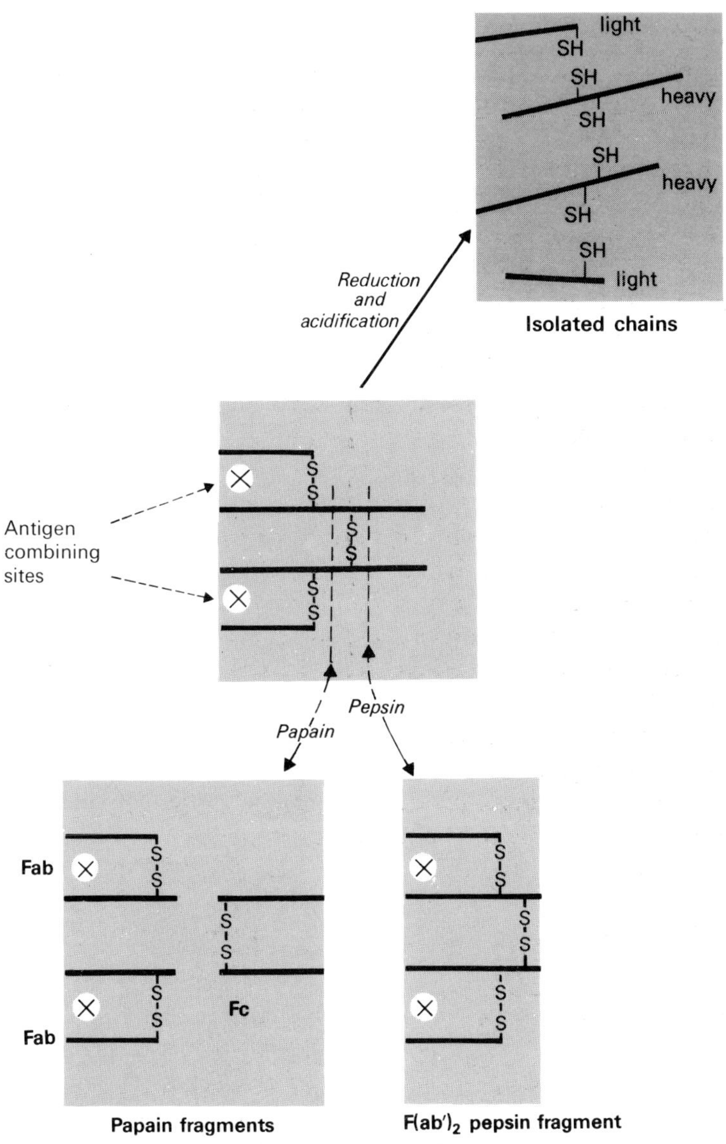

FIGURE 2.3. Degradation of immunoglobulin to constituent peptide chains and to proteolytic fragments showing divalence of pepsin $F(ab')_2$ and univalence of the papain Fab. After pepsin digestion the *p*Fc′ fragment representing the C-terminal half of the Fc region is formed. The portion of the heavy chain in the Fab fragment is given the symbol Fd.

fragments by proteolysis and reduction is represented in figure 2.3.

Purified IgG antibodies when visualized in the electron microscope by negative staining can be seen to be Y-shaped molecules whose arms can swing out to an angle of 180°

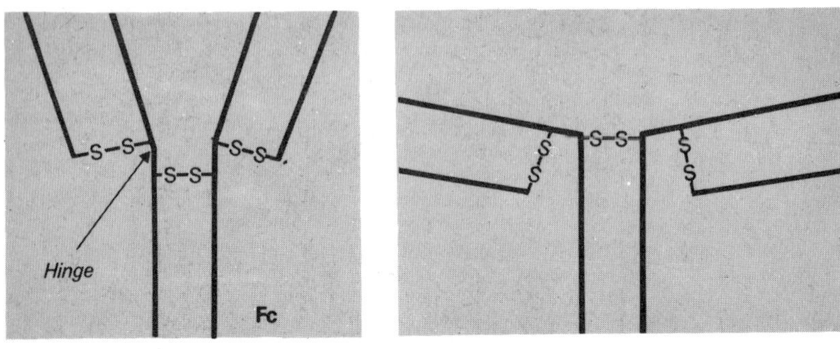

FIGURE 2.4. Illustrating the flexibility of the immunoglobulin molecule at the hinge region. Compare with conformation of immunoglobulin molecules in figure 2.5.

through the papain and pepsin sensitive region acting as a hinge (figure 2.4). Amino acid analysis of the hinge region has revealed an unusual feature—a large number of proline residues; because of its structure, proline prevents the peptide chain assuming α-helix conformation, and so this stretch of the chain is extended and accessible to proteolytic enzymes.

Elegant confirmation of the correctness of these general views on the structure of the antibody molecule has come from studies using a divalent hapten, bis-N-dinitrophenyl (DNP)-octamethylene-diamine:

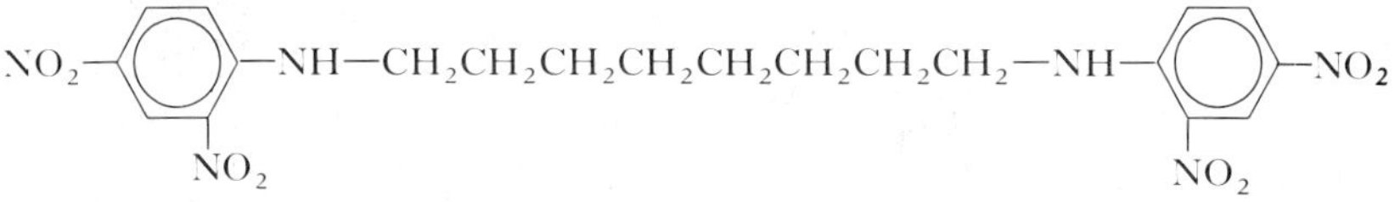

$$NO_2-C_6H_3(NO_2)-NH-CH_2CH_2CH_2CH_2CH_2CH_2CH_2CH_2-NH-C_6H_3(NO_2)-NO_2$$

where the two haptenic DNP groups are far enough apart not to interfere with each other's combination with antibody. When mixed with purified IgG antibody to DNP, the divalent hapten brings the antigen-combining sites on two different antibodies together end to end; when viewed by negative staining in the electron microscope a series of geometric forms are observed which represent the different structures to be expected if a Y-shaped hinged molecule with a combining site at the end of each of the two arms of the Y were to complex with this divalent hapten. Triangular trimers, square tetramers and pentagonal pentamers may be readily discerned (figure 2.5). The way in which these

FIGURE 2.5. (a)–(d) Electron micrograph (× 1,000,000) of complexes formed on mixing the divalent DNP hapten with rabbit anti-DNP antibodies. The 'negative stain' phosphotungstic acid is an electron-dense

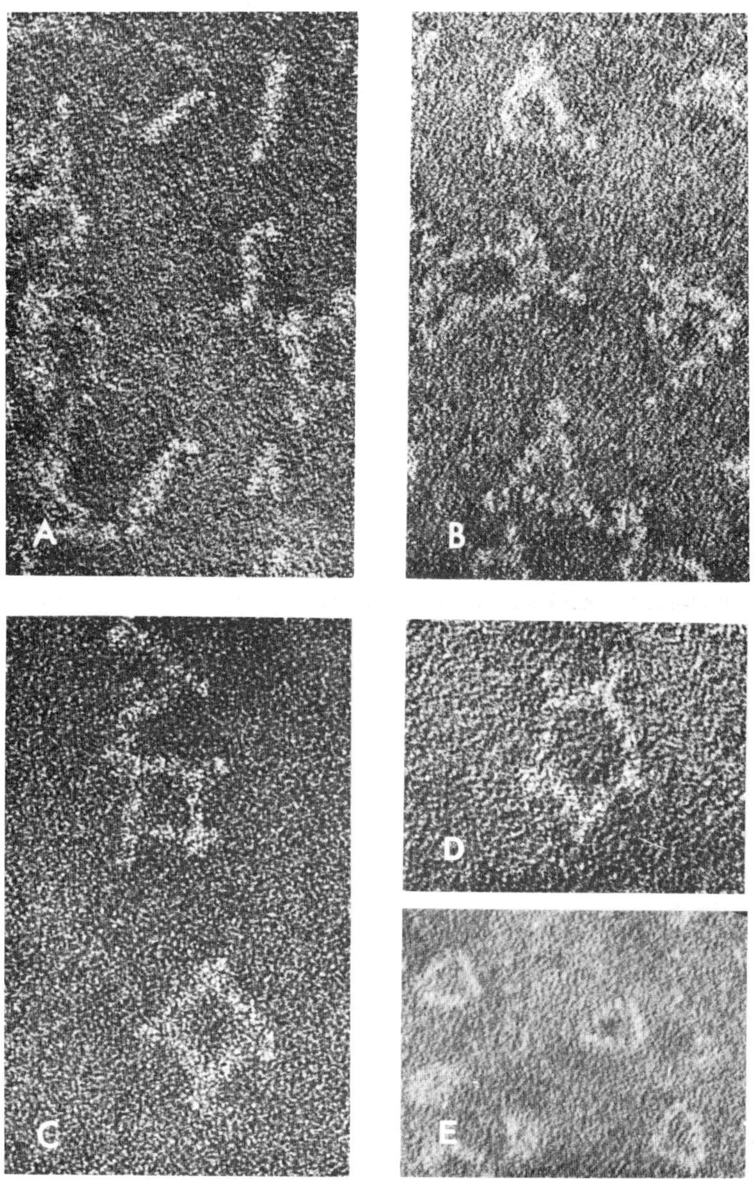

solution which penetrates in the spaces between the protein molecules. Thus the protein stands out as a 'light' structure in the electron beam. The hapten links together the Y-shaped antibody molecules to form (a) dimers, (b) trimers, (c) tetramers and (d) pentamers (cf. figure 2.6). The flexibility of the molecule at the hinge region is evident from the variation in angle of the arms of the 'Y'.

(e) As in (b); trimers formed using the $F(ab')_2$ antibody fragment from which the Fc structures have been digested by pepsin (× 500,000). The trimers can be seen to lack the Fc projections at each corner evident in (b). (After Valentine R.C. & Green N.M., *J.mol.Biol.* 1967, **27**, 615; courtesy of Dr. Green and with the permission of Acad. Press, N.Y.)

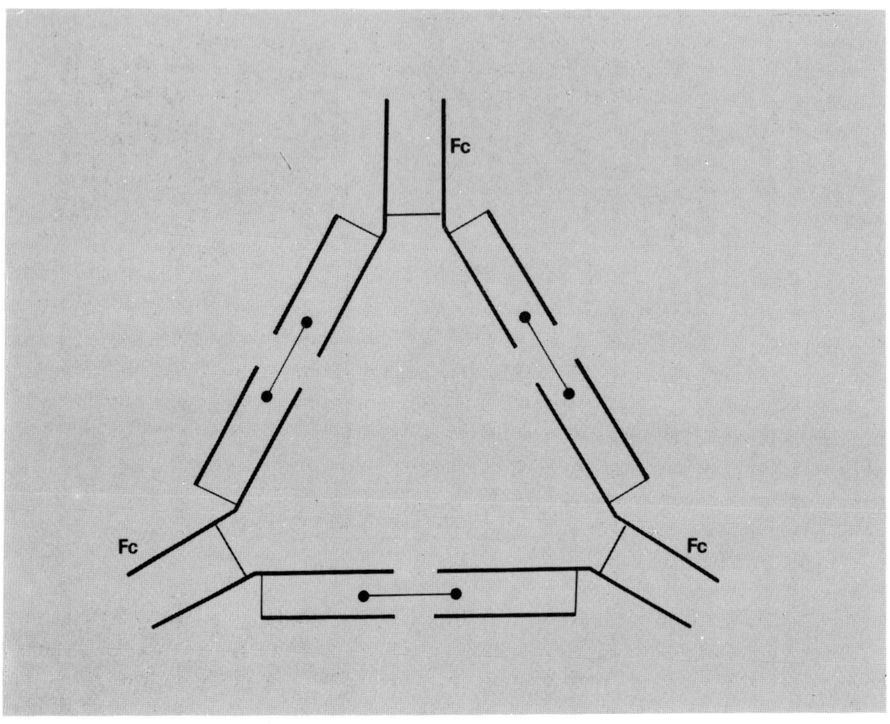

FIGURE 2.6. Three DNP antibody molecules held together as a trimer by the divalent hapten (●——●). Compare figure 2.5b. When the Fc fragments are first removed by pepsin, the corner pieces are no longer visible (figure 2.5e).

polymeric forms arise is indicated in figure 2.6. The position of the Fc fragment and its lack of involvement in the combination with antigen are apparent from the shape of the polymers formed using the pepsin $F(ab')_2$ fragment (figure 2.5e).

Variations in structure of the immunoglobulins

Any attempt to analyse the amino acid structure of the immunoglobulins in normal serum is bedevilled by the incredible number of different molecules present. This heterogeneity may be inferred from analysis by immunoelectrophoresis, the principle of which is explained in figure 2.7. It is evident that the immunoglobulins occur in different classes of molecules and also that they have a very wide range of electrophoretic mobilities within each class, ranging

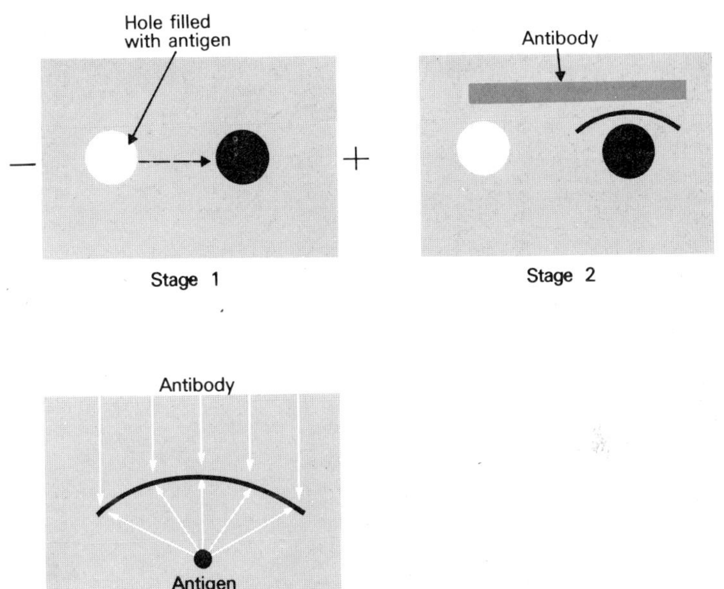

FIGURE 2.7. The principle of immunoelectrophoresis. *Stage 1 :* Electrophoresis of antigen in agar gel. Antigen migrates to hypothetical position shown. *Stage 2 :* Current stopped. Trough cut in agar and filled with antibody. Precipitin arc formed.

Because antigen theoretically at a point source diffuses radially and antibody from the trough diffuses with a plane front, they meet in optimal proportions for precipitation along an arc. The arc is closest to the trough at the point where antigen is in highest concentration.

in the case of IgG, from slow γ- to α_2-globulin (figure 2.8). This range of mobilities is due to different net charges on the different immunoglobulin molecules and is indicative of variations in amino acid structure (e.g. replacement of a neutral residue such as valine with a basic amino acid like lysine will tend to increase the net charge by $+1$). Even 'purified' antibodies directed against a simple hapten may show a wide spectrum of electrophoretic mobilities since, as mentioned in the previous chapter, they represent a variety of antibodies of varying degrees of fit for various shapes on the hapten surface.

The answer to this seemingly insoluble problem of analysing amino acid structure has come from study of the *myeloma proteins*. In the human disease known as multiple myeloma, one cell making one particular individual immunoglobulin divides over and over again in the uncontrolled way a cancer cell does, without regard for the overall requirement of the host. The patient then possesses enormous numbers

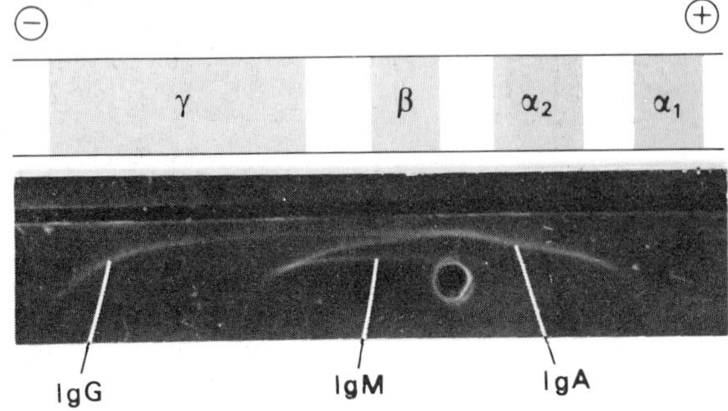

FIGURE 2.8. Major human immunoglobulin classes demonstrated by immunoelectrophoretic analysis of human serum using a rabbit antiserum in the trough. The position of the main electrophoretic globulin fractions are indicated. Three of the five major immunoglobulin classes can be recognized: immunoglobulin G (IgG), immunoglobulin A (IgA) and immunoglobulin M (IgM). The IgG precipitin arc extends from the γ region well into the α_2-globulin mobility range.

of identical cells derived as a clone from the original cell and they all synthesize the same immunoglobulin—the myeloma or M-protein—which appears in the serum, sometimes in very high concentrations. By purification of the myeloma protein we can obtain a preparation of an immunoglobulin having a unique structure. These myeloma proteins have been studied in two ways: amino acid analysis and the recognition of major characteristic groups on the molecules using specific antibodies produced in experimental animals.

STRUCTURAL VARIATION IN RELATION TO ANTIBODY SPECIFICITY

Amino acid analysis of a number of purified myeloma proteins has revealed that, within a given major immunoglobulin class such as IgG, the N-terminal portions of both heavy and light chains show quite considerable variations whereas the remaining parts of the chains are relatively constant in structure (figure 2.9). Each variable region has a basic overall amino acid structure which is common to a number of antibodies with differing specificities. They are said to belong to the same *subgroup* and to give an example, the heavy chain variable regions in a normal individual form three such subgroups (table 2.4, p. 46). This subgroup 'framework' structure cannot be related to antibody specifi-

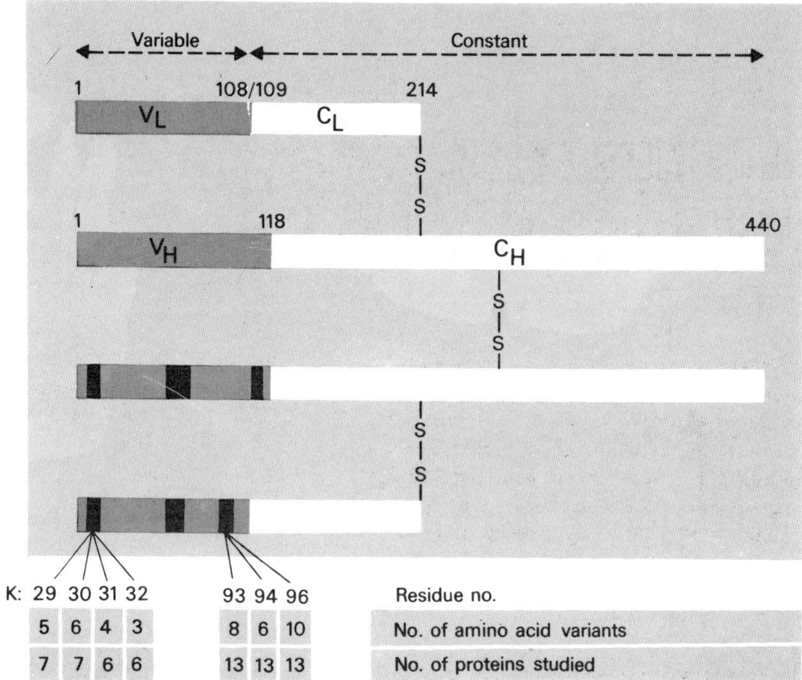

FIGURE 2.9. Showing the regions of IgG with relatively variable ( ) and constant (▭) amino acid composition. The terms '*V* region' and '*C* region' are used to designate the variable and constant regions respectively. 'V_L' and 'C_L' are generic terms for these regions on the light chain and 'V_H' and 'C_H' specify variable and constant regions on the heavy chain. The amino acid residues are numbered starting from the N-terminal end. C_L starts at residue 108 for κ-types and 109 for λ (see also figure 2.13). Examples are given of the degree of variation in amino acid residues seen in the hypervariable regions (▬).

city since so many different antibodies belong to the same subgroup. What is striking, however, is the hypervariability in amino acid residues at certain positions in the peptide chain. For example, when 13 myeloma light chains were sequenced, 8 different amino acids were found at residue number 93, 6 at residue 94 and 10 at residue 96 (figure 2.9). The most attractive view, supported by the latest X-ray analysis, is that these 'hot spots', three on the light and three on the heavy chain, lie relatively close to each other to form the antigen binding site (figures 2.10 & 2.15), their heterogeneity ensuring diversity in combining specificities through variation in the shape and nature of the surface they create (cf. p. 14). Thus each hypervariable region

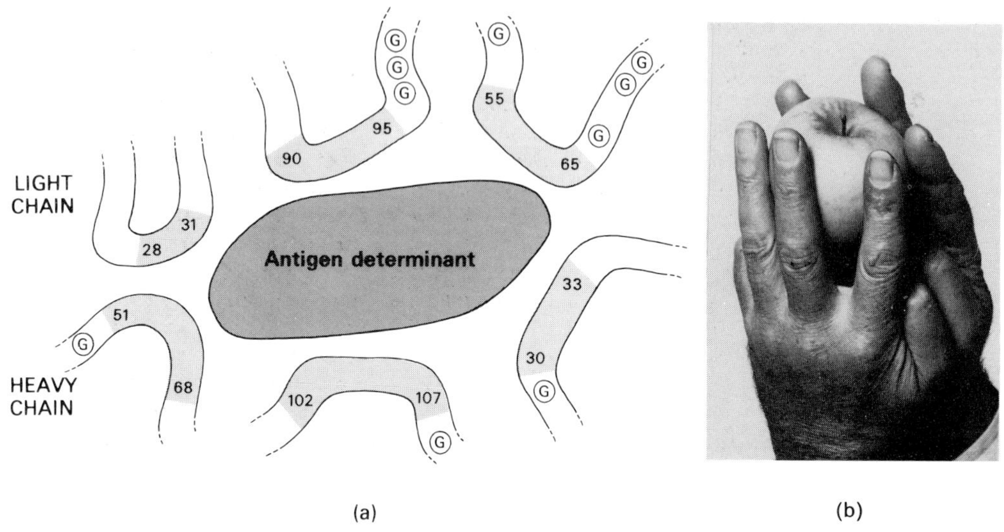

FIGURE 2.10. (a) 2-Dimensional representation of an antigen binding site formed by spatial apposition of peptide loops containing the hypervariable regions (hot spots: ▒) on light and heavy chains. Numbers refer to amino acid residues. Glycine residues (Ⓖ) are invariably present at the positions indicated whatever the specificity or animal species of the immunoglobulin. They are of importance in enabling peptide chains to fold back and form β-pleated sheet structures which enable the hypervariable regions to lie close to each other (figure 2.15). Wu and Kabat have suggested that the flexibility of bond angle in this amino acid is essential for the effective formation of a binding site. On this basis the greater frequency of invariant glycines on the light chain might indicate that coarse specificity for antigen binding was provided by the heavy chain and 'fine tuning' by the light chain. Through binding to different combinations of hypervariable regions and to different residues within each of these regions, each antibody molecule can form a complex with a variety of antigenic determinants (with a comparable variety of affinities). (b) A simulated combining site formed by apposing the 3 middle fingers of each hand, each finger representing a hypervariable loop. (Photograph by B.N.A. Rice.)

may be looked upon as an independent structure contributing to the complementarity of the binding site for antigen and perhaps one can speak of complementarity determinants.

That these variable regions on heavy and light chains both contribute to antibody specificity is suggested by experiments in which isolated chains were examined for their antigen combining power. In general, varying degrees of residual activity were associated with the heavy chains but relatively little with the light chains; on recombination, however, there was always a significant increase in antigen-binding capacity.

More direct attempts to identify the amino acid residues associated with the combining site have been made by Singer and others using a technique called 'affinity-labelling'. In this, a hapten is equipped with a chemically reactive side chain which will form covalent links with adjacent amino acids after combination of the hapten with antibody, so labelling residues in the neighbourhood of the combining site. A modification introduced by Porter and his colleagues utilizes a 'flick-knife' principle. The hapten with an azide side chain combines with its antibody and is then illuminated with ultraviolet light; this converts the azide to the reactive nitrene radical which will covalently link to almost any organic group with which it comes in contact (e.g. figure 2.11). The affinity label binds to both heavy and light chains in the hypervariable regions. There is no doubt that the electron microscopic studies with divalent hapten (cf. figures 2.5 and 2.6) show the antigen-combining sites to be associated with the N-terminal region of the molecule which at least bears out the overall view that the variable regions are implicated in antibody specificity.

VARIABILITY IN STRUCTURE UNRELATED TO ANTIBODY SPECIFICITY

Even the 'constant' portions of the immunoglobulin peptide chains which are not directly concerned in antigen binding show considerable heterogeneity. This has largely been analysed through the recognition of characteristic groupings on the molecules by use of specific antisera raised usually in other species. Let us consider, for example, studies on human immunoglobulin light chains.

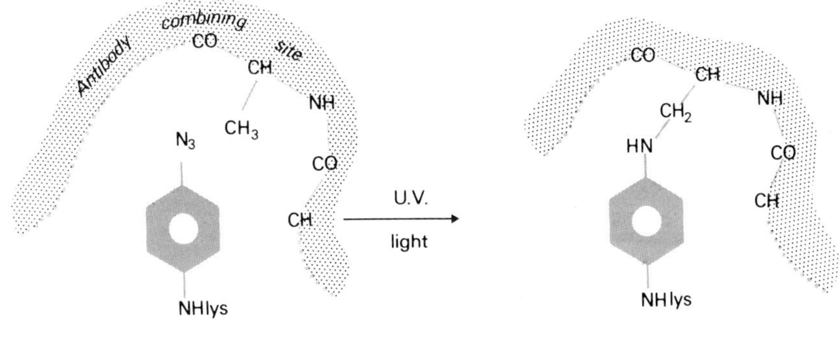

FIGURE 2.11 Affinity labelling: The hapten binds to its antibody and the azide group activated by ultraviolet light loses N_2 forming a reactive radical which combines with an adjacent amino acid—in this hypothetical example an alanine residue. Analysis of the protein after digestion would show the alanine to be labelled with the hapten and implicate this residue in the combining site. Studies by Fleet G.W.J., Porter R.R. & Knowles J.R. (*Nature* 1969, **224**, 511) indicate that the affinity label combines with heavy and light chains in a ratio of approximately 3·5 : 1.

Light chains

A convenient source of human material is the urinary Bence–Jones' protein which is found in a proportion of patients with myeloma. The Bence–Jones' protein represents a dimer of light chains derived from the pool used in the synthesis of the myeloma protein. By raising antisera in rabbits to a number of Bence–Jones' proteins it was found that light chains could be divided into two groups (called *kappa* (κ) and *lambda* (λ)) depending upon their reactions with the antisera. The Bence–Jones' light chains of the κ-group all gave precipitin reactions with anti-κ sera but no reaction with anti-λ sera. Parallel reactions were always obtained with the parent myeloma protein as would be expected if they were derived from light chains produced by one clone of myeloma plasma cells (figure 2.12). The reactions with normal serum show that molecules with κ- and λ-chains are present. They occur on different molecules and approximately 65 per cent of the immunoglobulin molecules in normal serum are of κ-type, the remainder being λ-type. It is of interest that myeloma proteins of type κ occur with nearly twice the frequency of type λ, suggesting that cells synthesizing molecules with λ-chains carry the same risk of becoming malignant as those making κ-chains. The $\kappa : \lambda$ ratio varies in different species.

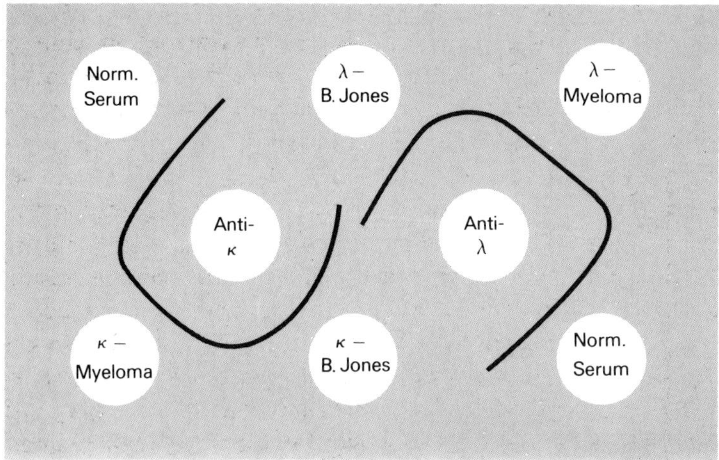

FIGURE 2.12. Precipitation reactions in agar-gel using antisera prepared against κ and λ Bence–Jones' proteins (urinary light chain dimers). The anti-κ reacted with κ but not λ light chains and gave reactions of 'identity' with the related myeloma protein and with normal serum. Parallel results were obtained with the anti-λ serum.

Similar studies using antisera prepared against normal and myeloma proteins have established the existence of *five* major types of heavy chain in the human, each of which gives rise to a distinct immunoglobulin class. As mentioned earlier these are IgG, IgA, IgM, IgD and IgE. But whereas each immunoglobulin class is associated with a particular type of heavy chain, they all have κ- and λ-light chains; thus each myeloma protein so far studied, whatever its class, has possessed light chains of either κ- or λ-specificity (but never of both together).

We have already considered the view that the variable portion of the immunoglobulin molecule is bound up with antibody specificity and all classes have been shown to have binding affinity for antigen associated with the Fab regions. What of the constant region, particularly the Fc part of the heavy chain backbone which makes no contribution to specificity? Almost certainly the Fc structure directs the *biological activity* of the antibody molecule. As will be seen below, it determines to some extent the distribution of the immunoglobulin throughout the body, e.g. the selective passage of IgG across the placenta and the secretion of IgA into the external body fluids. But also after combination with antigen a new or enhanced activity such as the ability to fix complement, or to bind effectively to macrophages may arise. It has been suggested that this occurs through an allosteric change in Fc conformation due to the opening of the 'hinge' Fc. However, the flexibility of the hinge makes this rather unlikely and physical measurements with nuclear magnetic resonance and electron spin probes only detect conformational changes in the Fab not the Fc region after complexing with antigen. The complement system (cf. p. 160) may be activated if the combination of antibody with antigen causes a shift in the relative spatial orientation of Fab and Fc fragments and permits access of the initiating complement component (C1) to the appropriate site in the Fc region; this contention is strengthened by the finding that IgG4 (a *sub*class variant of IgG, *vide infra*) with a very short hinge can only activate complement when the Fc is cleaved from the Fab. Secondary biological properties of antibodies which are mediated through interaction with cell surface receptors for the immunoglobulin Fc may depend upon greatly increased binding to the cell due to the multivalent Fc sites present in an immune complex (cf. bonus effect of multivalency, p. 15) or the cross-linking of Fc receptors by the complex, or both mechanisms. Each of these biological functions may require a different type of Fc structure and hence amino acid sequence. Thus the multiplicity of Fc structures as expressed in the different immunoglobulin classes and subclasses may be looked upon as a system which has evolved to provide antibodies with different biological capabilities in relation to antigens.

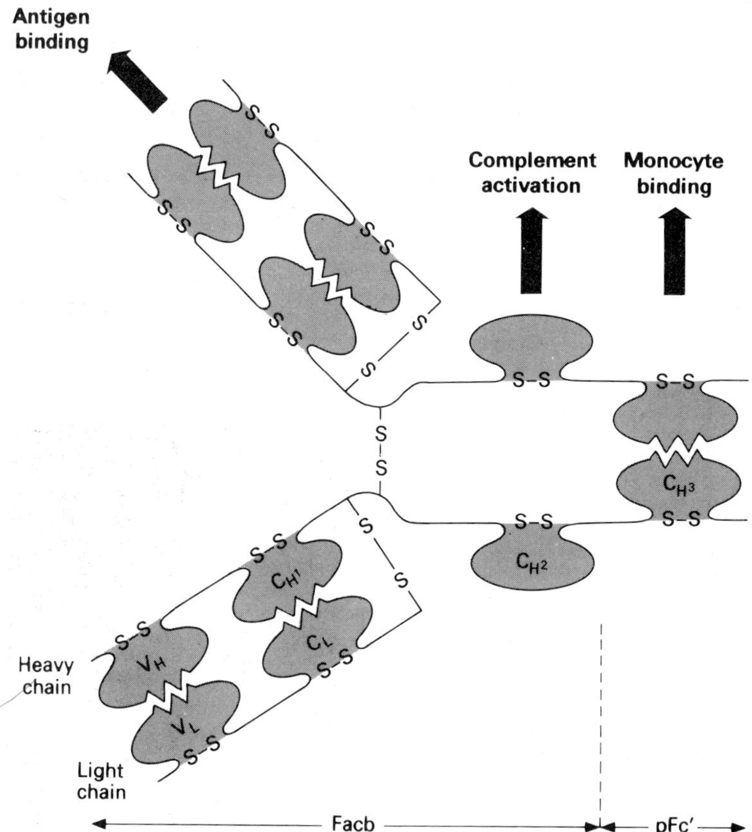

FIGURE 2.13. Immunoglobulin domains in IgG. Each loop in the peptide chain formed by an *intrachain* disulphide bond represents a single domain (shaded) and these are labelled V_H, C_{H^1} etc. as indicated. They show considerable homology (i.e. similarities in amino acid structure) but each domain appears to be specialized for a specific function as shown. The involvement of the C_{H^2} region in complement activation is indicated by the activity of the plasmin Facb fragment which contains the C_{H^2} domain, and the inactivity of the $F(ab')_2$ fragment which lacks it. The active site is a hydrophobic region near the hinge. The pepsin pFc′ fragment which bears the C_{H^3} domain can bind directly to the monocyte surface and inhibit the formation of Fc rosettes with antibody-coated red cells. Staphylococcal protein-A reacts at the interface between C_{H^2} and C_{H^3}.

In summary, the variable part provides specificity for binding antigen; the constant part is associated with different biological properties which vary from one immunoglobulin class to another, depending upon the primary structure, and which may require combination with antigen for their activation.

Immunoglobulin domains

In addition to the *interchain* disulphide bonds which bridge heavy and light chains, there are internal, *intrachain* disulphide links which form loops in the peptide chain (figure 2.13). As Edelman predicted, the loops are compactly folded to form globular domains (figure 2.15). These interact spatially through their hydrophobic regions (figure 2.14) and individual domains subserve separate functions.

Thus the variable region domains (V_L and V_H) are responsible for the formation of a specific antigen-binding site. The $C_{H}2$ region in IgG binds C1q to initiate the classical complement sequence (cf. p. 160) while adherence to the monocyte surface is mediated largely through the terminal $C_{H}3$ domain (figure 2.13).

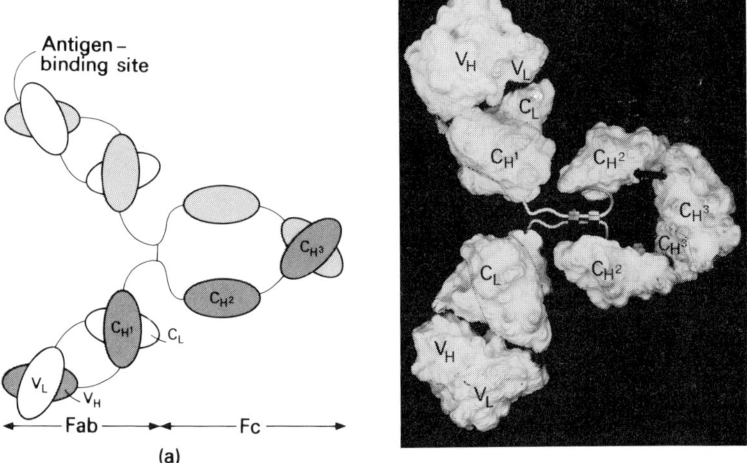

FIGURE 2.14. The disposition and interaction of Ig domains in IgG. (a) Diagram showing apposing domains making contact through hydrophobic regions (after Dr. A. Feinstein). These regions on the two complement fixing $C_{H}2$ domains are partly masked by carbohydrate and remain independent. This separation allows the formation of a hinge region which is extremely flexible both with respect to variation in the angle of the Fab fragments and their rotation about the hinge peptide chain. Thus combining sites in IgG can be readily adapted to spatial variations in the presentation of the antigenic epitopes. (b) Space filling model (courtesy of Dr. A. Feinstein).

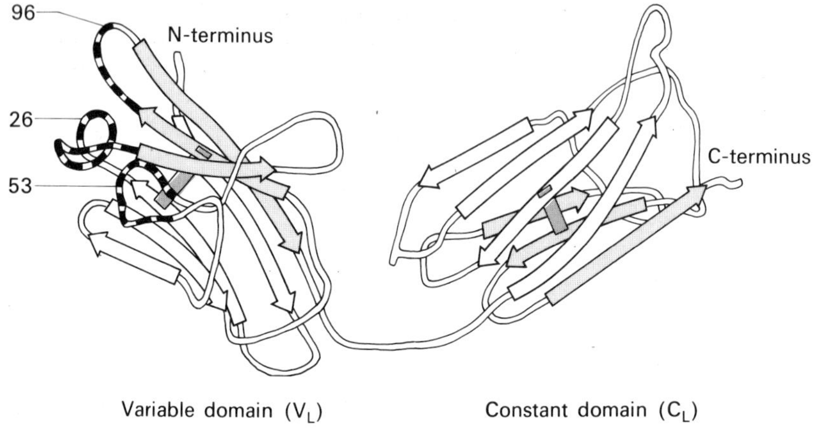

FIGURE 2.15. Structure of the globular domains of a light chain (from X-ray crystallographic studies of a Bence-Jones' protein by Schiffler *et al.*, *Biochemistry*, 1973, **12**, 4620). One surface of each domain is composed essentially of 4 chains arranged in an anti-parallel β-pleated structure (white arrows) and the other of 3 such chains (grey arrows); the dark bar represents the intra-chain disulphide bond. This structure is characteristic of all immunoglobulin domains. Of particular interest is the location of the hypervariable regions (▬▭▬▭▬) in 3 separate loops which are closely disposed relative to each other and form the light chain contribution to the antigen binding site (cf. figure 2.10). One numbered residue from each complementarity determinant is identified.

Comparison of immunoglobulin classes

The physical and biological characteristics of the five major immunoglobulin classes in the human are summarized in tables 2.1 and 2.2. The following comments are intended to supplement this information.

Immunoglobulin G

During the secondary response IgG is probably the major immunoglobulin to be synthesized. Through its ability to cross the placenta it provides a major line of defence against infection for the first few weeks of a baby's life which may be further reinforced by the transfer of colostral IgG across the gut mucosa in the neonate. IgG diffuses more readily than the other immunoglobulins into the extravascular body spaces where as the predominant species it carries the major burden of neutralizing bacterial toxins and of binding to micro-organisms to enhance their phagocytosis. The complexes of bacteria with IgG antibody activate complement thereby chemotactically attracting polymorphonuclear phagocytic cells (cf. p. 161) which adhere to the bacteria

TABLE 2.1. Physical properties of major human immunoglobulin classes

WHO Designation	IgG	IgA	IgM	IgD	IgE
Sedimentation coefficient	7*S*	7*S*, 9*S*, 11*S**	19*S*	7*S*	8*S*
Molecular weight	150,000	160,000 and dimer	900,000	185,000	200,000
Number of basic 4-peptide units	1	1, 2*	5	1	1
Heavy chains	γ	α	μ	δ	ε
Light chains $\kappa+\lambda$	$\kappa+\lambda$	$\kappa+\lambda$	$\kappa+\lambda$	$\kappa+\lambda$	$\kappa+\lambda$
Molecular formula†	$\gamma_2\kappa_2$, $\gamma_2\lambda_2$	$(\alpha_2\kappa_2)_{1-2}$ $(\alpha_2\lambda_2)_{1-2}$ $(\alpha_2\kappa_2)_2S$* $(\alpha_2\lambda_2)_2S$*	$(\mu_2\kappa_2)_5$ $(\mu_2\lambda_2)_5$	$\delta_2\kappa_2(\delta_2\lambda_2?)$	$\varepsilon_2\kappa_2\varepsilon_2\lambda_2$
Valency for antigen binding	2	2, 4	5(10)	2	2
Concentration range in normal serum	8–16 mg/ml	1·4–4 mg/ml	0·5–2 mg/ml	0–0·4 mg/ml	17–450 ng/ml‡
% total immunoglobulin	80	13	6	0–1	0·002
Carbohydrate content, %	3	8	12	13	12

* Dimer in external secretions carries secretory component—S.
† IgA dimer and IgM contain J chain.
‡ ng = 10^{-9} g.

through surface receptors for complement and the Fc portion of IgG (Fcγ); binding to the Fc receptor then stimulates ingestion of micro-organisms through phagocytosis. In a similar way, the extracellular killing of target cells coated with IgG antibody is mediated through recognition of the surface Fcγ by K cells bearing the appropriate receptors (cf. p. 227). The interaction of IgG complexes with platelet Fc receptors presumably leads to aggregation and vasoactive amine release but the physiological significance of Fcγ binding sites on other cell types, particularly lymphocytes, has not yet been clarified. Although unable to bind firmly to mast cells in human skin, IgG alone among the human immunoglobulins has the somewhat useless property of fixing to guinea pig skin. The thesis that the biological individuality of different immunoglobulin classes is dependent on the heavy chain constant regions, particularly the

TABLE 2.2. Biological properties of major immunoglobulin classes in the human

	IgG	IgA	IgM	IgD	IgE
Major characteristics	Most abundant Ig of internal body fluids particularly extra-vascular where it combats micro-organisms and their toxins	Major Ig in sero-mucous secretions where it defends external body surfaces	Very effective agglutinator; produced early in immune response—effective first line defence vs. bacteraemia	Most, if not all, present on lymphocyte surface	Protection external body surfaces Recruits anti-microbial agents Raised in parasitic infections Responsible for symptoms of atopic allergy
Complement fixation					
Classical	+ +	–	+ + +	–	
Alternative	–	±	–	–	
Cross placenta	+	–	–	–	–
Fix to homologous mast cells and basophils	–	–	–	–	+
Binding to macrophages and polymorphs	+	±	–	–	–

Fc, is amply borne out in relationship to the activities we have discussed such as transplacental passage, complement fixation and binding to various cell types, where function has been shown to be mediated by the Fc part of the molecule.

With respect to overall regulation of IgG levels in the body, the catabolic rate appears to depend directly upon the total IgG concentration whereas synthesis is largely governed by antigen stimulation so that in germ-free animals, for example, IgG levels are extremely low but rise rapidly on transfer to a normal environment.

Immunoglobulin A

IgA appears selectively in the sero-mucous secretions such as saliva, tears, nasal fluids, sweat, colostrum and secretions of the lung, genito-urinary and gastro-intestinal tracts where it clearly has the job of defending the exposed external surfaces of the body against attack by micro-organisms. It is present in these fluids as a dimer stabilized against

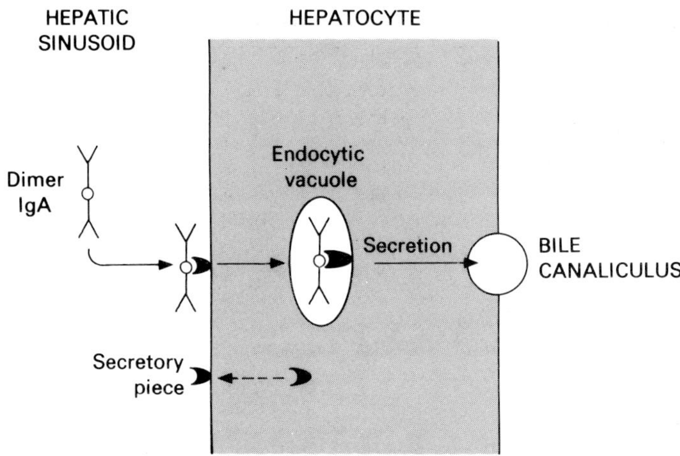

FIGURE 2.16. The mechanism of IgA secretion as exemplified by the transfer of circulating IgA into the bile. Dimeric IgA in the sinusoid binds to surface secretory piece thereby activating the uptake and secretion of the immunoglobulin. There is perhaps an analogy with the uptake of IgG into macrophages through stimulation of the surface IgG receptors.

proteolysis by combination with another protein—the secretory component which is synthesized by local epithelial cells and has a single peptide chain of molecular weight 60,000. The IgA is synthesized locally by plasma cells and dimerized intracellularly together with a cysteine-rich polypeptide called J-chain of molecular weight 15,000. If dimerization occurred randomly *after* secretion, dimers of mixed specificity would be formed which would not be as effective in combining with antigen as those of single specificity which would have a higher effective valency. The dimeric IgA binds strongly to secretory component present on the surface of the cell in which it was produced and the complex is then actively endocytosed, transported across the cytoplasm and secreted into the external body fluids (figure 2.16).

IgA antibodies function by inhibiting the adherence of coated micro-organisms to the surface of mucosal cells thereby preventing entry into the body tissues. Aggregated IgA binds to polymorphs and can also activate the alternative (p. 162) as distinct from the classical complement pathway which probably accounts for reports of a synergism between IgA, complement and lysozyme in the killing of certain coliform organisms. Human plasma contains relatively high concentrations of monomeric IgA and its role is still something of a mystery.

Immunoglobulin M

Often referred to as the macroglobulin antibodies because of their high molecular weight, IgM molecules are polymers of five 4-peptide subunits each bearing an extra C_H domain. As with IgA, polymerization of the subunits depends upon the presence of J-chain whose function may be to stabilize the Fc sulphydryl groups during Ig synthesis so that they remain available for cross-linking the subunits to give the structure shown in figure 2.17a. Under negative staining in the electron-microscope, the free molecule in solution assumes a 'star' shape but when combined as an antibody with an antigenic surface membrane it can adopt a 'crab-like' configuration (figures 2.17b and c). The theoretical combining valency is of course 10 but this is only observed on interaction with small haptens; with larger antigens the effective valency falls to 5 and this must be attributed to some form of steric restriction due to lack of flexibility in the molecule. IgM antibodies tend to be of relatively low affinity as measured against single determinants (haptens) but, because of their high valency, they bind with quite respectable avidity to antigens with multiple epitopes (bonus effect of multivalency p. 15).

For the same reason, these antibodies are extremely efficient agglutinating and cytolytic agents and since they appear early in the response to infection and are largely confined to the blood stream, it is likely that they play a role of particular importance in cases of bacteraemia. The isohaemagglutinins (anti-A, anti-B) and many of the 'natural' antibodies to micro-organisms are usually IgM; antibodies to the typhoid 'O' antigen (endotoxin) and the 'WR' antibodies in syphilis also tend to be found in this class. IgM would appear to precede IgG in the phylogeny of the immune response in vertebrates.

Immunoglobulin D

This class was recognized through the discovery of a myeloma protein which did not have the antigenic specificity of IgG, A or M, although it reacted with antibodies to immunoglobulin light chains and had the basic four-peptide structure. Among the different immunoglobulin classes it is uniquely susceptible to proteolytic degradation, and this may account for its short half-life in plasma (2·8 days). An exciting development has been the demonstration that

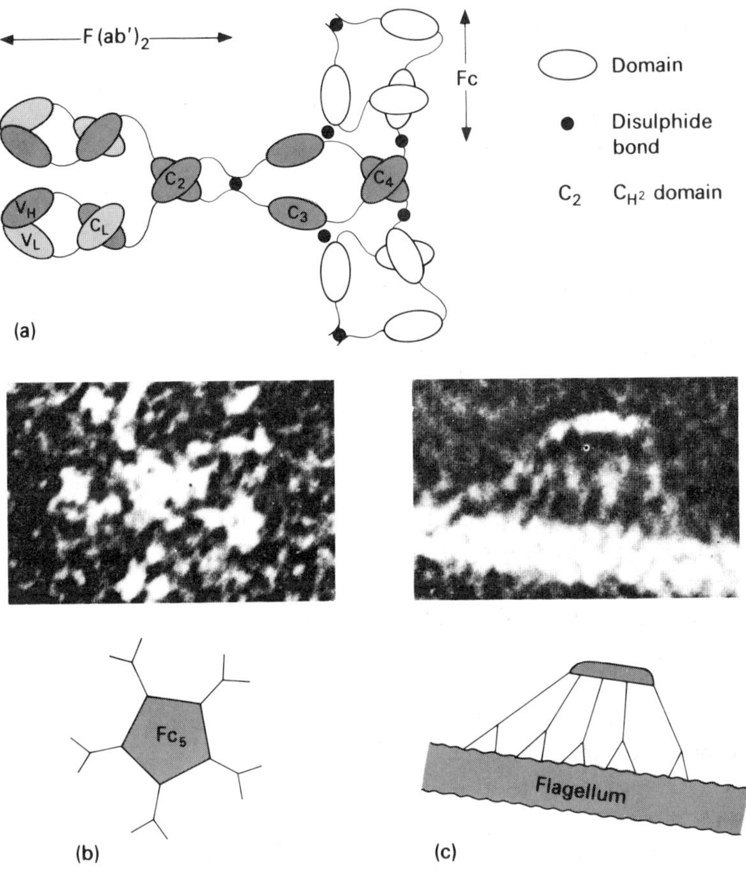

FIGURE 2.17. The structure of IgM: (a) The arrangement of domains in one of the 5 subunits showing how the pentamer is built up through the disulphide linkages between C_H3 and C terminal regions (after Hilschman & Feinstein). Without too much aggravation, I hope the reader will appreciate that the hinge region in IgG (cf. fig 2.14) is replaced by a rigid pair of extra domains (C_H2), while the C_H3 and C_H4 domains in IgM are structurally equivalent to the C_H2 and C_H3 regions respectively in IgG. (b) As shown by electron microscopy of a human Waldenström's macroglobulin in free solution adopting a 'star'-shaped configuration. (c) As revealed in an E.M. preparation of specific sheep IgM antibody bound to *Salmonella paratyphi* flagellum where the immunoglobulin has assumed a 'crab-like' conformation in establishing its links with antigen. With the $F(ab')_2$ arms bent out of the plane of the central Fc_5 region, the C_H3 complement binding domains are now readily accessible to the first component of complement (cf. p. 160). The Fc_5 constellation obtained by papain cleavage can activate complement directly. (Electron micrographs—kindly provided by Dr. A. Feinstein and Dr. E.A. Munn—are negatively stained preparations of magnification 2,000,000 ×, i.e. 1 mm represents 5 Å.)

nearly all the IgD is present on the surface of a proportion of blood lymphocytes together with IgM, and it seems likely that they may function as mutually interacting antigen receptors for the control of lymphocyte activation and suppression.

Immunoglobulin E

Only very low concentrations of IgE are present in serum and only a very small proportion of the plasma cells in the body are synthesizing this immunoglobulin. It is not surprising, therefore, that so far only six cases of IgE myeloma have been recognized compared with tens of thousands of IgG paraproteinaemias. IgE antibodies remain firmly fixed for an extended period when injected into human skin where they are probably bound to mast cells. Contact with antigen leads to degranulation of the mast cells with release of vasoactive amines. This process is responsible for the symptoms of hayfever and of extrinsic asthma when patients with atopic allergy come into contact with the allergen, e.g. grass pollen.

The main *physiological* role of IgE would appear to be protection of the external mucosal surfaces of the body by local recruitment of plasma factors and effector cells. Infectious agents penetrating the IgA defences would combine with specific IgE on the mast cell surface and trigger the release of vasoactive agents and factors chemotactic for granulocytes so leading to an influx of plasma IgG, complement, polymorphs and eosinophils (cf. p. 160). In such a context, the ability of eosinophils to damage IgG-coated helminths and the generous IgE response to such parasites would constitute an effective defence.

IMMUNOGLOBULIN SUBCLASSES

Antigenic analysis of IgG myelomas revealed further variation and showed that they could be grouped into four *subclasses* now termed IgG1, IgG2, IgG3 and IgG4. The differences all lie in the heavy chains which have been labelled $\gamma 1$, $\gamma 2$, $\gamma 3$ and $\gamma 4$ respectively. These heavy chains show considerable homology and have certain structures in common with each other—the ones which react with specific anti-IgG antisera—but each has one or more additional structures characteristic of its own subclass arising from differences in primary amino acid composition and in disulphide bridging. These give rise to differences in biological behaviour which are summarized in table 2.3.

Two subclasses of IgA have also been found. The IgA2 subclass is unusual in that it lacks interchain disulphide bonds between heavy and light chains. Class and subclass variation is not restricted to human immunoglobulins but is a feature of all the higher mammals so far studied; monkey, sheep, rabbit, guinea-pig, rat and mouse.

OTHER IMMUNOGLOBULIN VARIANTS

Isotypes

The heavy chain constant region structures associated with the different classes and subclasses are termed isotypic variants, i.e. they are all present together in the serum of a normal subject. Other examples are provided by the types and subtypes of the C_L domain and by the subgroups of the light and heavy chain variable regions (table 2.4).

TABLE 2.3. Comparison of human IgG subclasses

	IgG1	IgG2	IgG3	IgG4
% of total IgG in normal serum	65	23	8	4
Electrophoretic mobility	slow	slow	slow	fast
Spontaneous aggregation	—	—	+ + +	—
Gm allotypes	a,z,f,x	n	bo,b1,b3, g,s,t, etc.	
Ga site reacting with rheumatoid factor*	+ + +	+ + +	—	+ + +
Combination with staphylococcal A protein	+ + +	+ + +	—	+ + +
Cross placenta	+ +	±	+ +	+ +
Complement fixation (C1 pathway)	+ + +	+ +	+ + + +	±
Binding to monocytes	+ + +	+	+ + +	±
Binding to heterologous skin	+ +	—	+ +	+ +
Blocking IgE binding	—	—	—	+
Antibody dominance	Anti-Rh	Anti-dextran Anti-levan	Anti-Rh	Anti Factor VIII

* Other rheumatoid factors apparently react with Gm specific sites.

TABLE 2.4. Summary of immunoglobulin variants

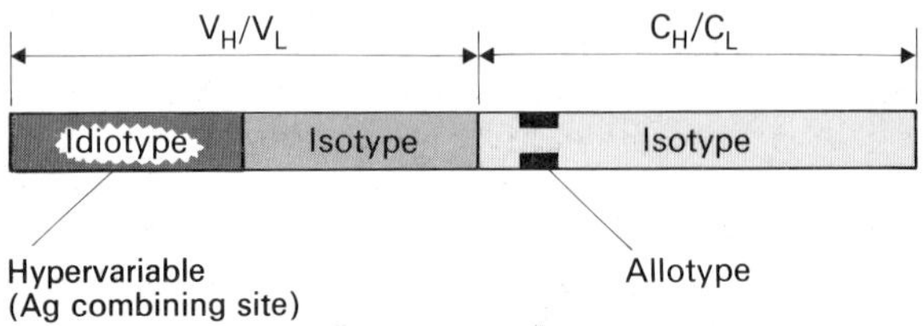

Type of variation	Distribution	Variant	Location	Examples
ISOTYPIC	All variants present in serum of a normal individual	Classes Subclasses Types Subtypes Subgroups	C_H C_H C_L C_L V_H/V_L	IgM, IgE IgA1, IgA2 κ, λ λOz^+, λOz^- $V_{\kappa I}$, $V_{\kappa II}$, $V_{\kappa III}$ V_{HI}, V_{HII}, V_{HIII}
ALLOTYPIC	Alternative forms: genetically controlled so not present in all individuals	Allotypes	Mainly C_H/C_L sometimes V_H/V_L	Gm groups (human) b4, b5, b6, b9 (rabbit light chains)
IDIOTYPIC	Individually specific to each immunoglobulin molecule	Idiotypes	Variable regions	Probably one or more hypervariable regions forming the antigen-combining site.

Allotypes

These represent yet a further type of variation which depends upon the existence of allelic forms (encoded by alleles or alternative genes at a single locus). In somewhat the same way as the red cells in genetically different individuals can differ in terms of the blood group antigen system A, B, O, so the Ig heavy chains differ in the expression of their allotypic groups. Typical allotypes are the Gm specificities on IgG (Gm = *marker* on Ig*G*) which are recognizable by the ability of the individual's IgG to block agglutination of red cells coated with anti-rhesus D bearing the Gm allotype by sera from patients with rheumatoid arthritis containing the appropriate anti-Gm rheumatoid factors. Allotypic differences at a given Gm locus usually involve one or two amino acids in the peptide chain. Take for example the Glm(a) locus on IgGl (table 2.3). An individual with this allotype would have the peptide sequence: Asp . Glu . Leu . Thr . Lys on each of his IgGl molecules. Another person whose IgGl was a-negative would have the sequence Met . Glu . Thr . Lys, i.e. two amino acids different. To date, 25 Gm groups have been found on the γ-heavy chains and a further 3 (the Km—previously Inv groups) on the κ constant region.

Allotypic markers have also been found on the immunoglobulins of rabbits and of mice using reagents prepared by immunizing one animal with an immune complex obtained with antibodies from another animal of the same species. As in other allelic systems, individuals may be homozygous or heterozygous for the genes encoding the markers. Take for example the b4, b5 allotypes on rabbit light chains: an animal of b^4b^4 genotype would express the b4 allotype whereas a rabbit of b^4b^5 genotype would express the b4 marker on one fraction and b5 on another fraction of its immunglobulin molecules.

Isoallotypes are horrendously small print: these are groups shared by 2 or more subclasses which are structurally anti-thetic to a Gm marker present in one class only, e.g. nGlm(a) is present on all IgG2 and IgG3 proteins but only on IgG1 molecules lacking Glm(a).

Idiotypes

We have seen that it is possible to obtain antibodies that recognize isotypic and allotypic variants; it is also possible to raise antisera which are specific for individual antibody molecules and discriminate between one monoclonal antibody and another or one myeloma protein and another independently of isotypic or allotypic structures. These individual or idiotypic determinants (Oudin) are located in the variable part of the antibody, almost certainly in the combining site and it seems likely that each hypervariable region could function as an idiotype. Thus in many cases, an anti-idiotypic serum directed against an anti-hapten antibody can block the binding of hapten. Anti-idiotypic sera which do not block are presumably directed to hyper-variable regions not concerned in the binding of that hapten (we know that small haptens do not fill the whole of the potential combining site of the antibody molecule). The existence of anti-idiotypes provides further support for the idea that each antibody has a unique structure. These antisera provide useful reagents, e.g. for demonstrating the same V region on different heavy chains and on different cells, for identification of specific immune complexes in patients' sera, for recognition of V_L type amyloid in subjects excreting Bence-Jones proteins, for detection of residual monoclonal protein after therapy and perhaps for selecting lymphocytes with certain surface receptors.

Summary

Immunoglobulins (Ig) have a basic 4 peptide structure of 2 identical heavy and 2 identical light chains joined by interchain disulphide links. Papain splits the molecule at the exposed flexible hinge region to give two identical univalent antigen binding fragments (Fab) and a further fragment (Fc). Pepsin proteolysis gives a divalent Ag binding fragment $F(ab')_2$ lacking the Fc.

There are perhaps 10^8 or more different Ig molecules in normal serum. Analysis of myeloma proteins which are homogeneous Ig produced by single clones of malignant plasma cells has shown the N terminal region of heavy and light chains to have a variable amino acid structure and the remainder to be relatively constant in structure. Each chain is folded into globular domains. The variable region domains bind Ag and 3 *hypervariable* loops on the heavy and 3 on the light chain form the Ag binding site. The constant region domains of the heavy chain (particularly the Fc) carry out a secondary biological function after the binding of Ag, e.g. complement fixation and macrophage binding.

In the human there are 5 major types of heavy chain giving 5 *classes* of Ig. IgG is the most abundant Ig particularly in the extravascular fluids where it combats micro-organisms and toxins; it fixes complement, binds to phagocytic cells and crosses the placenta. IgA exists mainly as a monomer (basic 4 peptide unit) in plasma, but in the seromucous secretions where it is the major Ig concerned in the defence of the external body surfaces, it is present as dimer linked to a secretory component. IgM is a pentameric molecule, essentially intravascular, produced early in the immune response. Because of its high valency it is a very effective bacterial agglutinator and mediator of complement dependent cytolysis and is therefore a powerful first line defence against bacteraemia. IgD is largely present on the lymphocyte and probably functions as an Ag receptor. IgE binds firmly to mast cells and contact with antigen leads to local recruitment of anti-microbial agents through degranulation of the mast cells and release of inflammatory mediators. IgE is of importance in certain parasitic infections and is responsible for the symptoms of atopic allergy. Further diversity of function is possible through subdivision of classes into subclasses based on structural differences in heavy chains present in each normal individual.

Allotypic structural variations are controlled by allelic genes and provide genetic markers. Idiotypic determinants unique to a given immunoglobulin are recognizable by anti-idiotypic antibodies and are associated with the hypervariable regions forming the Ag binding site.

Further reading

Benacerraf B. (ed) (1975) *Immunogenetics and Immunodeficiency* (Articles by B. Frangione on Ig structure and by H.G. Kunkel & T. Kindt on allotypes and idiotypes). MTP, Lancaster, England.

Edelman G.M. *et al.* (1969) Complete sequence of human IgG1. *Proc.Nat. Acad.Sci.*, **63**, 78.

Fongerean M. & Dansset J. (eds) (1980) *Progress in Immunology IV*. Academic Press, London.

Givol D. (1974) Affinity labelling and topology of the antibody combining site. In *Essays in Biochemistry* (eds Campbell P.N. & Dickens F.) **10**, 73. *Biochem.Soc.* London.

Glynn L.E. & Steward M.W. (eds) (1977) *Immunochemistry : an Advanced Textbook*, Wiley, Chichester

Leslie R.G.Q. & Cohen S. (1973) The active sites of immunoglobulin molecules. In *Essays in Fundamental Immunology 1*, page 1. Blackwell Scientific Publications, Oxford.

Moller E. (ed.) (1978) Immunoglobulin E. *Immunol. Rev.* **41**.

Poljak R.J. (1975) Three-dimensional structure, function and genetic control of immunoglobulin. *Nature*, **256**, 373.

3 The immune response I—Fundamentals

Two types of immune response

When antigen enters the body, two different types of adaptive immunological reaction may occur:

1. The synthesis and release of free antibody into the blood and other body fluids (*humoral immunity*). This antibody acts, for example, by coating bacteria to enhance their phagocytosis and by combination with and neutralization of bacterial toxins.
2. The production of 'sensitized' lymphocytes which are themselves the effectors of *cell-mediated immunity*. This confers protection against organisms such as the tubercle bacillus and viruses which are characterized by an ability to live and replicate *within* the cells of the host. In individuals immune to tubercle infection, the 'sensitized' lymphocytes interact with injected tuberculin antigen to produce the delayed type hypersensitivity skin response, well known as the Mantoux reaction. Cells of this type are also involved in the rejection of skin grafts.

Role of the small lymphocyte

The central importance of the lymphocyte for both types of immune response was established largely by the work of Gowans. By labelling the lymphocytes with radioisotope and following their fate in the body it could be shown that there is a pool of recirculating lymphocytes which pass from the blood into the lymph nodes, spleen and other tissues and back to the blood by the major lymphatic channels such as the thoracic duct (figure 3.1).

PRIMARY RESPONSE

When rats are depleted of their lymphocytes by chronic drainage of lymph from the thoracic duct by an indwelling cannula, they have a grossly impaired ability to mount a primary antibody response to antigens such as tetanus toxoid and sheep red blood cells, or to reject a skin graft. Immunological reactivity can be restored by injecting thoracic duct lymphocytes obtained from another rat. The same effect can be obtained if, before injection, the thoracic duct cells are first incubated at 37°C for 24 hours under conditions which kill off large and medium-sized cells and leave only the small lymphocytes. Thus the small lymphocyte is necessary for the primary response to antigen.

Transfer experiments have also shown that small lymphocytes can become antibody synthesizing cells (plasma cells) and effector cells in cell-mediated immunity transplantation reactions.

SECONDARY RESPONSE—MEMORY

An immunologically 'virgin' rat, i.e. one which has had no previous contact with a specific antigen, may be inoculated with small lymphocytes from a rat which has already

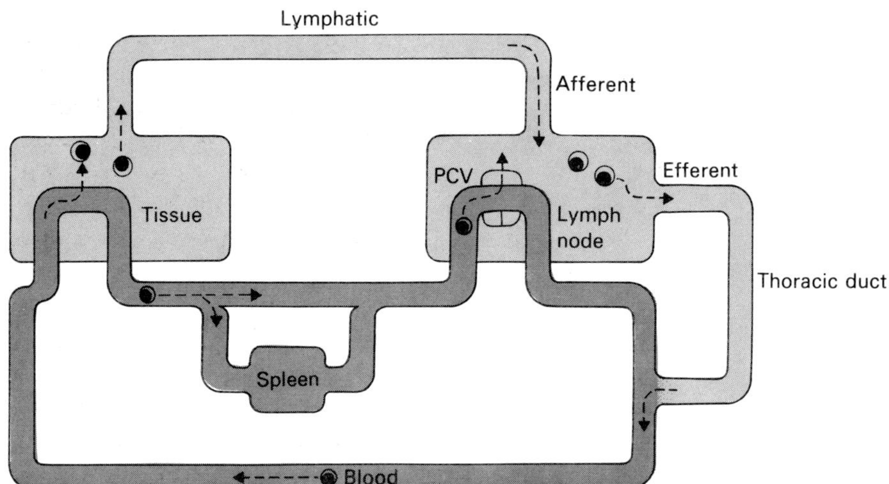

FIGURE 3.1. Traffic and recirculation of lymphocytes. Blood-borne lymphocytes enter the tissues and lymph nodes passing between the high cuboidal cells of the post-capillary venules (PCV) and leave via the draining lymphatics. The efferent lymphatics finally emerging from the last node in each chain join to form the thoracic duct which returns the lymphocytes to the blood stream where it empties into the left subclavian vein (in the human). In the spleen, lymphocytes enter the lymphoid area (white pulp) from the arterioles, pass to the sinusoids of the erythroid area (red pulp) and leave by the splenic vein.

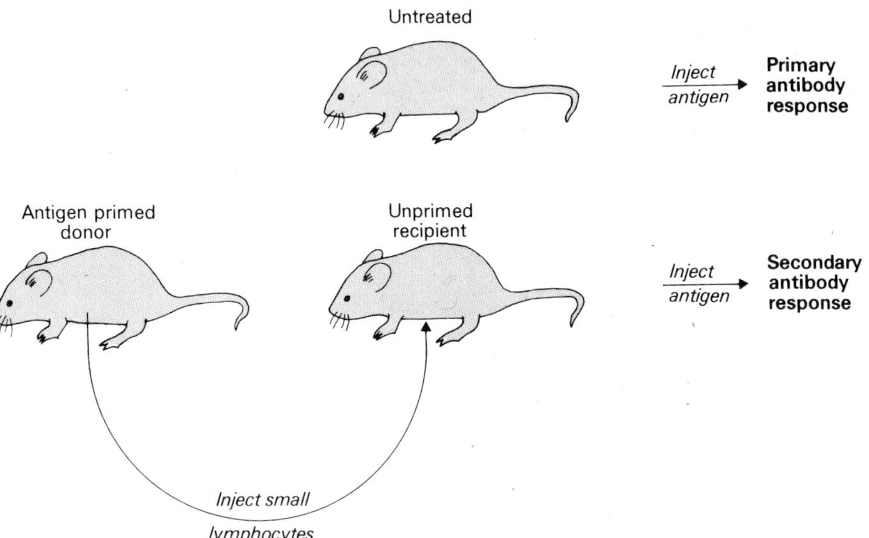

FIGURE 3.2. Transfer of immunological memory by small lymphocytes from primed donor rat. In these transfer experiments, genetically identical animals of the same strain are used to prevent complications arising from transplantation reactions between the transferred lymphocytes and the host.

given a primary response to that antigen. Challenge of the recipient rat with antigen leads to a secondary type response with the rapid production of high-titre antibodies. If the recipient had not been injected with small lymphocytes from the 'primed' donor, a primary response with the relatively slow development of lower titre antibodies would have been seen (figure 3.2). Thus the small lymphocytes carry the *memory* of the first contact with antigen.

In the primary response, the relatively small number of virgin cells specific for the antigen are induced to *proliferate*; some go on to produce antibody- or cell-mediated immunity while others form an expanded population of antigen-sensitive memory cells which are capable of a faster response to antigen (figure 3.3). This combination of increase in cell number and more rapid maturation after antigen triggering is responsible for the characteristically brisk and heightened course of the secondary antibody response.

The thymus

This gland is organized into a series of lobules made up essentially of a meshwork of epithelial cells within which are packed aggregates of lymphocytes. The outer cortical

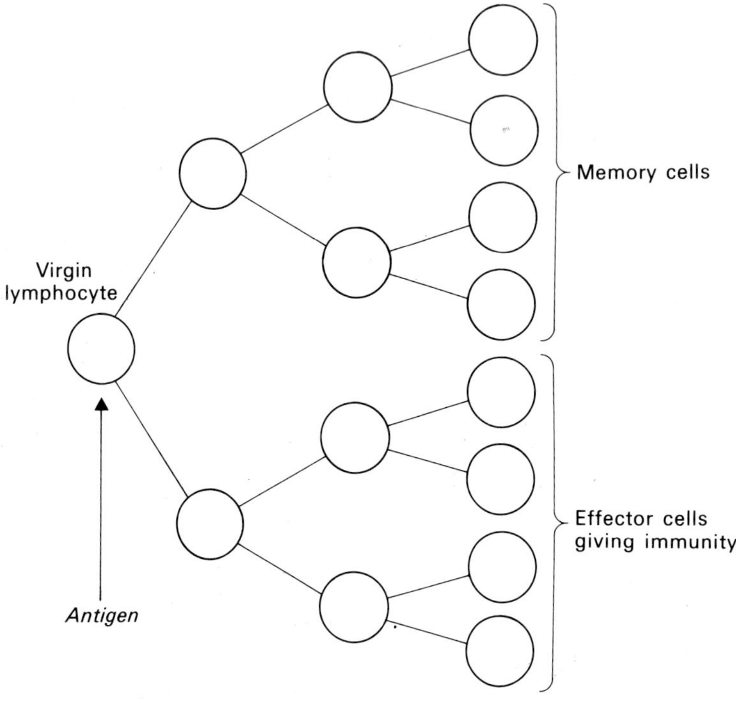

FIGURE 3.3. The cellular basis of the primary response. After stimulation by antigen the previously resting virgin lymphocyte proliferates and during these divisions the cells mature. Some become non-dividing memory cells and others the effector cells of humoral or cell-mediated immunity. Memory cells require fewer cycles before they develop into effectors and this shortens the reaction time for the secondary response. The expanded clone of cells with memory for the original antigen provides the basis for the greater secondary relative to the primary immune response. Priming with low doses of antigen can often stimulate effective memory without producing very adequate antibody sythesis.

area is densely populated with actively mitotic and some dying lymphoid cells and surrounds an inner medullary zone of prominent reticular dendritic and epithelioid cells with considerably fewer lymphocytes and isolated Hassall's corpuscles (figure 3.4). The occurrence of frequent thymic abnormalities in children with immunological deficiency disorders led to the suggestion that the thymus was related in some way to the development of immune responses (Good and colleagues). The relationship was clarified by Miller's demonstration that removal of the thymus gland in mice at birth led to:

(i) decrease in circulating lymphocytes;

(ii) severe impairment of graft rejection;

(iii) reduced humoral antibody response to some but not all antigens;

(iv) wasting after 1–3 months—probably a result of inability to combat infection effectively since neonatally thymectomized mice reared under germ-free conditions did not waste.

X-irradiation of adult mice destroys the ability of their lymphocytes to divide and hence their immunological responsiveness. This can be restored by injection of bone

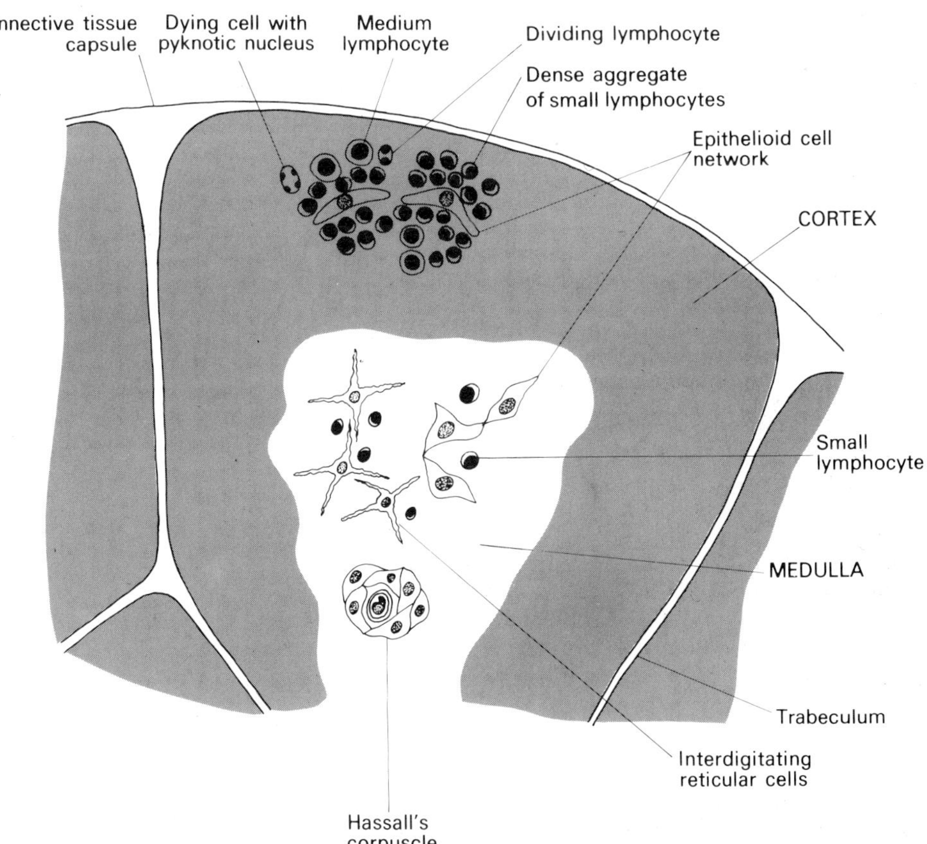

FIGURE 3.4. Features of a thymus lobule. The medulla is continuous and sends finger-like processes into each lobule. The meshwork of epithelioid cells forms an almost continuous cytoplasmic barrier around the blood vessels ('blood-thymus barrier'). Whorled, possibly degenerate aggregates of epithelial cells appear as the characteristic Hassall's corpuscles. Reticular dendritic cells are prominent in the medulla. The densely packed, rapidly dividing lymphocytes in the cortex are mostly immunologically immature and readily destroyed by cortisone; 90% are small, 1% large and the remainder are medium-sized. Lymphocytes in the medulla are more sparse and more cortisone resistant.

marrow cells. However bone marrow cells fail to restore X-irradiated adult mice which have been thymectomized; on the other hand mature cells from adult spleen or lymph node were effective. It is thus concluded that the thymus acts on primitive cells coming from the bone marrow to make them immunologically competent.

The Bursa of Fabricius

In chickens, another lymphoid organ termed the Bursa of Fabricius can be recognized. It is similar to the thymus and also embryologically derived from gut epithelium. Just as the thymus appears to act as a central lymphoid organ controlling the maturation of lymphocytes concerned largely with cell-mediated immunity, so the Bursa of Fabricius is responsible for the development of immunocompetence in cells destined to make humoral antibody. This differentiation of function may be readily seen from the results of the experiments documented in table 3.1: the thymus or bursa was removed from newborn chicks which were then irradiated to inactivate any competent lymphocytes which had already reached the peripheral tissues. After several weeks the chickens were tested and it was found that bursectomy had a profound effect on humoral antibody synthesis but did not unduly influence the cell mediated reactions responsible for tuberculin skin reactivity and graft rejection. On the other hand, as in the mice, thymectomy grossly impaired cell-mediated reactions and had some effect on antibody production.

TABLE 3.1. Effect of neonatal bursectomy and thymectomy on the development of immunological competence in the chicken (From Cooper M.D., Peterson R.D.A., South M.A. & Good R.A., *J.exp.Med.* 1966, **123**, 75, with permission of the editors)

All X-irradiated after birth	Peripheral blood lymphocyte count	Ig concn.	Antibody	Delayed skin reaction to tuberculin	Graft rejection
Intact	14,800	+ +	+ + +	+ +	+ +
Thymectomized	9,000	+ +	+	−	−
Bursectomized	13,200	−	−	+	+

Two populations of lymphocytes: T- and B-cells

Thus primitive lymphoid cells from the bone marrow appear to differentiate into two small lymphocyte populations:

(i) *T-lymphocytes*, processed by or in some way dependent on the thymus, and responsible for cell-mediated immunity;

(ii) *B-lymphocytes*, bursa-dependent, and concerned in the synthesis of circulating antibody.

Both populations on appropriate stimulation by antigen proliferate and undergo morphological changes (figure 3.5). The B-lymphocytes develop into the plasma cell series. The mature plasma cell (figure 3.6d & h) is actively synthesizing and secreting antibody and has a well-developed rough surfaced endoplasmic reticulum (figure 3.7c) characteristic of a cell producing protein for 'export'. T-lymphocytes transform to lymphoblasts (figure 3.6c) which in the electron microscope are seen to have virtually no rough-surfaced endoplasmic reticulum although there are abundant free ribosomes, either single or as polysomes (figure 3.7d). This high ribosome content makes them basophilic so that they show superficial resemblance to plasmablasts in the light microscope but no antibody can be detected in their cytoplasm nor in their secretions. However, they do elaborate a series of soluble factors which act largely through the macrophage in establishing cell-mediated immunity, the other arm of this response being provided by a subpopulation of activated T-lymphocytes which are cytotoxic for virus-infected cells (cf. p. 79).

The equivalent of the bursa in man and other mammals has not yet been clearly defined but experiments involving the culture of bone marrow or fetal liver *in vitro* make it seem likely that haemopoietic tissue itself provides the appropriate microenvironment for maturation of B-lymphocytes from precursor stem cells.

IDENTIFICATION OF B- AND T-LYMPHOCYTES

From the morphological standpoint it is difficult to differentiate T and B small lymphocytes at the light microscope level with conventional histological stains although some differences are now becoming apparent in their enzyme content and their ultrastructure (figure 3.6a & b, 3.7a & b). Fortunately the two populations differ strikingly in their surface markers (table 3.2) and these have been widely exploited.

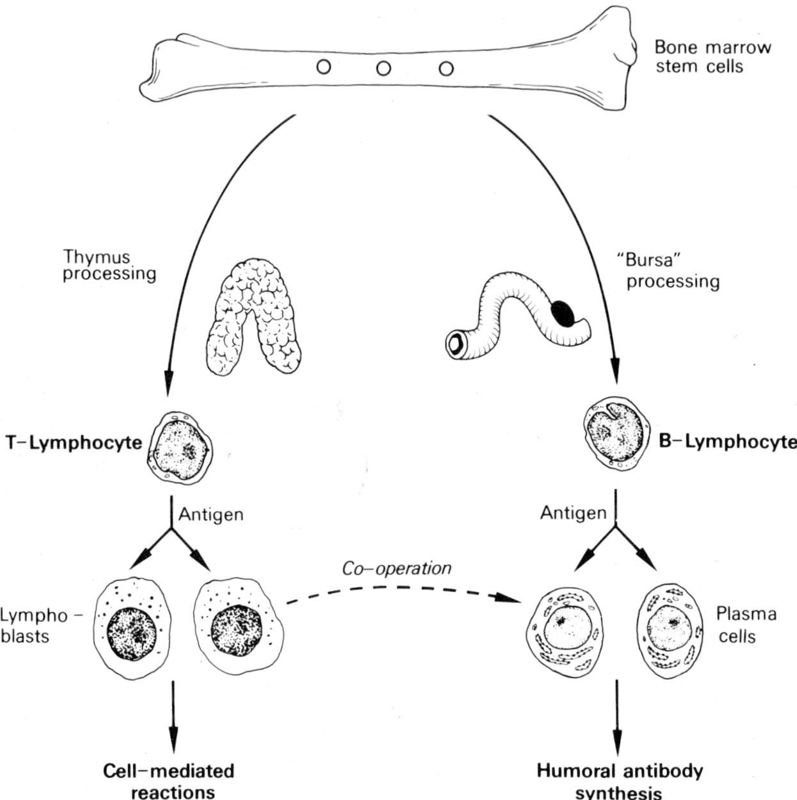

FIGURE 3.5. Processing of bone marrow cells by thymus and gut-associated central lymphoid tissue to become immunocompetent T- and B-lymphocytes respectively. Proliferation and transformation to cells of the lymphoblast and plasma cell series occurs on antigenic stimulation.

Immunoglobulins are readily demonstrable on the surface of B- but not T-lymphocytes using an immunofluorescent technique with reagents such as fluorescein-labelled anti-immunoglobulin light chain (cf. figure 3.9b); this has also been shown in the electron microscope using peroxidase coupled (figure 6.13) ^{125}I-labelled anti-Ig. Nearly all B-cells bear surface IgM, probably as monomer, but a proportion also stain with antisera directed against the Fc portion of other Ig classes particularly IgD. Antisera specific for the terminal heavy chain domain (*p*Fc′ cf. p. 36) stain more weakly suggesting attachment to the membrane through this region. The heavy chain of the surface IgM, which is present as a monomer, has an extra hydrophobic sequence relative to secreted pentameric IgM as revealed by its ability to bind detergent in the Fc region, to be labelled by lipophilic reagents and to insert itself into artificial membrane vesicles

TABLE 3.2. Tests for surface markers on B- and T-cells

Lymphocytes	Immunofluorescent staining for:		Rosette formation using sheep r.b.c. coated with:				Virus receptors	Approx. % of human blood lymphocytes
	Ig	Thy1 (θ)	Nothing	IgG	IgM	C3		
T	−	++	++*	+	++	±	Measles	70
B	++	−	−	++	±	++	EB	10–20

* Human T-cells.

(liposomes). It must be supposed that the hydrophobic sequence anchors the molecule to the surface membrane and that removal of this sequence by mRNA splicing can be suitably arranged should the cell be turned on for Ig secretion as an antibody forming cell. I would like now to make an exceedingly important point. As we will see later, *each lymphocyte is programmed to make Ig of only one specificity and it is this Ig, placed on the B-lymphocyte surface, which is used as a specific receptor for antigen.*

In some circumstances, a proportion of T-cells do stain for surface immunoglobulin. This is not a product of the T-cell itself but is acquired by adsorption and probably represents immune complexes binding to receptors for Ig Fc region which are displayed by some T-cells. These can be demonstrated by the formation of rosettes with red cells coated with IgG antibody; clusters of red cells surround the lymphocyte to which they bind through the Fc of the coating IgG. Other T-cells have Fcμ receptors (i.e binding sites for the Fc region of IgM heavy chains) and some features of these two subpopulations are contrasted in figures 3.6 and 3.7. Most if not all B-cells carry Fc receptors and form 'Fcγ-rosettes' (figure 3.8a). In addition, approximately one half of the B-lymphocytes and perhaps some T-cells form clusters with red cells coated with the third component of complement (C3; cf. 161) (figure 3.8b).

Interestingly, human T-cells can be persuaded to form so-called 'spontaneous' rosettes with uncoated sheep erythrocytes, a useful if fortuitous reaction without any immunological foundation. The T-lymphocyte membrane also possesses a specific discriminating antigen which is shared by brain. In the mouse this is recognized as the Thy1 isoantigenic system (watch for the old nomenclature—θ) which is acquired as the cells differentiate within the milieu of the thymus gland.

FIGURE 3.6. Light microscopy of cells involved in immune responses. (a) Small lymphocytes. Condensed chromatin gives rise to heavy staining of the nucleus. The cell on the left is a typical T-cell with receptors for IgM with a thin rim of cytoplasm. The other cell has more cytoplasm and azurophilic granules are evident; it bears receptors for IgG and sheep red cells and has therefore been defined as a T_G lymphocyte. Isolated platelets are visible. B-lymphocytes have a similar appearance. Giemsa stain × 2,500. (b) T_M lymphocytes. Acid esterase staining giving characteristic 'dot'-like appearance × 2,500. (c) Transformed lymphocyte (lymphoblast) following stimulation of lymphocytes in culture with a polyclonal activator. The large lymphoblasts with their relatively high ratio of cytoplasm to nucleus may be compared in size with the isolated small lymphocyte. One cell is in mitosis. May–Grünewald–Giemsa × 2,500. (d) Plasma cells. The nucleus is eccentric. The cytoplasm is strongly basophilic due to high RNA content. The juxta-nuclear lightly-stained zone corresponds with the Golgi region. May–Grünewald–Giemsa × 2,500. (e) Monocyte, showing 'horseshoe-shaped' nucleus and moderately abundant pale cytoplasm with well defined granules. A small lymphocyte with a more strongly-stained nucleus is shown for comparison. Staining for peroxidase is frequently positive. Giemsa × 5,000. (f) Four polynorphonuclear leucocytes (neutrophils) and one eosinophil. The multi-lobed nuclei and the cytoplasmic granules are clearly shown, those of the eosinophil being heavily stained. Leishman stain × 2,000. (g) Macrophages in monolayer cultures after phagocytosis of mycobacteria (stained red). Carbol–Fuchsin counterstained with Malachite Green × 1,000. (h) Plasma cells stained to show intracellular immunoglobulin using a fluorescein-labelled anti-IgG (green) and a rhodamine-conjugated anti-IgM (red) × 2,500. (a), (b), (c) and (g) were photographed by Dr. P.M. Lydyard. The material for (a) was supplied by Dr. K. McLennan and (g) by Dr. G. Rooke. (d) and (h) were given by Professor C. Grossi, (e) by Professor J. Stewart and (f) by Professor J.J. Owen.

FIGURE 3.7 (pp. 62–65). Electron microscopy of cells involved in immune responses (eosinophils may be seen in figure 7.12, mast cells in figure 8.6 and platelets in figure 9.10).

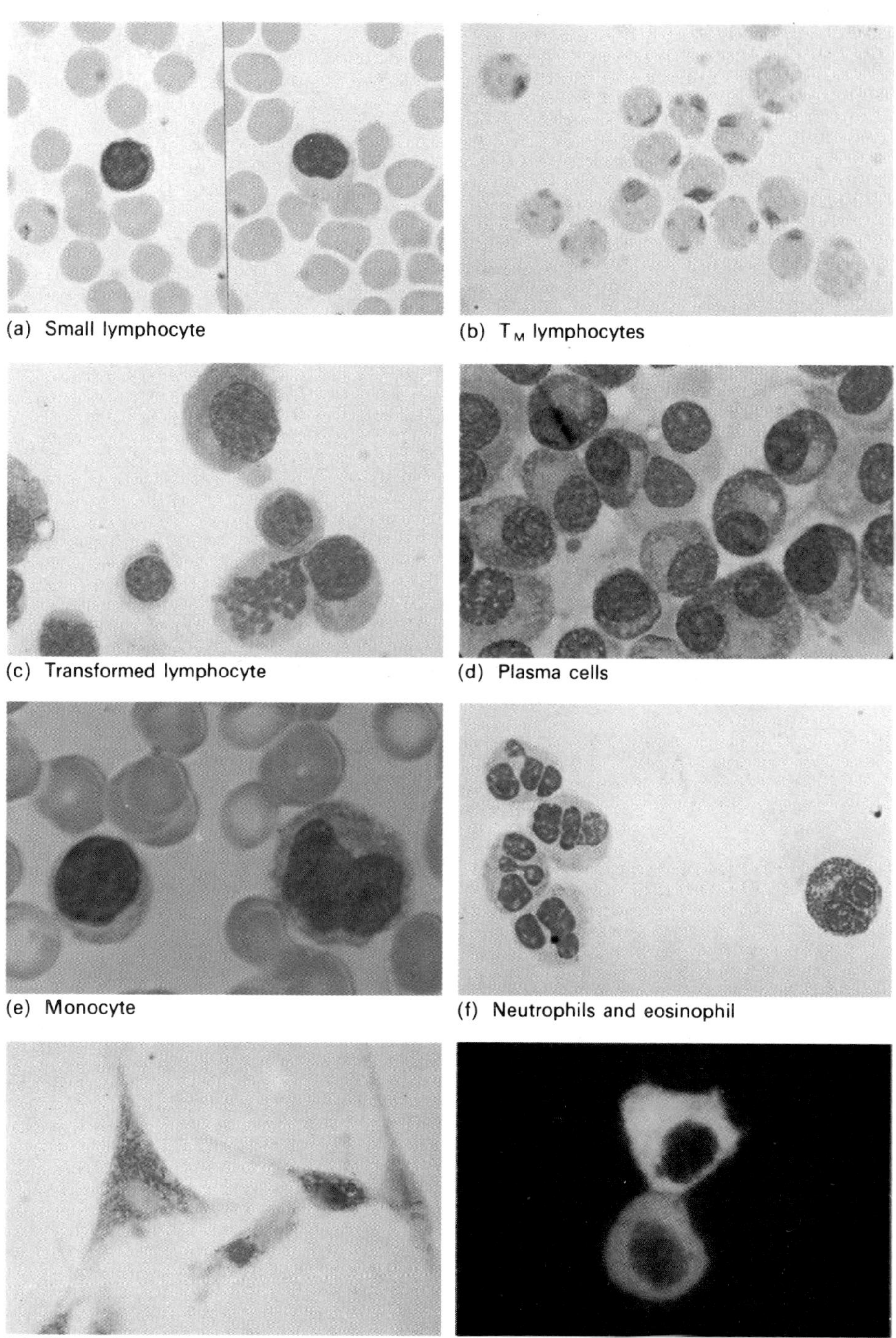

(a) Small lymphocyte

(b) T_M lymphocytes

(c) Transformed lymphocyte

(d) Plasma cells

(e) Monocyte

(f) Neutrophils and eosinophil

(g) Macrophages

(h) Plasma cells

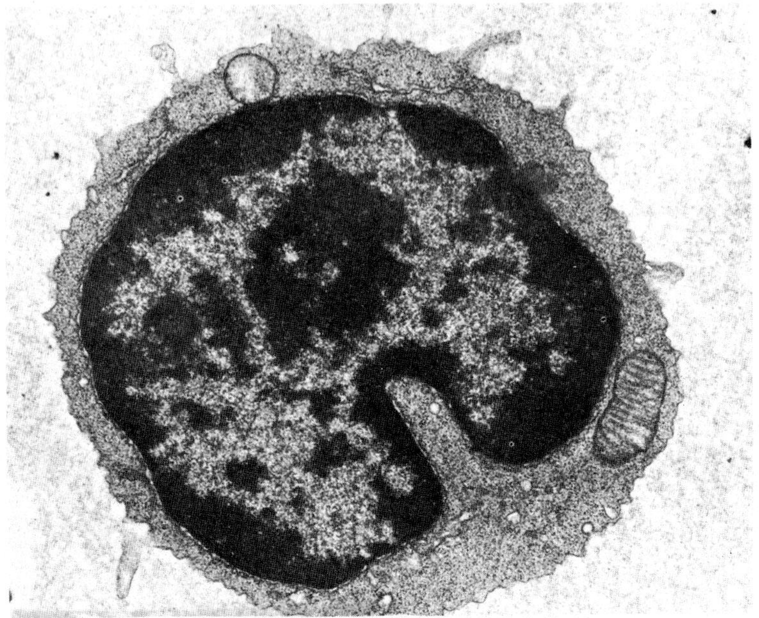

FIGURE 3.7. (a) Small T-lymphocyte with receptors for IgM. Indented nucleus with condensed chromatin, sparse cytoplasm: single mitochondrion shown and many free ribosomes but otherwise few organelles. ($\times$ 13,000). B-lymphocytes are essentially similar with slightly more cytoplasm and occasional elements of rough-surfaced endoplasmic reticulum.

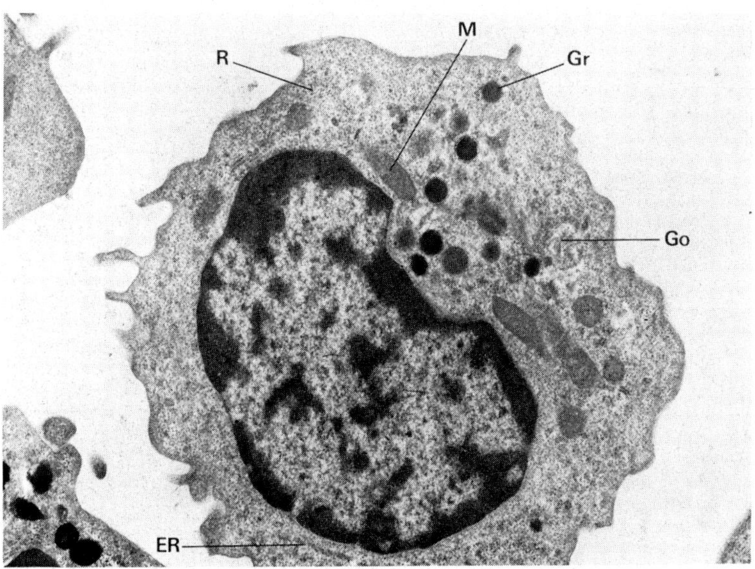

(b) T-lymphocyte with receptors for IgG ($\times$ 7,500). The more abundant cytoplasm contains several mitochondria (M), free ribosomes (R) with some elements of rough-surfaced endoplasmic reticulum (ER), prominent Golgi apparatus (Go) and characteristic membrane-bound electron-dense granules (Gr). The nuclear chromatin is less condensed than that of the T_M cell. (Courtesy of Drs. A. Zicca & C.E. Grossi.)

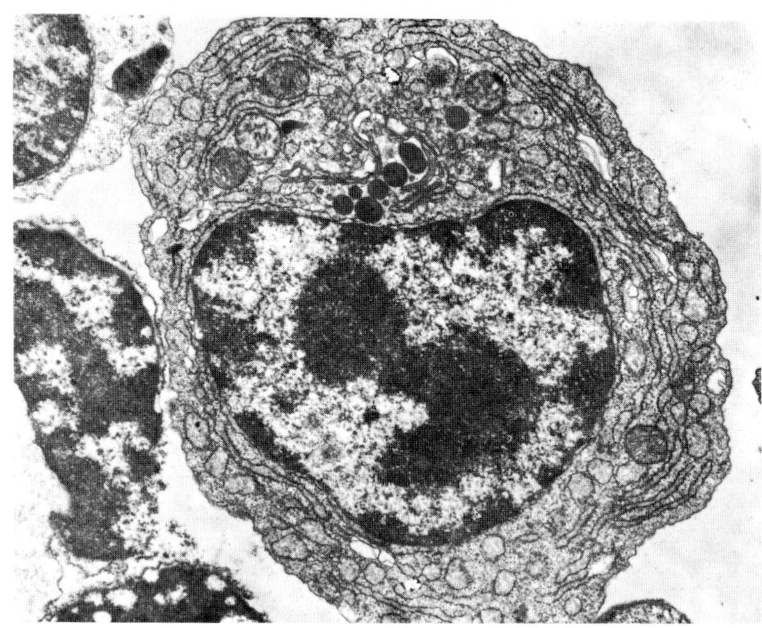

(c) Plasma cell (× 10,000). Prominent rough-surfaced endoplasmic reticulum associated with the synthesis and secretion of Ig.

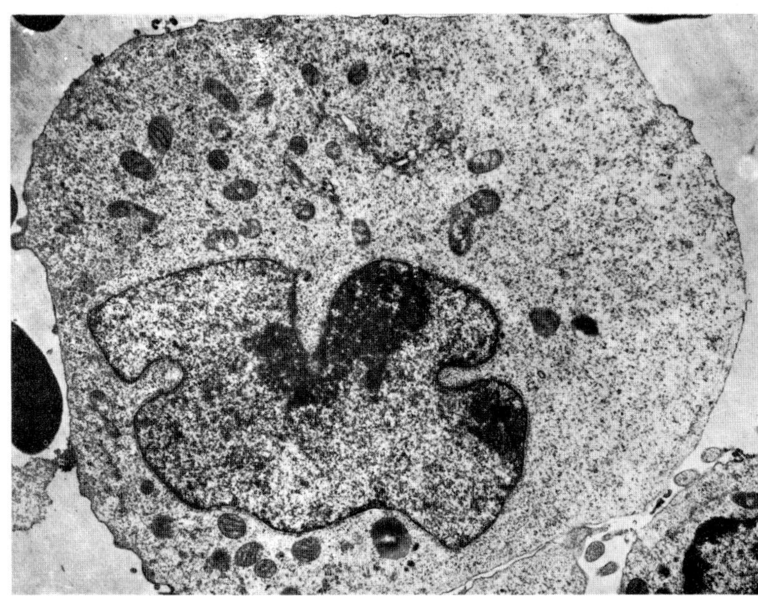

(d) Transformed lymphocyte (lymphoblast) (× 7,000). The nuclear chromatin is less condensed than in the small lymphocyte (a). The more extensive cytoplasm shows numerous mitochondria and free polyribosomes. (Courtesy Miss V. Petts.)

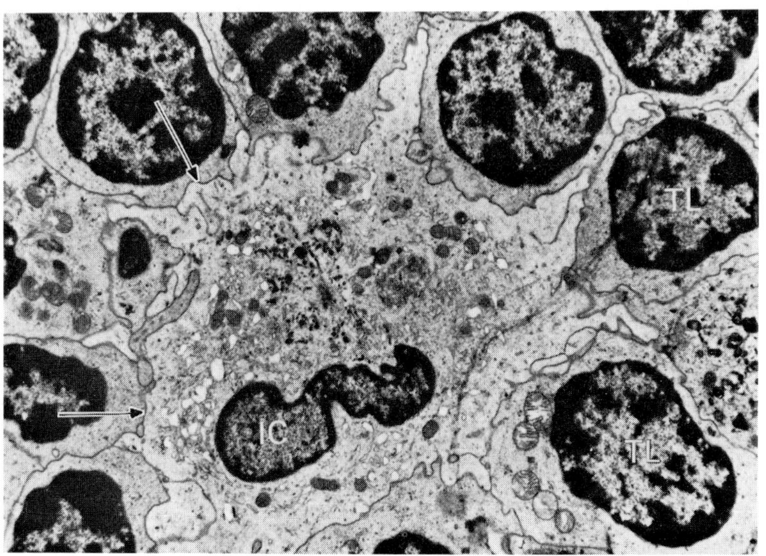

(e) Interdigitating cell (IC) in the thymus dependent area of the rat lymph node. This is thought to be an antigen-presenting cell derived from the Langerhans' cell in the skin which travels to the node in the afferent lymph as a 'veiled' cell bearing antigen on its profuse surface processes. Intimate contacts are made with the surface membranes (arrows) of the surrounding T-lymphocytes (TL). The cytoplasm of the IC contains relatively few organelles and does not show Birbeck granules (racket-shaped cytoplasmic organelles, characteristic of the Langerhans' cell), but these granules appear after antigenic stimulation. (× 2,000) (From E.W.A. Kamperdijk, E.Ch.H. Hoefsmit, H.A. Drexhage and B.H. Balfour; In 'Mononuclear Phagocytes', ed. III, R.v.Furth, editor. The Hague, Rijhoff Publishers, 1980: courtesy of authors and publishers.)

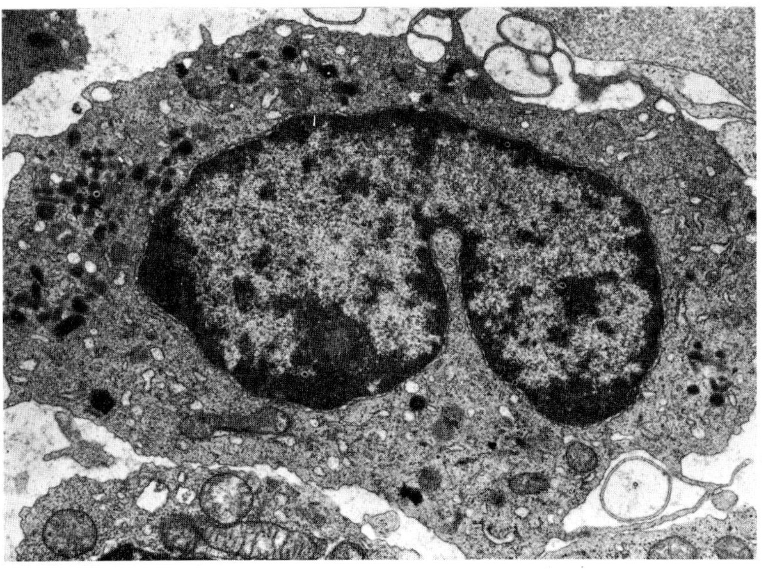

(f) Monocyte (× 10,000). 'Horseshoe' nucleus. Phagocytic and pinocytic vesicles, lysosomal granules, mitochondria and isolated profiles of rough-surfaced endoplasmic reticulum are evident.

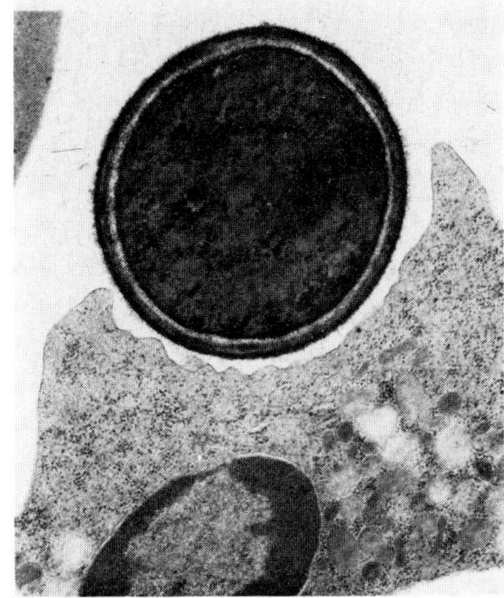

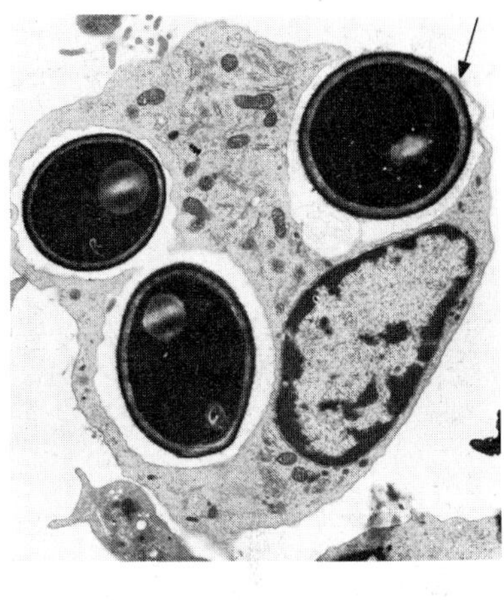

(g) (Left) Phagocytosis of *Candida albicans* by a polymorphonuclear leucocyte (Neutrophil). Adherence to the surface initiates enclosure of the fungal particle within arms of cytoplasm. Lysosomal granules are abundant but mitochondria are rare. (× 15,000) (h) (Right) Phagocytosis of *C. albicans* by a monocyte showing near completion of phagosome formation (arrowed) around one organism and complete ingestion of two others. (× 5,000) (Figs. 3.7 g–j courtesy of Dr. H. Valdimarsson.)

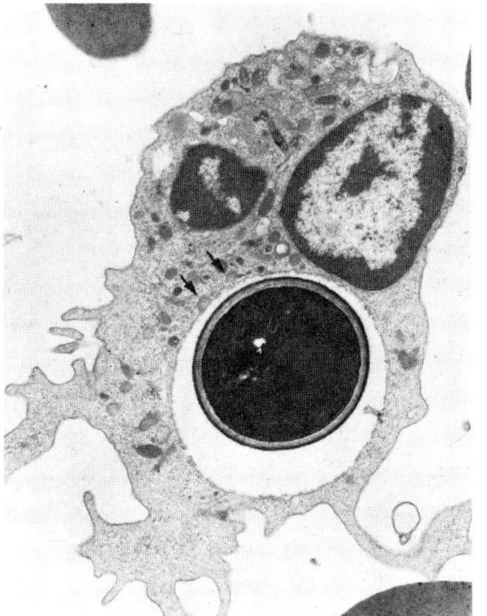

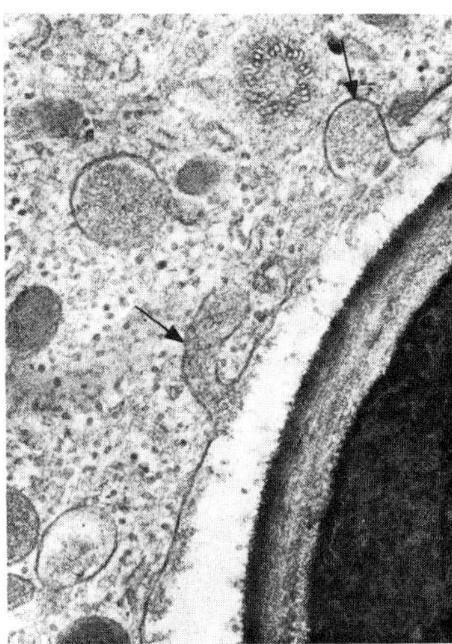

(i) (Left) Neutrophil 30 minutes after ingestion of *C. albicans*. The cytoplasm is already partly degranulated and two lysosomal granules (arrowed) are fusing with the phagocytic vacuole. Two lobes of the nucleus are evident. (× 5,000) (j) (Right) Higher magnification of (i) showing fusing granules discharging their contents into the phagocytic vacuole (arrowed). (× 33,000)

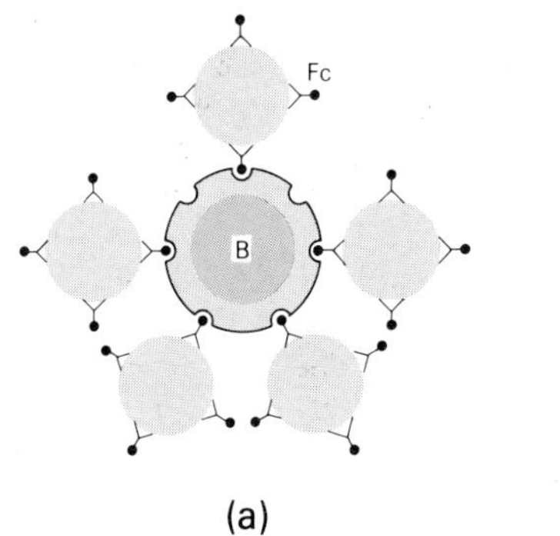

(a)

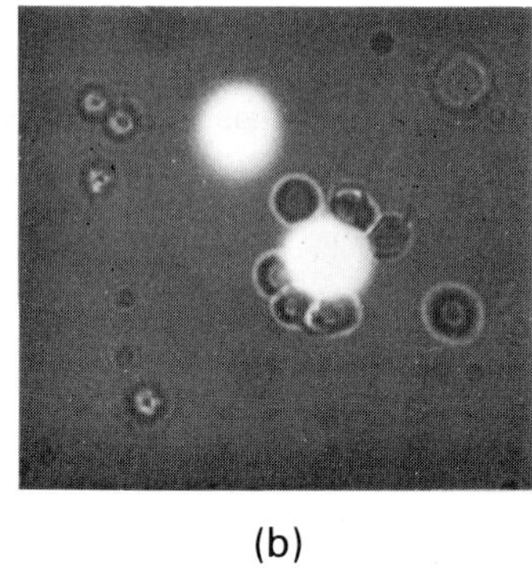

(b)

FIGURE 3.8. B-cell rosettes—(a) diagrammatic representation of rosette formed with IgG (Y) coated erythrocytes binding to the receptor for Fcγ; (b) cluster of C3 coated red cells around B-lymphocyte (visualized in u.v. light after staining with acridine orange). (Courtesy of Dr. A. Arnaiz-Villena.)

At the time of writing, the most popular means of enumerating lymphocyte populations in human blood is to use fluorescent anti-immunoglobulin for B-cells and spontaneous rosette formation with neuraminidase-treated sheep erythrocytes for T-cells. Values given by these two tests usually add up to a few per cent short of 100%; without giving anything away, the remaining lymphocyte-like cells, negative on both counts, are termed 'null-cells' (figure 6.15).

For the unwearying seeker after truth, the plot diversifies. Aside from the implication above that B-cells may exist as subpopulations, only one of which bears a C3 receptor, different subsets of murine T-cells have been defined by the allelic forms of two genetic loci, Ly1 and Ly2. Cells destined to subserve 'helper' and 'lymphokine' activity (p. 70 and p. 77 respectively) display the Ly1 phenotype on their surface; the precursors of cytotoxic and suppressor T-cells (p. 79 and 100) are Ly1,2, but essentially express only the Ly2 surface antigen as they become effector cells.

B- and T-cells can be separated by selective depletion of one or the other by rosette formation. For example, T-cells forming spontaneous sheep cell rosettes can be isolated by centrifugation over a 'density step' of Ficoll which holds back non-rosetting cells. T-lymphocytes can be recovered by mechanically disrupting the rosettes and recentrifuging over Ficoll to remove the sheep cells. Further fractionation may be effected by forming rosettes between the T-cells with Fcγ receptors and IgG-coated ox cells. Depletion of one population, say T-cells, by destruction with anti-T serum plus complement (cf. p. 157) has also been extensively employed. Another procedure involves affinity chromatography. B-lymphocytes can be selectively retained on solid phase columns to which anti-light chain is bound covalently, the effluent providing a T (+null-cell) population virtually free of Ig-bearing B-cells; the column-bound cells can be released by elution with IgG. The prize for elegance (and expense) must go to the fluorescence activated cell sorter (FACS) designed by Herzenberg and colleagues. Lymphocytes coated with fluorescently labelled antibodies directed against the surface antigens of one sub-population of cells, flow obediently in a single stream past a laser beam. Each fluorescent cell is charged and then separated from non-fluorescent and therefore uncharged cells in an electric field. The flow-through rate is approximately 10^4 cells/sec. The machine can also be used to measure the quantitative distribution of fluorescence within the lymphocyte population (flow cytofluorography). Passage down nylon wool columns depletes adherent T-cells and most B-lymphocytes.

LYMPHOCYTE SURFACE PHENOMENA

When viable B-lymphocytes are stained in the cold with a fluorescein-conjugated anti-Ig, the fluorescence is seen as patches on the cell surface (figure 3.9b). However, if the

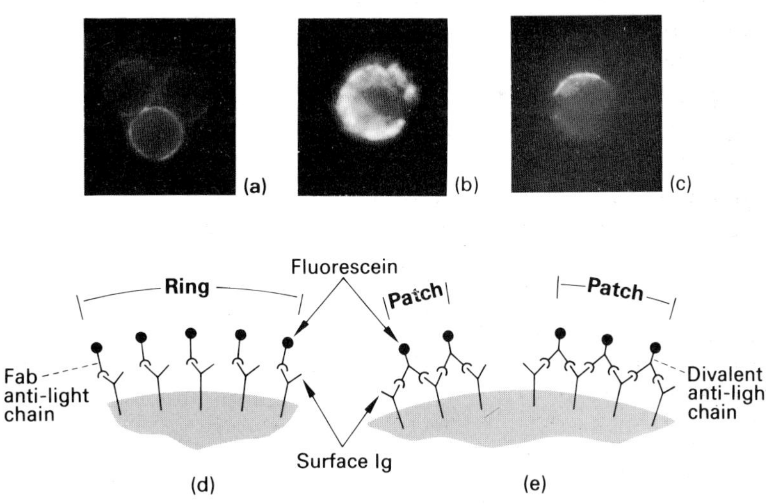

FIGURE 3.9. Patterns of immunofluorescent staining of B-lymphocyte surface immunoglobin using fluorescein-conjugated anti-Ig (cf. p. 152 for discussion of technique). Provided the reaction is carried out in the cold to prevent pinocytosis, the labelled antibody cannot penetrate to the interior of the viable lymphocytes and reacts only with surface components. (a) ring staining with monovalent (Fab) anti-Ig; (b) patch formation with whole anti-Ig; (c) cap formation on warming the cells in (b); (d) diagram of ring staining by monovalent anti-Ig; (e) diagram of patch formation by divalent anti-Ig. During cap formation, submembraneous myosin becomes redistributed in association with the surface Ig and induces locomotion of the previously sessile cell in a direction away from the cap. (Photographs kindly provided by Drs. A. Arnaiz-Villena & L. Hudson.)

experiment is repeated using monovalent (Fab) anti-Ig, a smooth ring of surface fluorescence is observed (figure 3.9a). The interpretation of these findings is that the lymphocyte surface immunoglobulins are floating freely in the plasma membrane (like icebergs in a sea of lipid) and are agglutinated into little patches by the divalent anti-Ig (figure 3.9d and e). If the lymphocytes are now allowed to warm up, the patches coalesce to form a cap over one pole of the cell (figure 3.9c) and the complexes are taken into the cytoplasm by endocytosis leaving the surface free of immunoglobulin. The cell will resynthesize its surface immunoglobulin within a few hours if washed and incubated at 37° in fresh medium.

When rabbit lymphocytes are cultured in the presence of anti-Ig for a minimum of 16–20 hours, they go on to transform into blast-like cells (cf. figure 3.6c) and divide. Activation also occurs with the divalent $F(ab')_2$ pepsin fragment derived from the anti-Ig but not the monovalent Fab with the strong implication that cross-linking and aggregation of surface Ig is an important step in B-lymphocyte stimulation which would normally be brought about by antigen combining with complementary surface Ig receptors on those lymphocytes capable of synthesizing the appropriate antibody. However the blast cells induced by such activation do not make antibody and current thinking is that in most circumstances an additional non-specific or 'second' signal (Bretscher & Cohn) is required particularly for the triggering of antibody production by thymus-dependent antigens (i.e. those antigens which provoke a grossly depressed response in animals deprived of T-lymphocytes by neonatal thymectomy or other means: cf. p. 55).

Cellular co-operation in the antibody response

THE ROLE OF MACROPHAGES

The mononuclear cells of the monocyte-macrophage series play a central role in the induction of the immune response with respect to the presentation of antigen to lymphocytes. Intimate cytoplasmic contacts between macrophages and lymphocytes have been observed cf. figure 3.7e and co-operative effects of macrophages for antibody production are clearly revealed by tissue culture studies showing that the antibody response to most antigens is largely abrogated when glass-adherent cells are first removed from the responding lymphoid cell population, and that this defect can be overcome by the addition of macrophages. Furthermore, antigens such as bovine serum albumin provoke a vastly superior antibody response when injected together with macrophages rather than as a free solution; interestingly the more thymus-dependent the response to a given antigen, the greater the enhancing effect due to macrophages. Antigen trapping and concentration of antigen at the cell surface for effective presentation to the lymphocyte seems to be important. Antigen-antibody complexes formed in antigen excess and containing the 3rd component of complement (C3b, p. 161) localize efficiently in lymphoid follicles where they persist on the surface of dendritic cells and trap antigen-specific B-cells to generate B-cell memory. In general, when antigen is taken up by macrophages, a proportion is degraded by phagocytic digestion while part is fixed to the cell surface where it is thought to be in a strongly immunogenic state in some form of association with the Ia antigens of the major histocompatibility complex (p. 97). Cells of the macrophage series adopt many morphological forms which vary greatly in their expression of these two mechanisms for handling antigens. Some, like the Kupffer cells of the liver, the alveolar macrophages or the lining cells of splenic cords, have well-developed lysosomal granules and are actively phagocytic. We may look upon them as 'professional phagocytes' destined for a life of microbe-crunching. In contrast with these men of violence, the dendritic macrophages of the lymph node cortex and skin (Langerhans' cells) are far more genteel; largely eschewing the degrading process of phagocytosis, they prefer to incorporate antigen into their surface membranes for the more aristocratic purpose of presentation to and activation of lymphocytes. Even the dendritic macrophages are specialized depending upon the particular lymphocyte subpopulation they serve.

CO-OPERATION BETWEEN T- AND B-CELLS

Attention has already been drawn to the fact that the antibody response to certain antigens is considerably depressed following neonatal thymectomy. However, we know from the work of Davies with chromosome (T6) marked thymus cells, that the T-lymphocytes do not themselves secrete antibody even though they actively divide after contact with antigen. This involvement of the T-lymphocyte in antibody synthesis without itself producing antibody is now seen to be due to a form of *co-operation* by the T-cell which helps the antigenic stimulation of B-lymphocytes to be more effective (figure 3.5). Using an irradiated mouse (which cannot itself make an immune response) as a 'living test-tube', Claman and his colleagues showed that thymocytes or bone marrow cells (containing B-cell precursors) injected together with sheep red cells gave only poor or modest antibody production. When T- and B-cells were injected together, there was a very marked increase in the number of cells engaged in antibody synthesis (table 3.3).

The cellular origin of the antibody-forming cells was elegantly demonstrated by Miller and his colleagues in co-operation experiments involving transfer of T-cells and bone marrow from genetically different mouse strains. The antibody-forming cells in the recipient spleen were studied *in vitro* by the Jerne plaque technique (p. 88) and could be inhibited only by an antiserum to the transplantation antigens of the strain providing the bone marrow *not* the thymus cells (figure 3.10).

At the molecular level, further light on the nature of co-operation has been shed by the experiments with carrier-hapten conjugates. The reader may recall that haptens are small groups which can combine with preformed antibody but fail to stimulate antibody synthesis unless coupled with an antigenic carrier (usually a protein; cf. p. 8). Both Mitchison and Rajewsky have shown that primed B-cells make a secondary antibody response to a hapten bound to protein carrier only when T-cells primed to the carrier ('helper cells') are also present (figure 3.11). In other words, when T-cells recognize and respond to carrier determinants, they help B-lymphocytes specific for the hapten

TABLE 3.3. Co-operation of bone marrow and thymus cells in production of antibody to sheep red cells in irradiated recipient

Irradiated recipient given antigen plus:	Antibody response
Spleen cells	+ + +
Thymocytes (T-cells)	±
Bone marrow (B-cells)	+
Thymocytes and bone marrow	+ + +

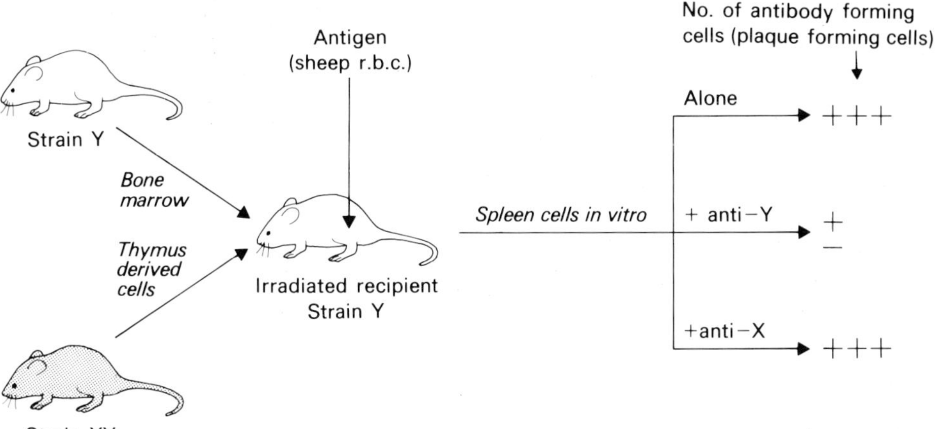

FIGURE 3.10. Bone marrow origin of antibody-forming cells. Antibody-forming cells were studied in the antigen stimulated recipient of a bone marrow/thymus mixture. Antibodies to the transplantation antigens of the strain providing bone marrow inhibited the plaque-forming cells whereas antibodies to the thymocyte donor were ineffective (based on Miller J.F.A.P. & Mitchell G.F., *J.exp.Med.* 1968, **128**, 821: in these studies thymus derived cells from the thoracic duct were used).

to develop into antibody-forming cells, presumably by providing the required second or accessory signal(s) discussed earlier (figure 3.12).

The mechanisms underlying co-operation are not yet clearly defined. They involve complex interactions between macrophages, T-cells and B-cells in which association of the carrier determinants with Ia antigens of the major histocompatibility complex is crucial (p. 97) and in which various soluble growth factors are implicated. Activated B-blasts produced during the limited antigen-specific first phase are driven by non-antigen specific growth factors (usually resulting from a specific antigenic stimulus; cf. p. 188) to divide extensively and mature to form an expanded clone of plasma cells (figure 3.13).

RELEVANCE TO ANTIGENICITY

When discussing the question of antigenicity in chapter 1 (p. 18) we were largely preoccupied with the factors governing the shape of the antigenic determinant and its fit with the antibody site without considering the initiation of an antibody response. If a single determinant binds to a B-lymphocyte surface receptor, no cross-linking will result

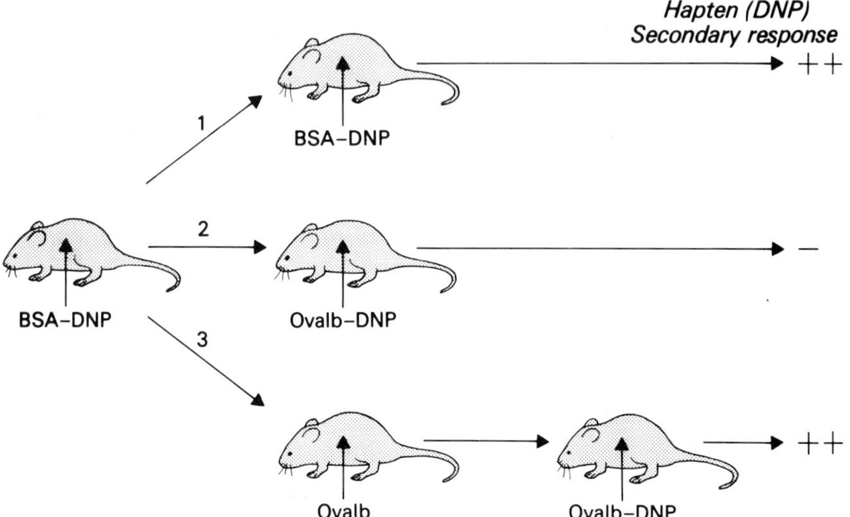

FIGURE 3.11. Carrier-hapten co-operation showing that a secondary response to the hapten (dinitrophenyl group—DNP) is only obtained when cells are primed to both carrier and hapten.

1. After priming with an injection of DNP linked to bovine serum albumin (BSA) as a carrier, later inoculation with the same BSA–DNP combination gives a secondary response to DNP.

2. If the primed animals are challenged instead with DNP on a different carrier, ovalbumin, there is no secondary response.

3. However, if animals primed with BSA–DNP are further primed with ovalbumin, challenge with Ovalb–DNP will now give a secondary response. Similar results can be obtained using lymphoid cell transfers from primed animals into irradiated recipients. The 'helper-cells' with specificity for the carrier can be shown to be T-cells by the use of anti-Thy1 serum or thymectomized donors.

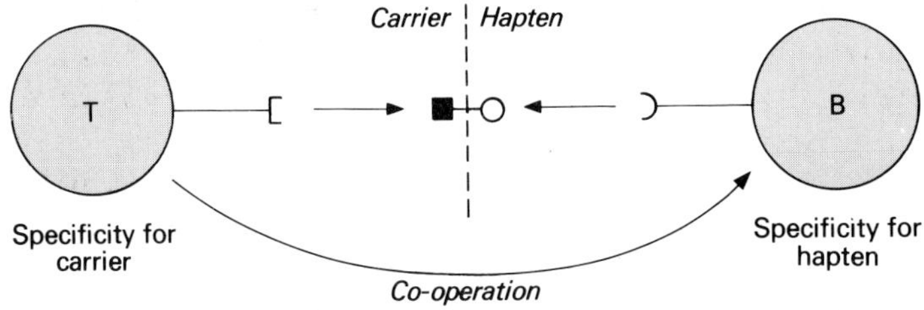

FIGURE 3.12. T-B *co-operation.* The T-cells on recognizing carrier determinants on the antigen provide a co-operative signal which enables B-cells that recognize hapten to mature into antibody-secreting plasma cells.

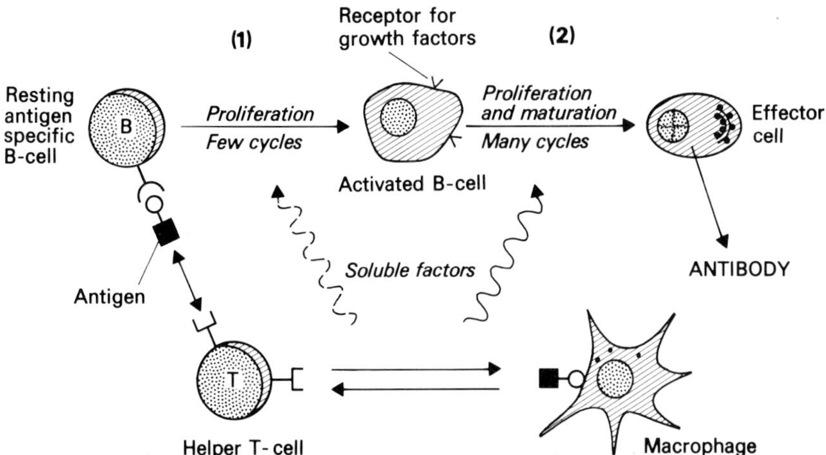

FIGURE 3.13. T-B co-operation in the response to a carrier (■)—hapten (○). STAGE 1—*Antigen-specific*: helper T-cells activated by macrophage processed antigen stimulate the resting B-cell, which has bound antigen through its hapten-specific Ig receptors, to transform after a small number of divisions to a blast cell with receptors for soluble growth factors. STAGE 2—*Non-antigen specific*: these soluble growth factors produced by interactions between the T-cell and macrophages (possibly different from the original type initially presenting the antigen) stimulate the blast cells to repeated division and maturation to become antibody-producing effector cells.

(figure 3.14a) and the cell will not be activated (remember the definition of a hapten—combines with antibody but won't stimulate antibody synthesis). Certain linear antigens which are not readily degraded in the body and which have an appropriately spaced, highly repeating determinant—pneumococcus polysaccharide, endotoxin, D-amino acid polymers and polyvinylpyrrolidine for example—are thymus independent in that they can stimulate B-cells directly without the need for T-cell help. They persist on the surface of the antigen-specific B-cell to which they bind with great avidity through their multivalent attachment (cf. p. 15) to the specific Ig receptors thereby causing cross-linking and the stimulation of IgM but not IgG antibody synthesis. Whether efficient cross-linking alone will trigger IgM-producing cells or whether these antigens provide a 'second signal' through the C3 receptor by activating the alternative complement pathway (p. 162), or through some innate ability to stimulate B-cells or macrophages non-specifically, is still open. Antigens which cannot fulfil the molecular requirements for direct stimulation must use their other determinants as carriers to evoke

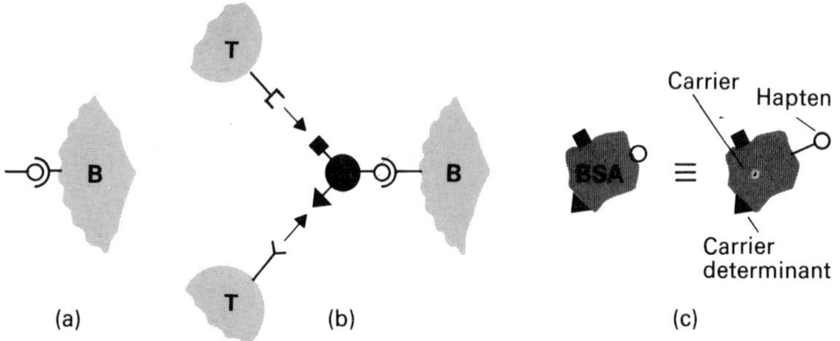

FIGURE 3.14. Response to a simple protein antigen looked at from the carrier-hapten standpoint. A small protein such as bovine serum albumin has several determinants but all are different, so that the molecule itself cannot cross-link B-cell receptors and therefore behaves as a monovalent hapten with respect to each determinant (cf. (a)). Only if other determinants can be recognized by T-cells can appropriate co-operation be provided for B-cell stimulation (b). Thus the determinants on the protein act in a 'carrier' function for each other (c).

T-cell co-operation. Such help from the T-cell must be even more essential for those cases where a determinant appears only once on each molecule thereby acting in effect as a monovalent hapten. This will usually be the case with proteins which have little or no symmetry such as bovine serum albumin where it will be appreciated that each determinant can only activate its specific B-cell by calling upon the carrier function of the others (figure 3.14c). To a first approximation larger molecules tend to be better antigens because they have more determinants capable of acting as carriers. Where an animal lacks T-cells capable of recognizing potential carrier determinants there will be a correspondingly poor response to the hapten even if hapten-specific B-cells are present.

The overall picture is still admittedly uncertain; very tentatively it might be said that cross-linking by certain multivalent antigens can trigger cells to produce IgM but that antigens which cross-link less effectively require a second signal normally provided by a T-cell recognizing carrier determinants (figure 3.15). T-cell participation also permits a switch to IgG antibody synthesis.

The cell-mediated immune response

Immunity to those infectious organisms which have developed the capacity for living and multiplying *within* the cells of the host is masterminded by the T-lymphocytes

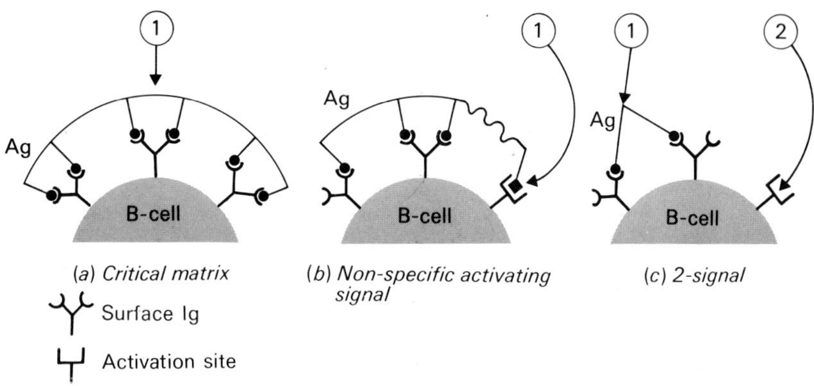

FIGURE 3.15. *Models of B-cell triggering*

(a) Critical matrix (Feldmann)—the antigen (Ag) provides a single activating signal 1 by forming a critically spaced matrix of Ig receptors bound to repeating determinants on the antigen. With thymus dependent antigens the antigen is presented in a multivalent form through binding to macrophages by T-dependent factors which recognize carrier determinants. The matrix is created by presenting the antigen in a multivalent form through binding to macrophages by cytophilic T-dependent factors with specificity for carrier determinants.

(b) One non-specific signal (Moller & Coutinho)—the Ig receptors on the B-cell passively focus the antigen which non-specifically activates the cell through some inherent property of the molecule (such as that which gives lipopolysaccharide its polyclonal activating powers). For thymus dependent antigens, the T-cell provides the activating signal by recognizing the carrier (cf. figure 3.14).

(c) 2-signal model Bretscher & Cohn)—signal 1 is provided by antigen binding to Ig receptors (many think that cross-linking may also be required) and by itself leads to inactivation of the cell, i.e. tolerance. However, the cell will become switched-on for antibody synthesis by the concurrent action of a second signal which may be provided through T-cell recognition of carrier or a polyclonal B-cell activator such as lipopolysaccharide. A major difference from the Moller–Coutinho model is that antigen binding by Ig receptors is considered as a purely passive event by the latter authors.

If one accepts that there are two populations of B-cells, B_{TD} which can co-operate with T-cells and B_{TI} which cannot, then it seems likely that the 2-signal model best fits the behaviour of B_{TD} cells since antihapten responses *in vitro* can be induced in primed cells by a mixture of anti-Ig antibodies (signal 1) plus soluble T-derived factor (signal 2), while hapten coupled to a thymus independent carrier (e.g. pneumo-coccus polysaccharide or autologus IgG) induces tolerance. The induction of IgM antibody-forming cells with a whole range of specificities by polyclonal activators such as lipopolysaccharide, and the triggering of specific IgM antibody synthesis by thymus-independent antigens like levan in circumstances where they are not polyclonal activators suggests that B_{TI} cells may be turned on by either the Moller/Coutinho or the matrix model respectively. Since the intracellular ratio of cGMP : cAMP seems to determine lymphocyte activation, is it possible that there are two alternative activating sites on these cells, one Ig and the other non-specific, such that one lowers cAMP while the other may increase cGMP?

independently of the B-cells. Thus infections with intracellular facultative parasites such as tubercle and leprosy bacilli, budding viruses like smallpox and parasites such as toxoplasma, pose serious problems for children with thymic insufficiency in contrast to infants with primary immunoglobulin deficiency who cope relatively well with these organisms. Support for this view is also afforded by studies on thymectomized and bursectomized chicks and by the demonstration that T-cells from mice which had recovered from infection with TB could passively confer immunity on previously uninfected animals into which they had been injected (cf. figure 7.7).

The T-cells are antigen-sensitive in that they show specificity for antigen in their response to carriers, in delayed hypersensitivity reactions and in their cytotoxicity for virally infected cells or allogeneic (cf. p. 79) targets. The fact that such cytotoxic cells can be specifically adsorbed onto fibroblasts bearing the transplantation antigens to which the animal was initially sensitized clearly indicates that T-cells do have surface receptors which recognize antigen although it must be said that the nature of these receptors is still hotly debated. The presence of binding sites on different T-lymphocytes for Fcγ and Fcμ led to the inevitable suggestion that the antigen receptors were nothing more than exogenously acquired cytophilic antibody and in some instances (e.g. the Thy1 positive cells from immunized mice which form rosettes with sheep erythrocytes) this is undoubtedly the case. Nonetheless, the ability of neonatally bursectomized chickens and of a-γ-globulinaemic children to mount specific cell-mediated hypersensitivity responses is powerful evidence that T-cells possess their own endogenous receptors independently of B-cells and their products, a view reinforced by the phenomena of selective T-cell tolerance (p. 107) and the deletion of specific T-helpers by 'suicide' with radioactive antigen.

The receptors are not conventional Ig molecules. Very sensitive techniques have failed to detect light chain determinants on the surface of T-cells from bursectomized chickens and so far, with the exception of anti-idiotypic sera, which are probably directed against the antigen-combining site, no anti-Ig serum has been able to block the killing of allogeneic targets by cytotoxic T-cells. These anti-idiotypic sera have provided evidence for common or closely similar combining sites on cytotoxic T-cells and antibodies directed against the same major histocompatibility (transplantation) antigen, and for shared idiotypes on helper T-cells and antibodies with specificity for a given bacterial antigen determinant. In the latter case, the gene encoding the helper T-cell idiotype is found to be on the same chromosome and close to the cluster of genes for the Ig heavy chains. The present tentative view is that the receptor has a molecular weight of 150,000 daltons and consists of 2 chains, each of which uses an Ig heavy chain variable region gene (cf. p. 132) linked to a constant region gene different from those coding for conventional heavy chain peptides. A curious feature of the receptor is its ability to recognize antigen in association with a constituent of the major histocompatibility complex (p. 97).

The T-cell receptor is triggered by antigen on the surface of an appropriate macrophage where it may be present in a special 'processed' form in association with Ia. The cell membrane becomes activated and the signal is transmitted to the interior of the cell where the nucleus of the small lymphocyte with its compact chromatin becomes derepressed; the cell transforms into a large blast cell and proliferates in response to macrophage—derived growth factors rather like the later stages of B-cell differentiation (figure 3.13). One subpopulation of the stimulated T-cells releases a number of soluble factors, another develops cytotoxic powers while a further proportion become memory cells; together, these phenomena form the basis of cell-mediated immunity.

THE TWO ARMS OF THE CELL-MEDIATED RESPONSE

Proliferation of the stimulated T-cells provides the mechanism for amplification of the cell-mediated immune response which depends upon these two major effector mechanisms—the generation of cytotoxic cells and the release of biologically active soluble factors (termed 'lymphokines' by Dumonde) which modulate the behaviour of other cells, particularly the mononuclear phagocytes (monocytes and macrophages) (figure 3.16).

Lymphokines

The supernatant fluid recovered after stimulating sensitized lymphocytes with antigen possesses several biological activities some of which have been ascribed to different molecular species. These lymphokines have molecular weights of the

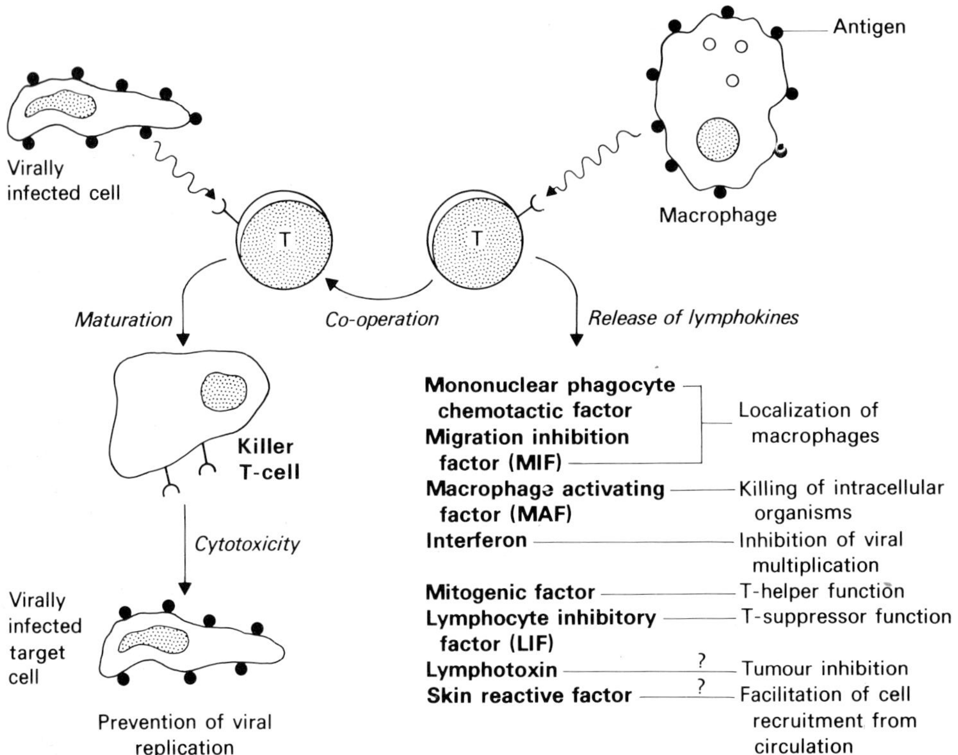

FIGURE 3.16. The cell-mediated immune response. This operates through the generation of cytotoxic T-cells and the release of lymphokines through the stimulation of two distinct T-subpopulations. Different lymphokines may be produced by different lymphocyte subsets. The intense proliferation induced by antigenic stimulation has not been shown but is an essential factor in the amplification of the response.

order of 20,000–80,000. Among them is a group which directly influence the movement and activity of macrophages. *Macrophage chemotactic factor* causes an accumulation of mononuclear phagocytes at the site of antigen-mediated lymphokine release; this can be demonstrated in Boyden chambers where monocytes or macrophages move across Millipore membranes into the chamber containing higher concentrations of factor. Once attracted, the cells are discouraged from leaving by macrophage *migration inhibition factor* (MIF); interaction with the cells appears to involve a fucose residue on MIF and a useful control for its assay is abrogation of a positive test by added fucose. Stimulation by *macrophage activating factor* (MAF) produces significant morphological changes with a ruffling of the surface membrane which gives the cell an 'angry' appearance, and leads to an increase in lysosomal enzyme content and a heightened ability to kill off ingested intracellular organisms. The movement of monocytes from blood vessels into the extra-vascular spaces is facilitated by another lymphokine, the *skin reactive factor* which also increases capillary permeability. *Immune interferon*, which inhibits intracellular viral replication, is present in lymphokine supernatants but it is not clear whether it is synthesized by T-cells or is secondarily released from activated macrophages.

Two lymphokines, *mitogenic factor* and *lymphocyte inhibitory factor* (LIF), with opposite effects on the proliferation of lymphocytes could well be related to T-helper and suppressor effects respectively. *Lymphotoxin*, although only mildly cytolytic for certain cultured cell lines, showed quite marked cytostatic activity and one is tempted to postulate a role in the constraint of tumour growth. Other biological activities which have been ascribed to lymphokines include effects on the migration and adhesiveness of polymorphs and eosinophils and on the aggregation of platelets.

Cytotoxic T-cells

Viral infection can generate a population of killer T-cells which are specifically cytotoxic for host cells infected with that virus. Similarly, a graft from a genetically dissimilar member of the same species (allogeneic graft) provokes the formation of cytotoxic T-cells directed against target cells bearing the major histocompatibility antigens of the donor. The first stage in this interaction, which may be followed *in vitro*, involves intimate binding of effector to target through recognition of the transplantation antigens by surface receptors; this stage is Ca^{2+} independent and cytochalasin B sensitive. Within a matter of minutes, a change occurs in the target cell, a 'kiss of death' so to speak, which leads irrevocably to cytolysis; this phase is Ca^{2+} dependent and cytochalasin insensitive. Thus by carrying out the binding step in the absence of Ca^{2+} and then allowing cytolysis to proceed by adding Ca^{2+} and cytochalasin (which inhibits cell movement and prevents binding to further target cells), each cytotoxic cell should theoretically lyse only one target. Enumeration of cytotoxic T-cells in this way by counting the number of killed allogeneic targets gives an estimate of approximately 1% of the spleen lymphocytes. This high proportion of cells committed to each major histocompatibility specificity is striking and implies a special relationship between T-cells and such antigens. In this context it should be noted that effective killing is only seen when the T-cells are sensitized to the major histocompatibility antigens or a determinant (e.g. viral) recognized in association with these antigens (cf. p. 279).

The anatomical basis of the immune response

The complex cellular interactions which form the basis of the immune response take place within the organized architecture of peripheral, or secondary, lymphoid tissue which includes the lymph glands, spleen and unencapsulated tissue lining the respiratory, alimentary and genito-urinary tracts.

LYMPH NODE

The encapsulated tissue of the lymph node contains a meshwork of reticular cells and their fibres organized into sinuses. These act as a filter for lymph draining the body tissues and possibly bearing foreign antigens which enters the subcapsular sinus by the afferent vessels and diffuses past the lymphocytes in the cortex to reach the medullary sinuses and thence the efferent lymphatics (figures 3.1 and 3.17).

B-cell areas

The follicular aggregations of B-lymphocytes are a prominent feature of the cortex. In the unstimulated node they are present as spherical collections of cells termed *primary nodules* but after antigenic challenge they form *secondary follicles* (figure 7.17) which consist of a corona or mantle of concentrically packed small B-lymphocytes surrounding a pale-staining *germinal centre* which contains large, often proliferating, lymphoid cells, scattered conventional reticular macrophages and the specialized dendritic macrophages with elongated cytoplasmic processes and few if any lysosomes. Germinal centres are greatly enlarged in secondary antibody responses and it is reasonable to regard them as important sites of B-cell memory. Following antigenic stimulation, differentiating plasmablasts appear and become plasma cells in the medullary cords of lymphoid cells which project between the medullary sinuses.

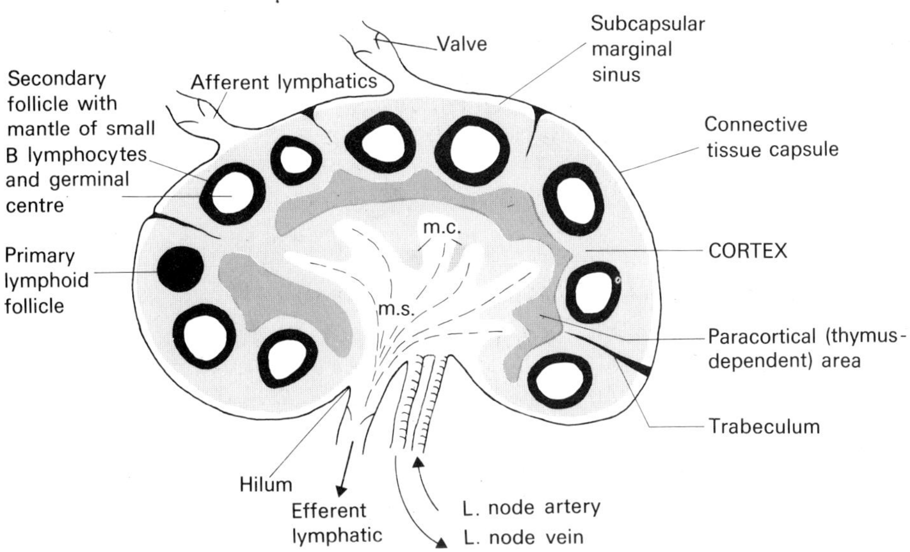

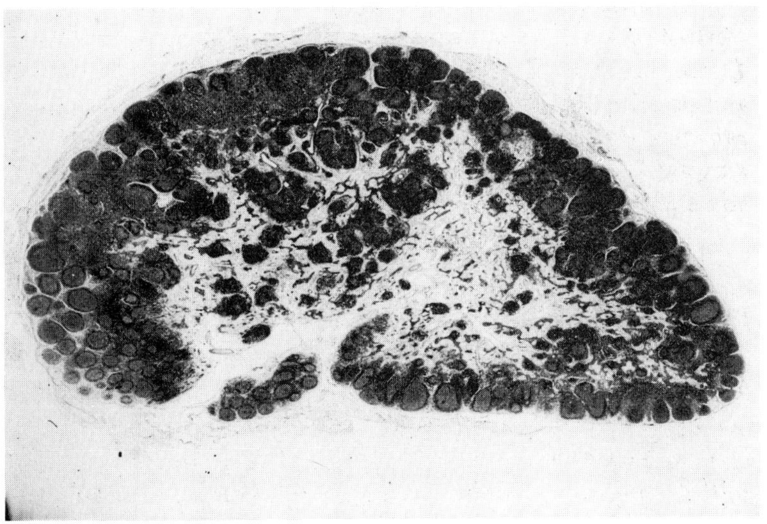

FIGURE 3.17. A human lymph node (a) (top) diagrammatic representation (b) (bottom) low power view of histological section, × 10. (Photographed by Dr. P.M. Lydyard.)

T-cell areas

Compartmentation of the two major lymphocyte populations occurs in that T-cells are largely confined to a region of the node referred to as the paracortical (or thymus-dependent) area (figure 3.17); if one looks at nodes taken from children with selective T-cell deficiency (figure 7.17) or neonatally thymectomized mice, the paracortical region is seen to be virtually devoid of lymphocytes. Furthermore, when a T-cell-mediated response is elicited in a normal animal, say by a skin graft or by painting chemicals such as picryl chloride on the skin to induce contact hypersensitivity, there is a marked proliferation of cells in the thymus-dependent area and typical lymphoblasts are evident. In contrast, stimulation of antibody formation by the 'thymus-independent' antigen pneumococcus polysaccharide leads to proliferation in the cortical lymphoid follicles with development of germinal centres while the paracortical region remains inactive reflecting the inability to develop cellular hypersensitivity to the polysaccharide. As would be expected, nodes taken from children with congenital hypogammaglobulinaemia associated with failure of B-cell development are conspicuously lacking in primary and secondary follicular structures. This segregation of B- and T-lymphocyte areas tends to favour models of co-operation which involve soluble factors rather than antigen-bridging of T- and B-cells but the separation of cell types is not absolute.

Lymphocyte traffic

Lymphocytes enter the node through the afferent lymphatics and by passage across the specialized cuboidal epithelium of the postcapillary venules (cf. figure 3.1). This traffic of lymphocytes between the tissues, the blood stream and the lymph glands enables antigen-sensitive cells to seek the antigen and to be recruited to sites at which a response is occurring, while the dissemination of memory cells and their progeny enables a more widespread response to be organized throughout the lymphoid system. Thus, antigen-reactive cells are depleted from the circulating pool of lymphocytes within 24 hours of antigen first localizing in the lymph nodes or spleen; several days later, after proliferation at the site of antigen localization, a peak of activated cells appears in the thoracic duct. When antigen reaches a node in a primed animal, there is a dramatic fall in the output of cells in the efferent lymphatics, a phenomenon described variously as 'cell shutdown' or 'lymphocyte trapping' and which probably results from the antigen-induced release of a T-cell soluble factor (cf. the lymphokines, p. 78); this is followed by an output of activated blast cells which peaks at around 80 hours.

On a fresh section of spleen, the lymphoid tissue forming the white pulp is seen as circular or elongated grey areas within the erythrocyte-filled red pulp consisting of splenic cords lined with macrophages and venous sinusoids. As in the lymph node, T- and B-cell areas are segregated (figure 3.18). The spleen is a very effective blood filter removing effete red and white cells and responding actively to blood-borne antigens, the more so if particulate. Plasmablasts and mature plasma cells are present in the marginal zone extending into the red pulp.

UNENCAPSULATED LYMPHOID TISSUE

The respiratory, alimentary and genito-urinary tracts are guarded immunologically by subepithelial accumulations of lymphoid tissue which are not constrained by a connective tissue capsule. These may occur as diffuse collections of

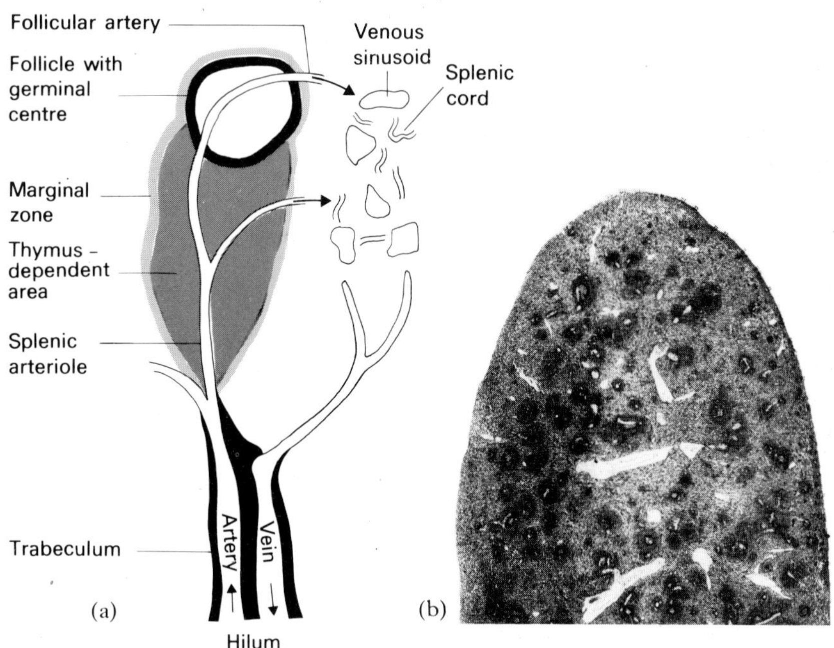

FIGURE 3.18. Human spleen (a) Diagrammatic representation. The lymphoid cells form a sheath around the arterioles (white pulp). The remainder (red pulp) consists of splenic cords and venous sinusoids filled with erythrocytes. (b) Low power view of histological section, × 35. (Photographed by Dr. P.M. Lydyard.)

lymphocytes, plasma cells and phagocytes throughout the lamina propria of the intestinal wall with only isolated solitary follicles (figure 3.19a) or as more clearly organized tissue with well-formed follicles (figure 3.19b). In man, the latter includes the lingual, palatine and pharyngeal tonsils, the small intestinal Peyer's patches and the appendix. It has been suggested that the unencapsulated lymphoid tissue forms a separate interconnected system, the mucosal-associated lymphoid tissue (MALT), within which cells committed to IgA or IgE synthesis may circulate.

In the gut, cells leave the Peyer's patches, presumably after antigenic stimulation, and ultimately drain into the blood from the thoracic duct and pass into the lamina propria where many become IgA-forming cells. This maturation of antibody-forming cells at a site distant from that at which antigen triggering has occurred is seen in the lymph node where plasma cells develop in the medullary cords and the spleen where they are found predominantly in the marginal zone. My guess is that this movement of cells acts to prevent the generation of high local concentrations of antibody in the region of the macrophage-processed antigen so avoiding neutralization of the antigen and premature shutting off of the immune response.

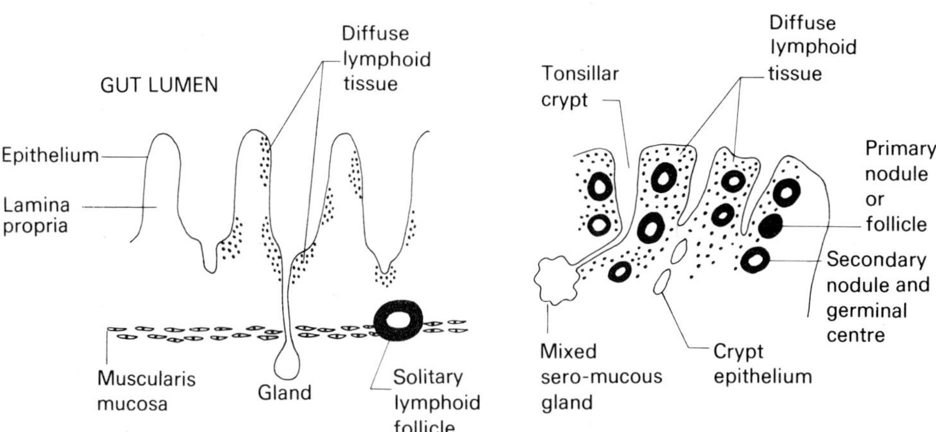

FIGURE 3.19. Unencapsulated lymphoid tissue.

Another tissue in the human which can support very active antibody synthesis is the bone marrow.

Summary

T-lymphocytes, which mature under the influence of the thymus, mediate cellular immunity and B-lymphocytes, which mature in the bone marrow in mammals (Bursa of Fabricius in birds), become antibody-forming cells responsible for humoral immunity. T- and B-cells are recognized by different surface markers: human T-cells form rosettes with sheep erythrocytes and B-cells have surface Ig which functions as a receptor for antigen.

Macrophages present antigen on their surface for reacting with and triggering antigen-sensitive lymphocytes. In the thymus dependent response to a hapten linked to an immunogenic carrier, T-cells reacting to the carrier help B-cells to be triggered by the hapten to form anti-hapten antibody. In the response to a typical protein, one determinant is like a hapten and the remaining determinants act as carrier. Combination of the antigen with B-cell Ig receptor provides a signal which tolerizes the B-cell unless it is activated by a second signal produced by the T-cell as a result of carrier stimulation. Poorly digested, linear, highly polymeric antigens can stimulate IgM-producing B-cells directly without T-cell help and are termed thymus independent antigens.

Cell-mediated immunity which provides the main defence against intracellular organisms, depends upon the interaction of antigen with specific receptors (not conventional Ig) on the surface of T-lymphocytes. One subpopulation of T-cells elaborates soluble factors (lymphokines) whose main function is to recruit and activate cells of the mono-nuclear phagocyte system; another population becomes cytotoxic for target cells bearing the antigen.

The immune response occurs most effectively in structured secondary lymphoid tissue. The lymph nodes filter and screen lymph flowing from the body tissues while spleen filters the blood. B- and T-cell areas are separated. B-cell structures appear in the lymph node cortex as primary follicles or secondary follicles with germinal centres after antigen stimulation; T-cells occupy the paracortical area; plasma cells synthesizing antibody appear in medullary cords which penetrate the macrophage lined medullary sinuses.

Lymphoid tissue guarding the G.I. tract is unencapsulated and somewhat structured (tonsils, Peyer's patches, appendix) or present as diffuse cellular collections in the lamina propria. Together with the subepithelial accumulations of cells lining the respiratory and genito-urinary tracts, they form the so-called mucosal associated lymphoid tissue system.

Further reading

See references at the end of chapter 4.

4 The immune response II—Further aspects

Synthesis of humoral antibody

DETECTION OF ANTIBODY-FORMING CELLS

Immunofluorescence

Cells containing antibody within their cytoplasm can be identified by the 'sandwich' technique (see figure 6.11c). For example, a cell making antibodies to tetanus toxoid if treated first with the antigen will subsequently bind a fluorescein labelled anti-tetanus antibody and can then be visualized in the fluorescence microscope (cf. figure 3.6h).

Plaque techniques

Antibody secreting cells can be counted by diluting them in an environment in which the antibody formed by each individual cell produces a readily observable effect. In one of the most widely used techniques, developed from the original method of Jerne and Nordin, the cells from an animal immunized with sheep erythrocytes are suspended together with an excess of sheep red cells within a shallow chamber formed between two microscope slides. On incubation the antibody-forming cells release their immunoglobulin which coats the surrounding erythrocytes. Addition of complement (cf. p. 157) will then cause lysis of the coated cells and a plaque clear of red cells will be seen around each antibody-forming cell (figure 4.1). Direct plaques obtained in this way largely reveal IgM producers since this antibody has a high haemolytic efficiency. To demonstrate IgG synthesizing cells it is necessary to increase the complement binding of the erythrocyte-IgG antibody complex by first adding a rabbit anti-IgG serum; this develops the 'indirect plaques' and can be used to enumerate cells making antibodies in different immunoglobulin subclasses, provided the appropriate rabbit antisera are available. The method can

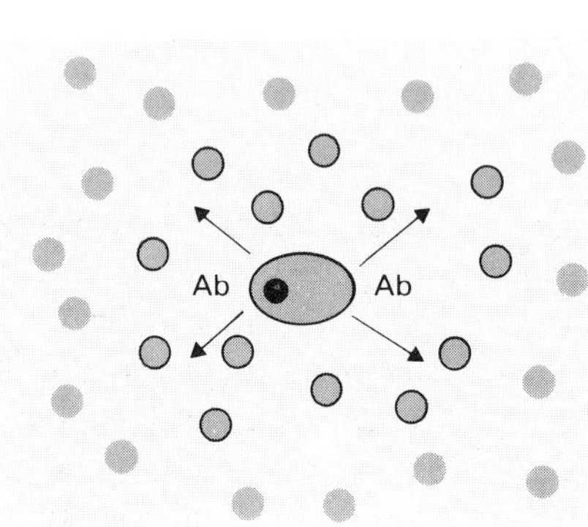

Secreted antibody coats surrounding red cells

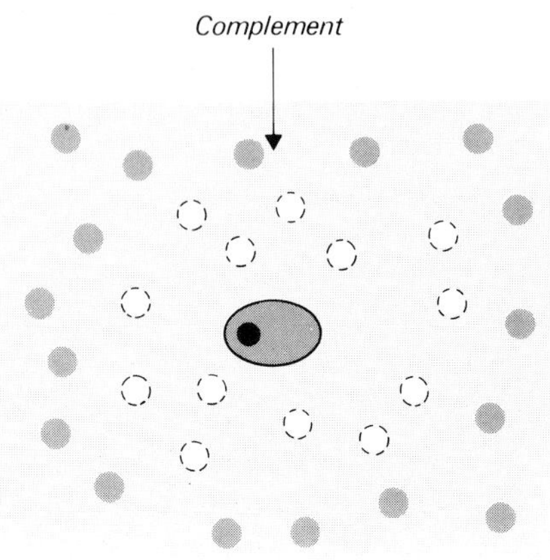

Coated erythrocytes lysed on adding complement to form plaque with antibody-forming cell at centre

(a)

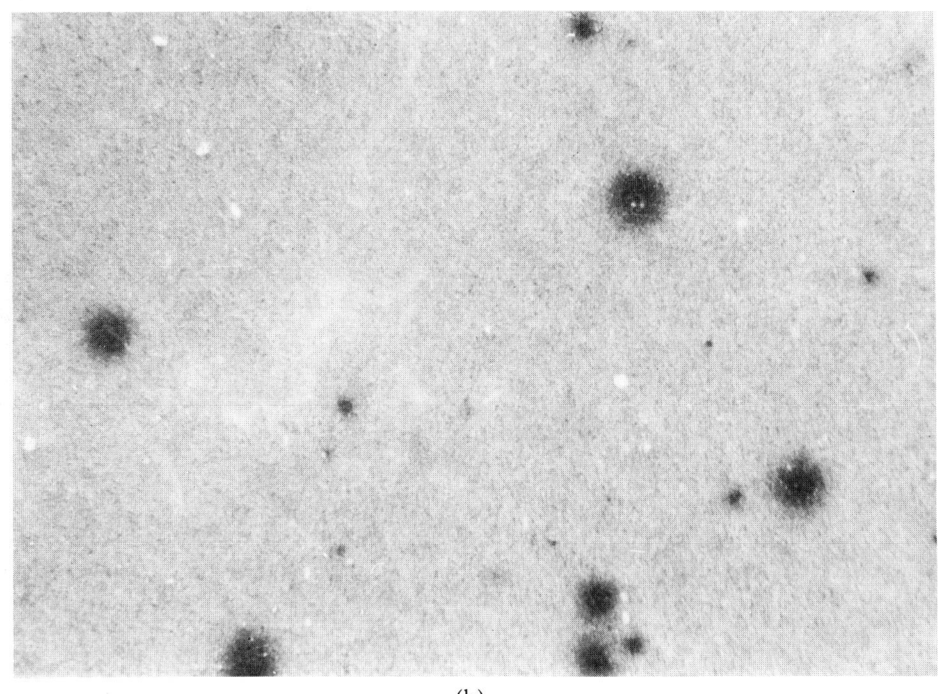

(b)

FIGURE 4.1. Jerne plaque technique for enumerating antibody-forming cells (Cunningham modification). (a) The direct technique for cells synthesizing IgM haemolysin is shown. The indirect technique for visualizing cells producing IgG haemolysins requires the addition of anti-IgG plus complement in the final stage. The difference between the plaques obtained by direct and indirect methods gives the number of 'IgG' plaques. (b) Photograph of plaques which show as circular dark areas under dark-ground illumination (courtesy of Mr. C. Shapland, Ms. P. Hutchings & Dr. D. Male).

be extended by coating an antigen such as pneumococcus polysaccharide onto the red cell, or by coupling hapten groups to the erythrocyte surface.

PROTEIN SYNTHESIS

In the normal antibody-forming cell there is a rapid turnover of light chains which are present in slight excess. Defective control occurs in many myeloma cells and one may see excessive production of light chains or complete suppression of heavy chain synthesis. Interchain disulphide bridges may form while the heavy chains are still attached to the ribosomes (figure 4.2) but the sequence in which the intermediates arise varies with the nature of the immunoglobulin. Using 'pulse and chase' techniques with radioactive amino acids it was found that the build-up of both light and heavy chains proceeds continuously starting from the N-terminal end. Furthermore, isolation of the mRNA for each type of chain has shown them to be of appropriate size to allow synthesis of the complete peptides. The evidence is, therefore, against the view that either chain can be formed by joining together two

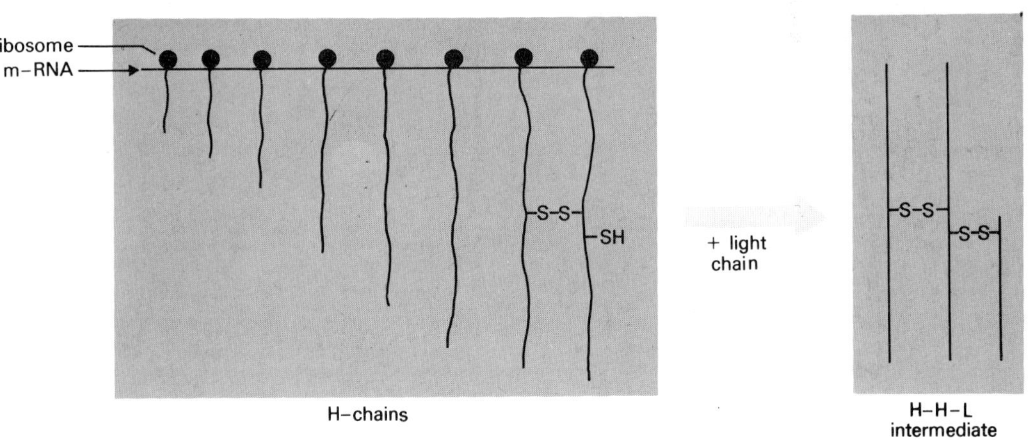

FIGURE 4.2. Synthesis of mouse IgG2a immunoglobulin. As the H-chains near completion, adjacent peptide chains can spontaneously cross-link through their constant regions. It is thought that the light chains may aid release of the terminal chains from the ribosome by forming the L–H–H molecule. Combination with a further light chain would yield the full immunoglobulin L–H–H–L (based on Askonas B.A. & Williamson A.R., *Biochem. J.* 1968, **109**, 637). The order in which the interchain disulphide bridges are formed varies in different immunoglobulins depending on the relative strengths of the bonds as assessed by susceptibility to reduction.

preformed lengths of peptide and it is now thought that the messenger regions for variable and constant regions are spliced together before leaving the nucleus.

ABNORMAL IMMUNOGLOBULIN SYNTHESIS

In chapter 2 we discussed the production of unique monoclonal immunoglobulins in multiple myeloma where there is an uncontrolled proliferation of a single clone of Ig-producing plasma cells. IgG, IgA, IgD and IgE myeloma has been reported in frequencies which parallel their serum concentration; Waldenström's macroglobulinaemia represents a closely comparable situation involving monoclonal IgM production. The myeloma or 'M' component in serum is recognized as a tight band on paper electrophoresis (all molecules in the clone are of course identical and have the same mobility) and as an abnormal arc on immunoelectrophoresis with a 'bump' caused by the monoclonal protein (figure 4.3a and b). 'M' bands have been found in the sera of a number of individuals who have no clinical signs of myeloma; the comparative rarity with which invasive multiple myeloma develops in these people and the constant

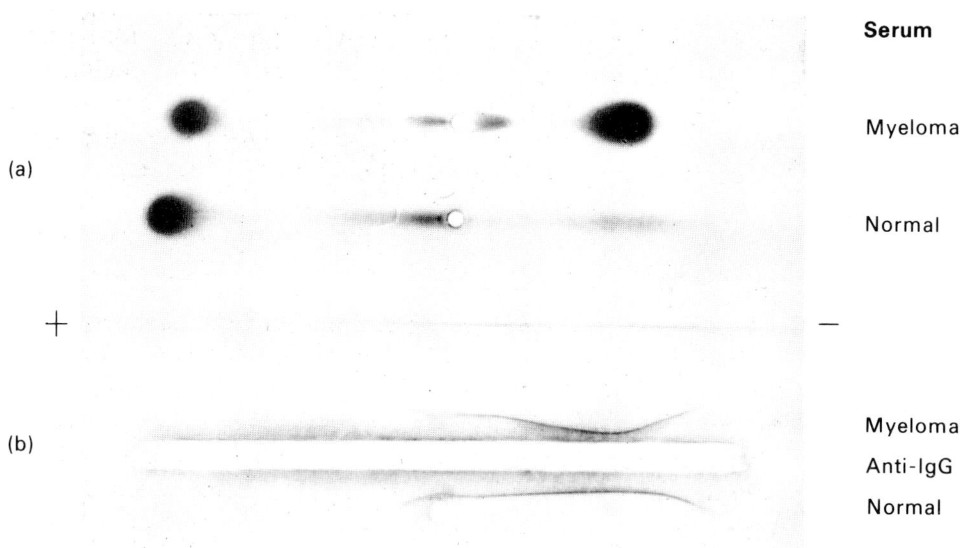

FIGURE 4.3. Myeloma serum with an 'M' component. (a) Agar gel electrophoresis showing strong band in γ-globulin region. (b) Immunoelectrophoresis against anti-IgG serum revealing the 'bump' or 'bow' in the precipitin arc. (Courtesy Dr. F.C. Hay.)

level of the monoclonal protein over a period of years suggests the presence of benign tumours of the lymphocyte-plasma cell series.

Amyloid Between 10 and 20% of patients with myeloma develop widespread amyloid deposits which contain the variable region of the myeloma light chain. Being identical, the variable region fragments polymerize and form the characteristic amyloid fibrils which are recognizable by their green birefringence on staining with Congo Red. Other components in amyloid have not yet been characterized. The fibrils are relatively resistant to digestion and accumulate in the ground substance of connective tissue where they can lead to pathological changes in the kidneys, heart and brain. Amyloid can also be formed secondarily to chronic inflammatory conditions such as rheumatoid arthritis and familial Mediterranean fever but in this case involves the polymerization of a unique substance, Amyloid A (AA) protein derived from the N-terminal part of a serum precursor (SAA) of molecular weight 90,000. SAA behaves as an acute phase protein in that its concentration increases rapidly in response to tissue injury or inflammation. Levels rise with age and the minority of individuals with high values are the most likely to develop amyloid.

Heavy chain disease is a rare condition in which quantities of abnormal heavy chains are excreted in the urine—γ-chains in association with malignant lymphoma and α-chains in cases of abdominal lymphoma with diffuse lymphoplasmacytic infiltration of the small intestine. The amino acid sequences of the N-terminal regions of these heavy chains are normal but they have a deletion extending from part of the variable domain through most of the $C_{H}1$ region so that they lack the structure required to form cross-links to the light chains. One idea is that the defect arises through faulty coupling of *V* and *C* region genes (cf. p. 131).

MONOCLONAL ANTIBODIES

A fantastic technological revolution has been achieved by Milstein and Köhler who devised a technique for the production of 'immortal' clones of cells making single antibody specificities by fusing normal antibody-forming cells with an appropriate B-cell tumour line. These so-called 'hybridomas' are selected out in a tissue culture medium which fails to support growth of the parental cell types, and by successive dilutions or by plating out, single clones can be established. These clones can be propagated in spinner culture or grown up in the ascitic form in mice when quite prodigious titres of monoclonal antibody can be attained. Remember that even in a good antiserum over

90% of the Ig molecules have little or no avidity for the antigen, and the 'specific antibodies' themselves represent a whole spectrum of molecules with different avidities directed against different determinants on the antigen. What a contrast is provided by the monoclonal antibodies where all the molecules produced by a given hybridoma are identical: they have the same Ig class and allotype, the same variable regions, structures, idiotypes, affinities and specificities. Furthermore, they have the advantage that, theoretically, all laboratories throughout the world can use the same reagent since the cell line should be immortal (please God or whoever). Their potential defies the imagination; the separation of individual cell types with specific surface markers (lymphocyte subpopulations, neural cells, etc.), diagnosis of lymphoid and myeloid malignancies, tissue typing, radioimmunossay, serotyping of micro-organisms, the fine structure of the antibody combining site and the basis for variability, immunological intervention with passive antibody, anti-idiotype inhibition or 'magic bullet' therapy with cytotoxic agents coupled to antitumour specific antibody—these and many other areas will all be transformed by hybridoma technology.

Activated T-cells have been fused with T-lymphoma lines to generate hybridomas producing individual suppressor factors for example and the technique is clearly not just confined to cells of immunological importance. Further excitement stems from the description of human cell hybridomas, an advance on the previously available technology in which antigen-enriched lymphocytes are transformed to cell-lines by polyclonal stimulation with EB virus.

IMMUNOGLOBULIN CLASSES

The synthesis of antibodies belonging to the various immunoglobulin classes proceeds at different rates. Usually there is an early IgM response which tends to fall off rapidly. IgG antibody synthesis builds up to its maximum over a longer time period. On secondary challenge with antigen, the time course of the IgM response resembles that seen in the primary though the peak may be higher. By contrast the synthesis of IgG antibodies rapidly accelerates to a much higher titre and there is a relatively slow fall-off in serum antibody levels (figure 4.4). The same probably holds for IgA and in a sense both these immunoglobulin

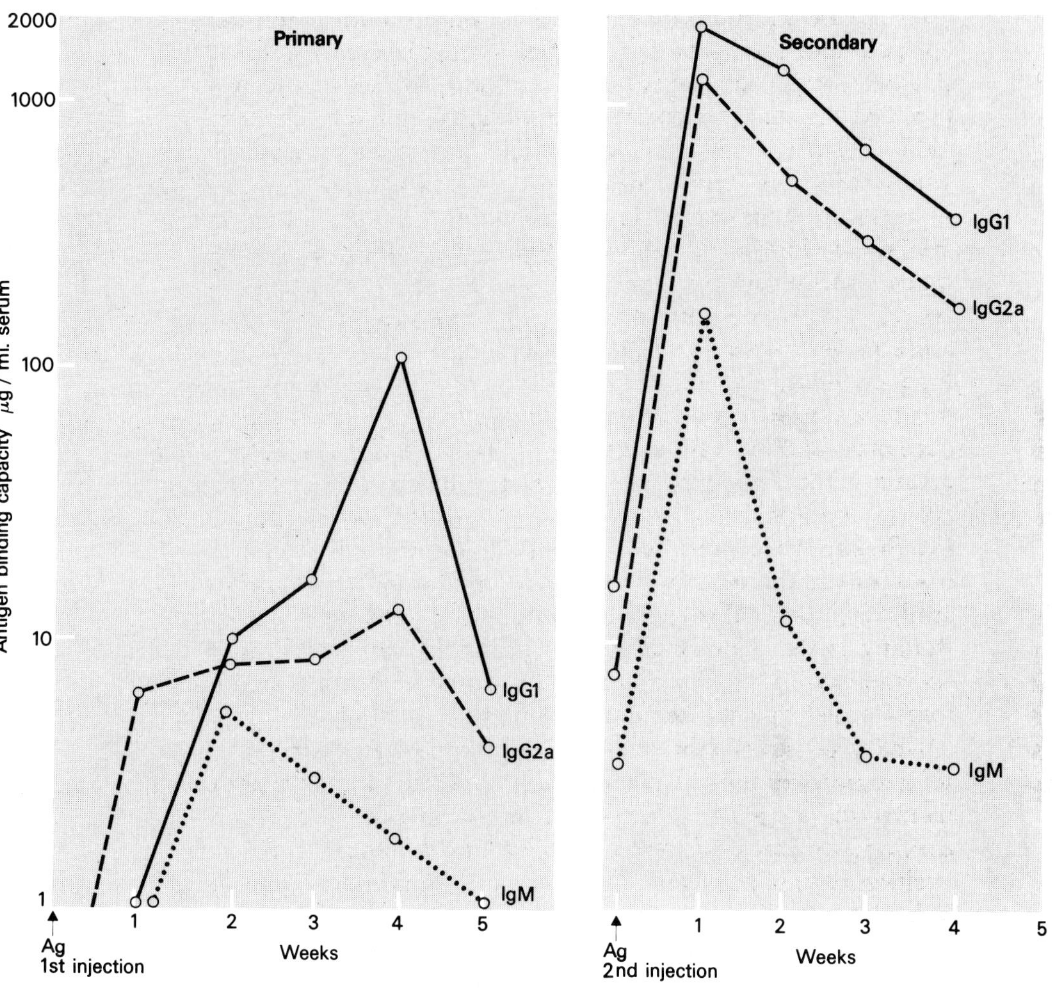

FIGURE 4.4. Synthesis of antibodies in different mouse immunoglobulin classes during the primary and secondary responses to bovine serum albumin. Using more sensitive methods such as agglutination or plaquing, IgM is found to be the first antibody class to be stimulated in the primary response. (Data kindly provided by Dr. G. Torrigiani.)

classes provide the main *immediate* defence against future penetration by foreign antigens.

There is evidence that individual cells can switch over from IgM to IgG production. Several days after immunization with salmonella flagella, isolated cells taken into microdrop cultures were shown to produce IgM and IgG immobilizing antibodies. In another study it was shown that antigen challenge of irradiated recipients receiving relatively small numbers of lymphoid cells, produced splenic foci of cells each synthesizing antibodies of different heavy chain class bearing a single idiotype; the common idiotype suggests that each focus is derived from a single precursor cell whose progeny can form antibodies of different class.

Antibody synthesis in certain classes shows considerable dependence upon T-co-operation in that the responses in T-deprived animals are strikingly deficient; such is true of mouse IgG1, IgE and part of the IgM antibody responses and of IgM memory. Immunopotentiation by complete Freund's adjuvant, a water-in-oil emulsion containing antigen in the aqueous phase and a suspension of killed tubercle bacilli in the oily phase (p. 202), seems to occur, at least in part, through the activation of helper T-cells which stimulate antibody production in T-dependent classes. The prediction from this that the response to T-independent antigens (e.g. pneumococcus polysaccharide p. 73) should not be potentiated by Freund's adjuvant is borne out in practice; furthermore, as would be expected, these antigens evoke primarily IgM antibodies and poorly defined immunological memory as do T-dependent antigens injected into thymectomized hosts. Thus in rodents at least the switch from IgM to IgG appears to be under some degree of thymus or T-cell control. Another class-specific effect which must be mentioned is the tremendous enhancement of IgE responses by helminths and even by soluble extracts derived from them.

Genetic control of the antibody response

GENES AFFECTING GENERAL RESPONSIVENESS

Mice can be selectively bred for high or low antibody responses through several generations to yield two lines, one of which consistently produces high titre antibodies to a variety of antigens and the other, antibodies of relatively low titre (Biozzi & colleagues). Of the order of 10 different genetic loci are concerned, one or more of which affect macrophage behaviour. The two lines are comparable in their ability to clear carbon particles or sheep erythrocytes from the blood by phagocytosis, but macrophages from the high responders retain a far higher proportion of added antigen in an undegraded (and presumably) immunogenic form on their surface (cf. p. 69). On the other hand, the low responders survive infection by *Salmonella typhimurium* better and their macrophages support much slower replication of listeria (cf. p. 185) suggesting a dichotomy in the ability of macrophages to subserve humoral as compared with cell-mediated immunity.

IMMUNE RESPONSE LINKED TO IMMUNOGLOBULIN GENES

In a number of cases where an antigen induces virtually a monoclonal response (e.g. type C streptococcal carbohydrate in rabbits), breeding experiments have shown that the capacity to produce this clone and its idiotype is inherited and is linked to the genetic markers for the immunoglobulin constant region, i.e. there is a gene coding for the variable region of the antibody and it occurs on the chromosome carrying the genes for the constant region. These findings would lead one to suppose that in general we inherit genes which enable us to make particular antibodies and that the capacity to produce an antibody response is limited by the repertoire of specificities encoded by the genes on this chromosome.

IMMUNE RESPONSE LINKED TO THE MAJOR HISTOCOMPATIBILITY COMPLEX

One genetic region in higher vertebrates termed the major histocompatibility complex (MHC) exerts a predominant influence on the survival of grafts within each species by controlling the synthesis of antigens which provoke intense immunological rejection (see p. 256). The MHC antigens are highly polymorphic (literally 'many shapes') due to the existence of several *alternative* genes (alleles) at each locus, each coding for a different antigen. It has been found that the antibody responses to a number of thymus-dependent antigenically simple substances are determined by genes—the so-called immune response or Ir genes—which are linked chromosomally to the MHC. Thus in mice, where the MHC is referred to as the H-2 region, all strains belonging to the H-2^b group respond well to the synthetic branched polypeptide antigen (T,G)-A--L (a polylysine backbone with side chains of polyalanine randomly tipped with mixed tyrosine and glutamyl residues), whereas mice of H-2^k specificity which bear a different set of allelic genes in the H-2 region, respond poorly. We say that mice of the H-2^b haplotype (i.e. a particular set of H-2 genes) are high responders to (T,G)-A--L because they possess the appropriate Ir gene. With another synthetic antigen, (H,G)-A--L, having histidine in place of tyrosine, the position is reversed, the 'poor (T,G)-A--L responders' now giving a good antibody response and the 'good (T,G)-A--L responders' a weak one showing that the capacity of a particular strain to give a high or low response varies with the individual antigen (Table 4.1). These relationships are only apparent when antigens of highly restricted structure are studied because the response to each single determinant is controlled by an Ir gene and it is highly unlikely that the different determinants on a complex antigen will all be associated with consistently high or consistently low responder Ir genes; rather would one expect an average of randomly high and low responder genes since the various determinants on most thymus dependent complex antigens are structurally unrelated. Thus H-2 linked immune responses have been observed not only with relatively simple polypeptides, but also with transplantation antigens from another strain and autoantigens where merely one or two determinants are recognized as foreign by the host. With complex antigens, H-2 linkage is only seen when the dose administered is so low that just one immunodominant determinant is recognized by the immune system. In this way, reactions controlled by Ir genes are distinct from the overall responsiveness to a variety of complex antigens which is a feature of the Biozzi mice (above).

TABLE 4.1. H-2 linked immune responses to synthetic polypeptide antigens.

Antigen	Antibody response	
	$H\text{-}2^b$	$H\text{-}2^k$
(T,G)-A--L	High	Low
(H,G)-A--L	Low	High

See text for definition of terms used.
After McDevitt H.O. & Sela M. (1965), *J. Exp. Med.* **122**, 517.

H-2I gene control of T-B co-operation

The I region containing the Ir genes has been localized within the H-2 complex close to the H-2K end (figure 4.5). Antisera raised between strains have identified several Ia antigens (i.e. antigens encoded by I region genes) which broadly correspond with 5 genetic subregions, I-A, I-B, I-J, I-E and I-C; each subregion is multi-allelic and gives rise to a number of different gene products certain of which may endow their host with high responder and others with low responder status to restricted determinants.

The Ir genes do not appear to affect B-cell triggering by T-independent antigens but rather control the co-operative response to T-dependent antigens. Ia determinants are largely expressed on the surface of B-cells and macrophages, particularly the dendritic variety. Antigens 'processed' by macrophages are presented to T-cells in some form of association with the surface Ia. Helper T-lymphocytes recognize this antigen-Ia complex in much the same way that cytotoxic T-cells have to recognize antigen on the target cell associated with other MHC products, H-2D and H-2K (cf. figure 9.16, p. 280). The primed helper cells could then be triggered by an Ia-bearing B-cell which had bound the antigen to its surface Ig receptors since it would recognize the same antigen-Ia combination it first saw on the macrophage. The activated T-helper would then presumably deliver the 'second signal' (p. 71) required for B-cell induction (figure 4.6). If the Ia product is unable to present antigen effectively or if the T-cells cannot recognize the Ia-antigen complex, the animal will be a poor responder; it is difficult to distinguish these two possibilities. An Alternative explanation for an H-2 linked poor response to a given antigen is provided by Ebringer's 'cross-tolerance' hypothesis which postulates that in these cases, a low response is the result of a similarity in shape between the antigen and the individual's own H-2 products (or H-2 plus minor surface determinants?), to which of course the animal is already tolerant.

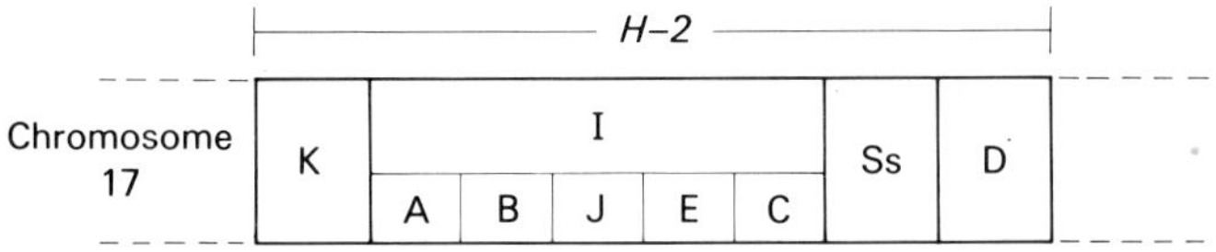

FIGURE 4.5. The major histocompatibility complex in the mouse (H-2). The sub-regions of I are designated I-A, I-B etc.

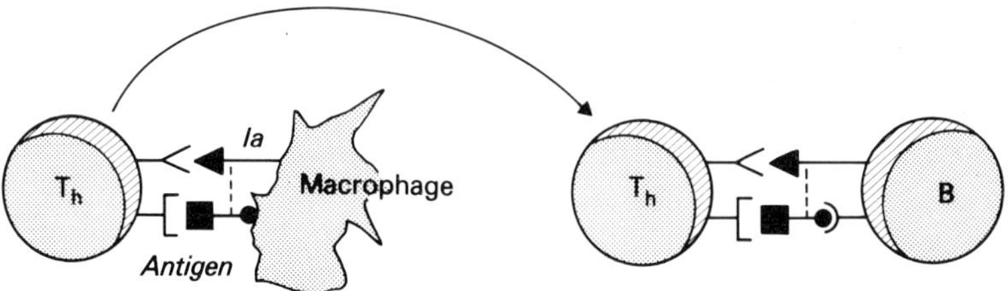

(a) Induction of helper T-cells

(b) Effector phase of T co-operation

FIGURE 4.6. H-2 linked immune response gene product (Ia) and T-B co-operation. Experimentally it can be shown that T-helper cells are most effective when the B-cells bear the same Ia specificity as the macrophages used for priming the T-cells. (a) The T-helpers are stimulated by antigen presented by the macrophage in some form of association (- - - - -) with Ia; (b) they can then co-operate with B-cells displaying the same Ia-antigen complex (although in this case the antigen is bound by surface Ig receptors). Other studies indicating the presence of I-A specificities on soluble 'helper' factors suggest the existence of further mechanisms of Ir gene involvement.

Other circumstances may also lead to poor antibody responses associated with the MHC. In some instances, low responders carry an I-J gene concerned in the synthesis of dominant amounts of a T-suppressor factor (see below) which acts to limit T-cell co-operation.

Factors influencing the genetic control of the antibody response are summarized diagrammatically in figure 4.7.

Regulation of the immune response

In addition to the genetic factors influencing the immune response discussed above, feedback mechanisms must operate to limit antibody production otherwise after antigenic stimulation we would become overwhelmed by the responding clones of antibody forming cells and their products, a clearly unwelcome state of affairs as may be clearly seen in multiple myeloma where control over lymphocyte proliferation is lost. Since antigen is needed to drive the division and differentiation of lymphocytes, the concentration of antigen must be a major regulating factor. As antigen is catabolized by body enzymes and neutralized or blocked by antibody so will its concentration fall and its ability to sustain the immune response be progressively weakened. The role of antibody in diverting antigen to immunogenically inoffensive sites in the body to prevent primary sensiti-

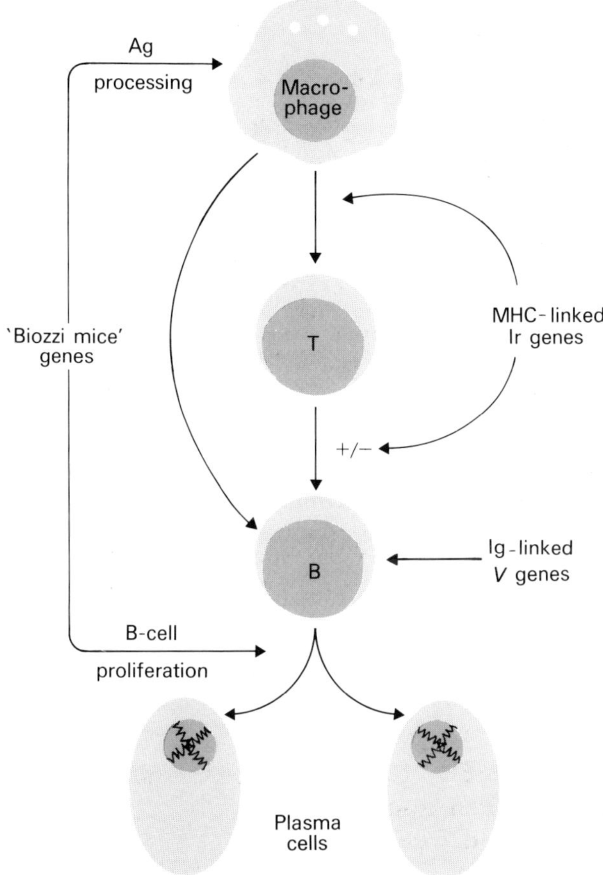

FIGURE 4.7. Genetic control of the antibody response.

zation is clearly evident from the protection against rhesus immunization afforded by administration of anti-D to mothers at risk (p. 229) and the inhibitory effect of maternal antibody on the peak titres obtained on vaccinating infants. Removal of circulating antibody by plasmapheresis during an ongoing response leads to an increase in synthesis, whereas injection of preformed IgG antibody markedly hastens the fall in the number of antibody-forming cells suggesting that such antibodies must exert an important feedback control on overall synthesis. It is unlikely that this is achieved by simple neutralization of antigen since whole IgG is overwhelmingly more effective than its $F(ab')_2$ fragment in switching off the reaction; perhaps an ability to bind simultaneously to macrophage Fc receptors enables the IgG to combine with immunogenic surface antigen more persistently and so block interaction with lymphocyte receptors.

T-cells provide a distinct regulatory system. Not only can they amplify the B-cell response through their helper activity, but there is now a body of evidence showing there to be a separate T-cell population with a *suppressor* function. If mice are made unresponsive by injection of a high dose of sheep red cells, their T-cells will suppress specific antibody formation in normal recipients to which they have been transferred (Gershon's 'infectious tolerance'; figure 4.8). Adult thymectomy in the mouse leads to a fall in the suppressor T-cell population, thereby increasing the response to T-independent antigens and preventing the fall-off in IgE antibody to haptens coupled with Ascaris extracts which occurs in intact animals. Furthermore, thymocytes from a young New Zealand Black (NZB) mouse can suppress autoantibody formation when injected into older diseased mice.

Helper and suppressor T-cells in the mouse have been distinguished in several ways. Suppressors are more vulnerable to adult thymectomy, x-irradiation and cyclophosphamide, and bind to sepharose-linked histamine-albumin conjugates, supposedly through surface histamine receptors. Unlike T-helpers, they can be depleted by passage down immunosorbent columns containing the specific antigen and whereas helpers are of phenotype Ly1 (cf. p. 66), suppressors are Ly2 and bear I-J determinants. In general terms the helper cells may be looked upon as inducers of the effector cells for humoral and cell-mediated immunity and it now

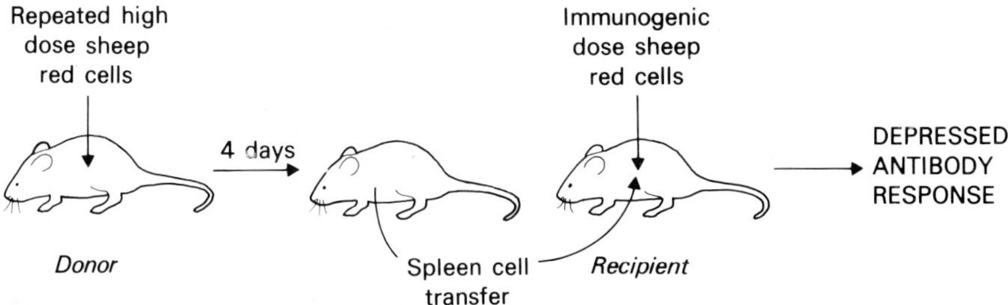

FIGURE 4.8. Demonstration of T-suppressor cells. Spleen cells from a donor injected with a high dose of antigen, depress the antibody response of a syngeneic animal to which they have been transferred. The effect is lost if the spleen cells are first treated with anti-Thy1 serum plus complement showing that the suppressors are T-cells (after Gershon R.K. & Kondo K. (1971) *Immunology* **21**, 903: in these studies mice were thymectomized, irradiated and reconstituted with bone marrow and thymocytes).

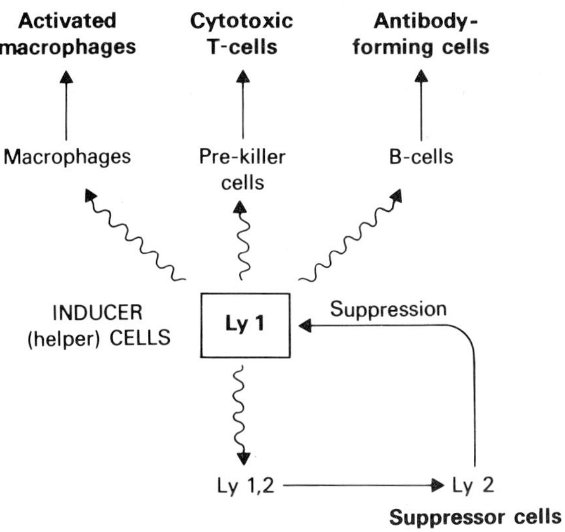

FIGURE 4.9. Immunoregulatory feedback circuit showing the central position of Ly1 cells in the induction (⁓⁓▸) of T-dependent responses and in the generation of T-supressors which in turn inhibit the Ly1 cells. A proportion of Ly1 cells express the Qa-1 antigen encoded by genes which map between the H-2D and TL loci (cf. figure 9.4). Both Ly1:Qa-1^+ and Ly1:Qa-1^- are involved in optimal collaboration with B-cells but only the former are able to generate suppressors; thus the balance between Qa-1^+ and Qa-1^- subsets may strongly influence the outcome of a given immune response (after Cantor H. & Gershon R.K.).

appears that they are also responsible for the generation of T-suppressors which exert negative feedback control on the helper cells (figure 4.9). There is evidence that this suppression is mediated by antigen. In the first place, soluble antigen-specific I-J positive suppressor factors have been well characterized. Secondly, experiments with lysozyme suggest that one determinant on the molecule can suppress the response to all the other determinants and it is not easy to see how a T-helper reacting with one epitope can be influenced by a T-suppressor directed against another structurally different epitope on the same molecule unless the two types of T-cell communicate in some way through the antigen itself. However, interaction can also occur through recognition of an idiotype on the T-helper receptors by an anti-idiotype on the suppressors and this will be discussed further in the next section.

Non-antigen specific T-suppression can also occur. Mouse T-lymphocytes when stimulated by the polyclonal activator concanavalin A (cf. p. 244) in culture are able to inhibit a variety of antibody responses. In the human, T-cells with receptors for Fcγ (IgG Fc) suppress the help given by T-cells with Fcμ receptors for the polyclonal stimulation of B-cells by pokeweed mitogen (cf. p. 244) and these findings may have relevance for the immunosuppressive action of IgG antibody described above and the stimulatory effect of IgM reported by Henry & Jerne. It has also been shown that immunoglobulin synthesis by normal B-lymphocytes following pokeweed stimulation in culture can be blocked by T-cells from a small proportion of patients with acquired hypo-γ-globulinaemia, with the clear implication that immunoglobulin production in the patient was restricted by active suppressor T-cells. This polyclonal B-cell inhibition contrasts with the antigen-specific suppression seen for example in the high dose sheep cell experiment mentioned above, and it seems that both non-specific and antigen-specific soluble suppressor factors can be demonstrated, mirroring the situation with T-helper factors. It has been postulated that a crowding out of acceptor sites on the macrophage by such molecules could be responsible for *antigenic competition*, the situation in which one T-dependent antigen can block the response to another. Awareness of this phenomenon in vaccination programmes involving more than one antigen is of self-evident importance.

IDIOTYPIC NETWORKS

The hypervariable loops on the immunoglobulin molecule which go to form the antigen combining site have individual characteristic shapes which can be recognized by the appropriate antibodies as idiotypic determinants (cf. p. 47). There are hundreds of thousands, if not more, different idiotypes in one individual, virtually all of them present in very low concentrations at birth and therefore unlikely to produce self-tolerance.

Jerne reasoned that the great diversity of idiotypes would to a considerable extent mirror the diversity of antigenic shapes in the external world. Thus if lymphocytes can recognize a whole range of foreign antigenic determinants, they should be able to recognize the idiotypes on other lymphocytes. They would therefore form a large network or series of networks depending upon idiotype—anti-idiotype recognition between lymphocytes of the various T- and B-subsets (figure 4.10) and the response to an external

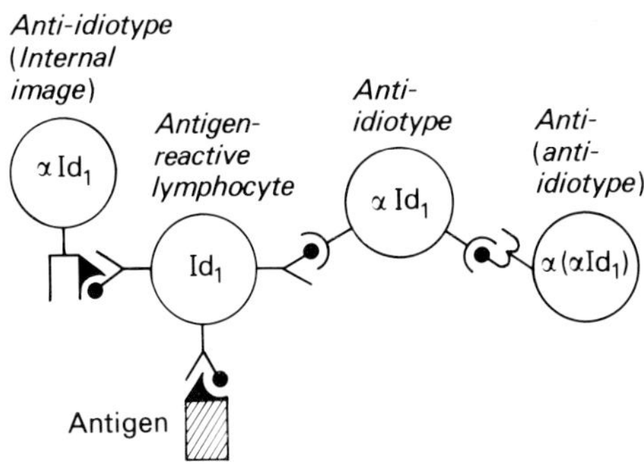

FIGURE 4.10. Elements in an idiotypic network. T-helper, T-suppressor and B-lymphocytes recognize each other through idiotype—anti-idiotype reactions; either stimulation or suppression may result. One of the anti-idiotype sets may bear an idiotype of similar shape to (i.e. provides an *internal image* of) the antigen. The same idiotype (●) may be shared by two receptors of different specificity (since the several hypervariable regions provide a number of potential idiotypic determinants and a given idiotype does not always form part of the epitope binding site), so that the anti-(anti-Id_1) does not necessarily bind the original antigen. This explains the paradoxical finding by Oudin & Cazenave that not all the Ig molecules bearing a given idiotype formed in the response to an antigen can function as specific antibody. The finding of Id_1 on the anti-(anti-Id_1) would suggest that the network does not branch significantly at each level. Complexes in antibody excess stimulate anti-idiotype in contrast with antigen excess complexes which establish immunological memory (cf. p. 69).

antigen perturbing this network would be conditioned by the state of the idiotypic interactions.

There is no doubt that the elements to form an idiotypic network are all there. A whole variety of auto-anti-idiotypes have been generated experimentally and they have been identified during the course of antigen-induced responses. Anti-idiotypic specificities have been associated with both T-helpers and suppressors and Eichman has shown that quite small amounts of anti-idiotypic antibodies can stimulate or inhibit an idiotype response depending on the Ig class of the anti-idiotype. Although outbred rabbits rarely produce the same idiotype (Id_1) in the response to a given antigen, they can be made to do so by preimmunization with anti-idiotype (αId_1) (see figure 4.10); the anti-(αId_1) suppresses the αId_1 clone and so allows the Id_1 clone to emerge in response to antigenic stimulation.

It is difficult to assess the extent to which idiotype networks control the immunological system. Is there a complete dynamic network in which messages are constantly passing between all cells including those in a 'resting phase', or are interactions limited largely to the immediate anti-idiotype partners, and then only during clonal expansion of cells bearing the antigen-reactive idiotype? What is the relative importance of antigen and anti-idiotype in regulation of the immune response? Since the body cannot help making anti-idiotypic responses there is bound to be some contribution from the network. However, the dominant effect of one lysozyme determinant in suppressing the response to all other epitopes (see above) and the inhibitory effect of a monoclonal antigen-specific suppressor factor on T-help provided by the whole carrier molecule, speaks for a major regulatory role of antigen because lymphocytes reacting with *different* determinants on the same molecule can be linked through the antigen itself but not through an idiotype network. It is worth noting that anti-Id may enable immune responses to 'tick-over' for extended periods after the complete elimination of antigen. The network provides interesting opportunities for immunological intervention: to give one example, Binz & Wigzell have conditioned rats to accept a skin graft by autoimmunization with the idiotype of the Ig V region receptor for the transplantation antigen concerned. It might even be feasible to immunize people against certain infections with a monoclonal anti-idiotype should this prove easier to obtain in bulk than the microbial

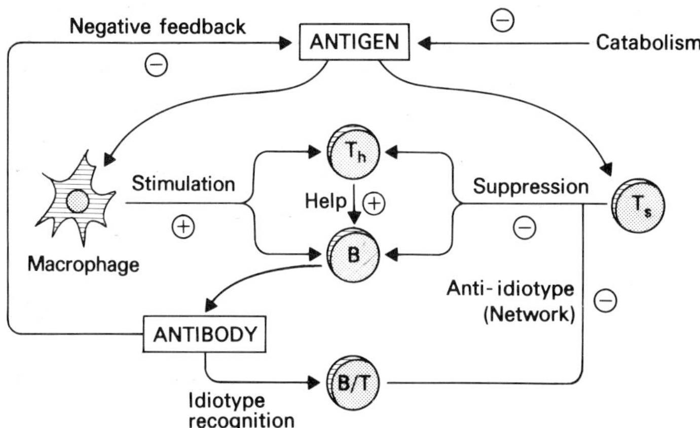

FIGURE 4.11. Regulation of the immune response T_h = T-helper cell; T_s = T-suppressor cell. T-help for cell-mediated immunity will be subject to similar regulation. Some of these mechanisms may be interdependent; for example one could envisage anti-idiotypic antibody acting in concert with a suppressor T-cell by binding to its Fc receptor, or suppressor T-cells with specificity for the idiotype on T_h or B-cells.

antigen itself and if successful, the strategy could be extended to tumour-associated antigens.

At this stage, if the reader is feeling a little groggy, try a glance at figure 4.11 which attempts a summary of the main factors currently thought to modulate the immune response.

Immunological tolerance

AT BIRTH

Over 20 years ago Owen made the intriguing observation that non-identical (dizygotic) twin cattle, which shared the same placental circulation and whose circulations were thereby linked, grew up with appreciable numbers of red cells from the other twin in their blood; if they had not shared the same circulation at birth, red cells from the twin injected in adult life would be rapidly eliminated by an immunological response. From this finding Burnet & Fanner conceived the notion that potential antigens which reach the lymphoid cells during their developing immunologically immature phase in the perinatal period can in some way specifically suppress any future response to that antigen when the animal reaches immunological maturity. This, they considered, would provide a means whereby unresponsiveness to the body's own constituents ('self') could be established and thereby enable the lymphoid cells to make the important distinction between 'self' and 'non-self'. On this basis, any foreign cells introduced into the body around the perinatal period should trick the animal into treating them as 'self' components in later life and the studies of Medawar and his colleagues have shown that *immunological tolerance* or unresponsiveness can be artificially induced in this way. Thus neonatal injection of CBA mouse cells into newborn A strain animals suppresses their ability to immunologically reject a CBA graft in adult life (figures 4.12 and 4.13). Tolerance can also be induced with soluble antigens; for example, rabbits injected with bovine serum albumin at birth fail to make antibodies on later challenge with this protein.

IN THE ADULT

It is now recognized that tolerance can be induced in the adult as well as the neonate, although in general much

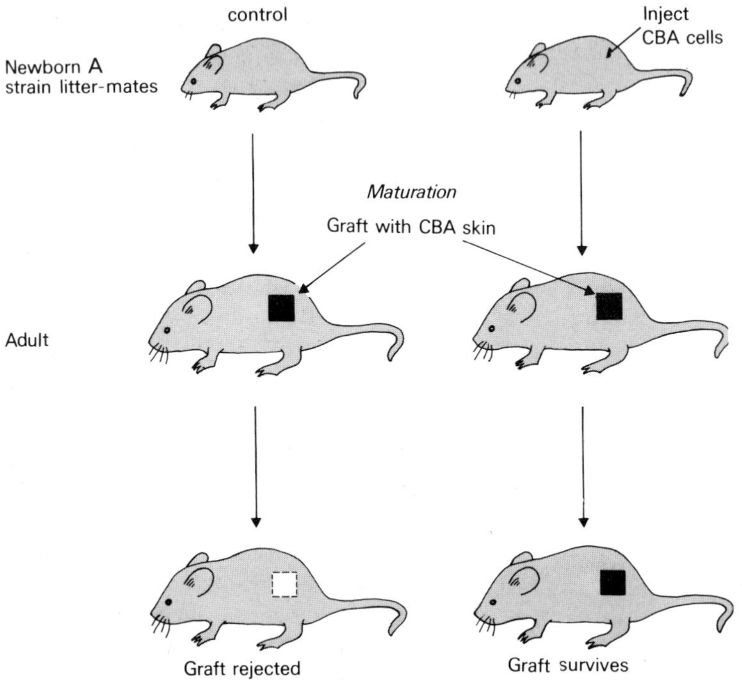

FIGURE 4.12. Induction of tolerance to foreign CBA skin graft in A strain mice by neonatal injection of antigen (after Billingham R., Brent L. & Medawar P.B.).

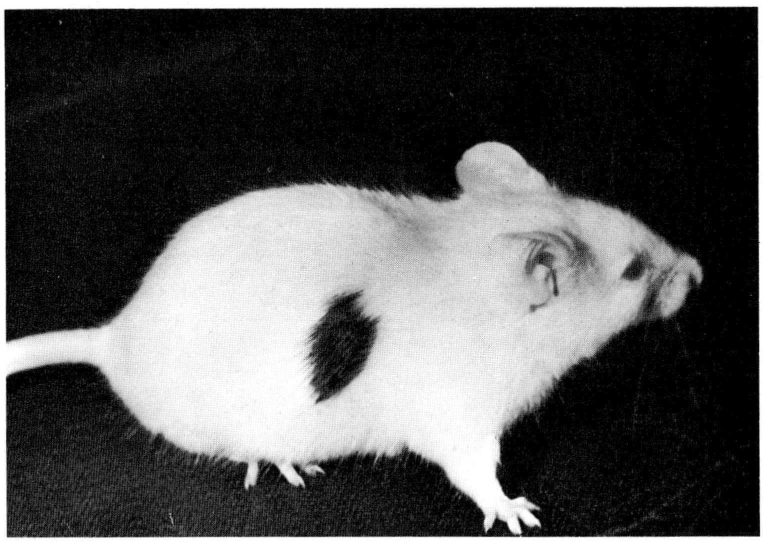

FIGURE 4.13. CBA skin graft on fully tolerant A strain mouse showing healthy hair growth eight weeks after grafting (courtesy of Professor L. Brent).

higher doses of antigen are required. Surprisingly, repeated injection of *low* doses of certain antigens such as bovine serum albumin (BSA) which are weakly immunogenic, established a state of tolerance as revealed by a poor antibody response on challenge with BSA in a strongly antigenic form (in complete Freund's adjuvant—see p. 202). It was shown subsequently that this 'low zone tolerance' could also be achieved with more powerful antigens provided an immunosuppressive drug such as cyclophosphamide were given to inhibit antibody synthesis during the low dose treatment.

Thus, there is a 'low zone' and a 'high zone' in terms of antigen predosage for tolerance induction. Elegant studies by Weigle and co-workers have pinpointed the T-cell as the target for tolerance at low antigen levels while both B- and T-lymphocytes are made unresponsive at high antigen dose (Table 4.2). Thus, for 'thymus-dependent' antigens at dose levels where the T-cells play a major co-operative role in antibody formation, the overall immunological performance of the animal will reflect the degree of reactivity of the T-cell population. In other words, the T-cells guide the reaction and when they are tolerant the B-cells will not respond.

Protein antigens are more tolerogenic (able to induce tolerance) when in a soluble rather than an aggregated or particulate form which can be readily taken up by macrophages and it seems that molecules are more likely to be tolerogenic if they escape processing by macrophages before

TABLE 4.2. Effect of antigen dose on tolerance induction in T- and B-cells

mg tolerogen administered	% Tolerance induced		
	T-cells	B-cells	Donor spleen
0.1	96	9	62
0.5	99	56	97
2.5	99	70	99

After induction of tolerance to aggregate-free human IgG in mice, the reactivity of thymocytes and bone marrow cells (containing B-cells) was assessed by transfer to irradiated recipients with either bone marrow or thymus respectively from normal donors. The degree of tolerance induced in the donor is shown in the final column. Low antigen doses tolerize the T-cells. B-cells become unresponsive at higher doses. The T-cell activity largely dictates the response of the spleen as a whole (from Chiller J.M., Habicht G.S. & Weigle W.O. (1971) *Science*, **171**, 813).

presentation to the lymphocyte. Persistence of antigen is required to maintain tolerance. In Medawar's experiments the tolerant state was long-lived because the injected CBA cells survived and the animals continued to be chimaeric (i.e. they possessed both A and CBA cells). With non-living antigens such as BSA, tolerance is gradually lost, the most likely explanation being that in the absence of antigen, newly recruited immunocompetent cells which are being generated throughout life, are not being rendered tolerant. Since recruitment of newly competent T-lymphocytes is drastically curtailed by removal of the thymus, it is of interest to note that the tolerant state persists for much longer in thymectomized animals.

MECHANISMS

Genetic unresponsiveness If an animal lacks the genetic programmes which enable it to recognize certain self-determinants it will be 'immunologically silent'. This would be the case if there are no genes coding for the appropriate lymphocyte receptors; analysis of the experimentally induced autoantibody response to cytochrome c suggests that only those parts of the molecule which show species variation are autoantigenic whereas the highly conserved regions do appear to be silent. It is conceivable that unresponsiveness might arise from an inability to present certain self-components on the surface of a macrophage in an immunogenic form in association with Ia.

Clonal deletion The exceptional vulnerability of the neonate to tolerance induction has led to the suggestion that during lymphocyte development, the cell goes through a phase in which contact with antigen leads to death or permanent inactivation. In support of this view, the surface Ig of very early B-cells can be capped at much lower concentrations of anti-IgM than are required by adult cells and remarkably, after endocytosis of the caps, the surface receptors are resynthesized by the adult cells but not by the early B-lymphocytes which are now effectively aborted through their inability to 'see' antigen. In Medawar's experiments it has been argued that tolerance is a result of T-suppressor activity rather than clonal deletion. However, animals made fully tolerant by neonatal injection of donor cells are devoid of mixed lymphocyte (p. 258) and cytotoxic T-cell reactivities against donor antigens and do not possess cells which suppress these reactivities in lymphocytes from a normal mouse of the same strain. Also, tolerance can be abrogated by the transfer of normal syngeneic (same strain) lymphocytes, which should not be possible if T-suppressor cells were dominant.

T-suppression Low zone tolerance to protein antigens has been shown in at least one case to be mediated by T-suppressors directed against T-helpers and a suppressor mechanism will probably prove to be the most common basis for this phenomenon. The inferior immunogenicity of soluble as distinct from aggregated or particulate antigen, may be ascribed to weak stimulation of T-helpers through poor macrophage processing in contrast to effective activation of suppressor cells which do not require macrophage presentation. T-suppression has been recognized to be a major factor in transplantation tolerance in *adults* induced by a cocktail of donor antigen, pertussis vaccine and anti-lymphocyte serum.

Helplessness T-cells are more readily tolerized than B-cells and, as a result, a number of self-reacting B-cells are present in the body which cannot be triggered by T-dependent self-components since the T-cells required to provide the necessary T-B help are already tolerant—you might describe the B-cells as helpless. If we think of the determinant on a self-component which combines with the receptors on a self-reacting B-cell as a hapten and another determinant which has to be recognized by a T-cell as a carrier (cf. figure 3.14), then tolerance in the T-cell to the carrier will prevent the provision of T-cell help and the B-cell will be unresponsive. There are further consequences of helplessness, because if the self-reactive determinants cross-link B-cell receptors in the absence of T-cell signals, the B-cell should become tolerized as predicted by the 1 and 2 signal hypothesis of Bretscher and Cohn (p. 75); in fact, B-cell tolerance to haptenic determinants is readily produced when the hapten is presented to the B-cell on a thymus-independent carrier or on a carrier such as autologous IgG, to which the individual is already tolerant.

It is likely that self-tolerance involves all these mechanisms to varying degrees and that while clonal deletion is of prime importance early in life, T-suppression becomes a dominant factor later (figure 4.14). It should be stressed that these terms early and late apply to the life of the lymphocyte not

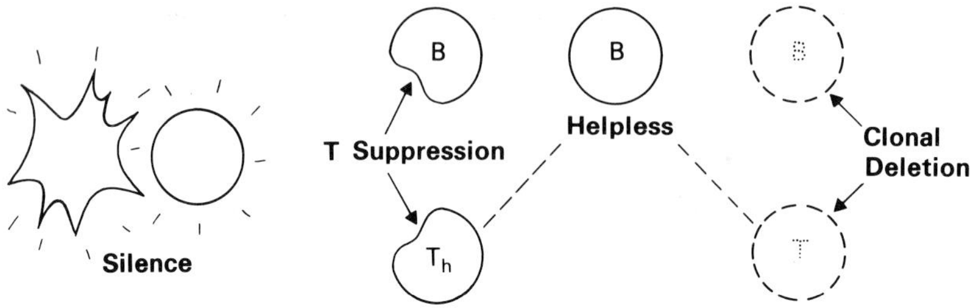

FIGURE 4.14. Mechanisms of self-tolerance.

of the host. If an adult is irradiated and reconstituted with immature lymphocytes in the form of bone marrow cells, the animal behaves as a neonate with respect to the ease of tolerance induction with low doses of antigen.

Ontogeny of the immune response

Haemopoiesis originates in the early yolk sac but as embryogenesis proceeds, this function is taken over by the fetal liver and finally by the bone marrow where it continues throughout life. The haemopoietic stem cell which gives rise to the formed elements of the blood and the cells of the lymphoreticular system (figure 4.15) can be shown to be multipotent, to seed other organs and to renew itself through the creation of further stem cells.

Stem cells attracted to the thymus by a chemotactic factor, differentiate within the microenvironment of the epithelioid cells where they proliferate extensively and acquire characteristic early T-cell markers (figure 4.16). Under the influence of the epithelioid cells, and in some cases also the dendritic reticular cells of the medulla, the thymocytes differentiate further to form distinct functional subpopulations with the competence to respond in the mixed lymphocyte reaction (p. 258), mediate allograft cytotoxicity (p. 79), generate carrier-specific help for B-cells and produce lymphokines for cell-mediated immunity ('delayed-type hypersensitivity' cells); cortisone-sensitive cells with potential suppressor function appear in the cortex. The ability to recognize self-MHC specificities which provide the basis for haplotype restricted T-cell responses to antigen (p. 279) is also acquired at this stage. Some cells move directly from the cortex into the periphery and others (future helper and delayed-type hypersensitivity cells which must learn to react with macro-

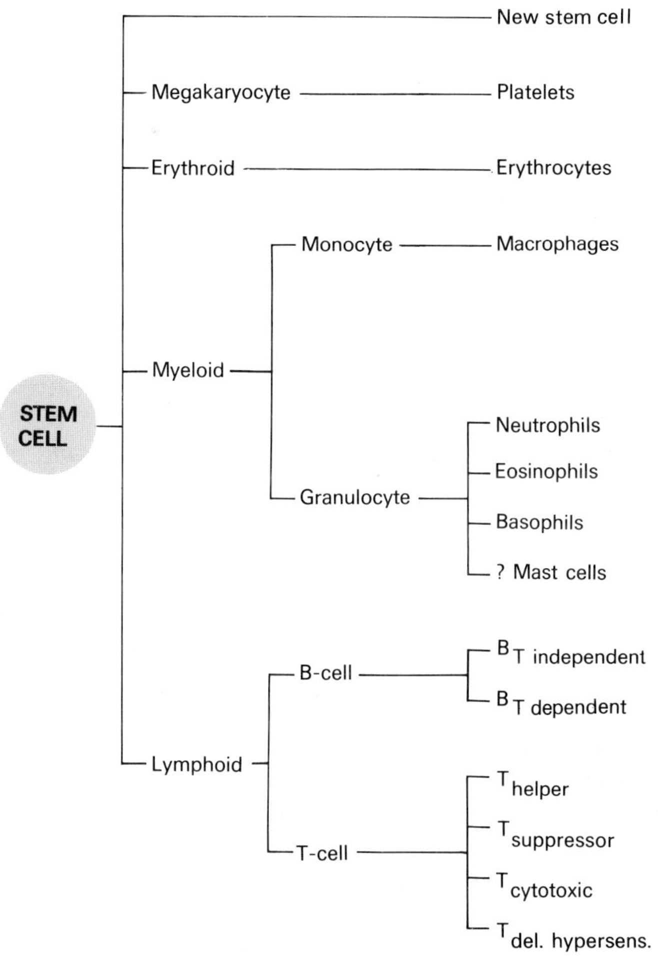

FIGURE 4.15. The multipotent haemopoietic stem cell. The classification of B- and T-cell subsets is still tentative as is the relationship between basophils and mast cells.

phages?) migrate to the medulla, a proportion staying there for a curiously long time.

Earlier experiments on the partial restitution of immunocompetence in thymectomized females through pregnancy were taken to imply that a soluble thymic product (derived from the fetal thymuses) was responsible, at least in part, for the influence of the gland on T-cell maturation. Several different soluble thymic extracts have been prepared and active preparations isolated usually on the basis of their ability to promote the appearance of T-cell differentiation markers (Thy1 in the mouse, sheep cell receptors in the human) on

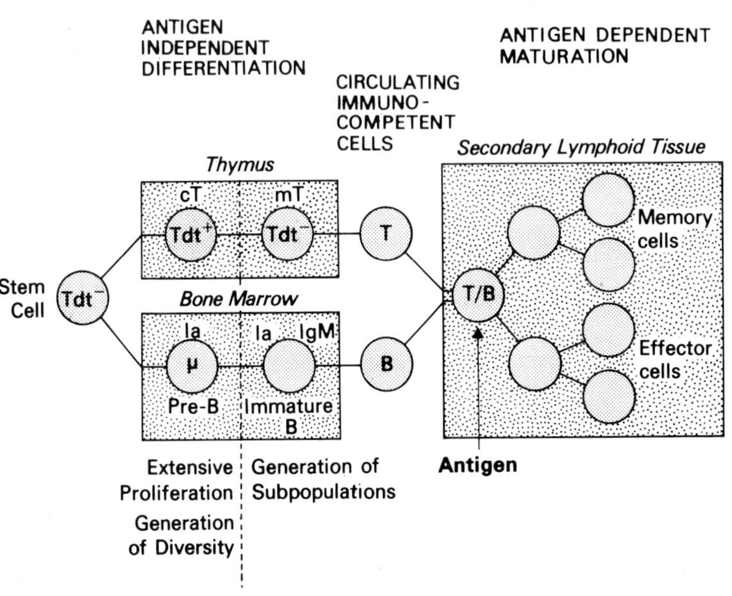

FIGURE 4.16. Differentiation and maturation of human B- and T-cells. Tdt = Terminal deoxynucleotidyl transferase; cT = cortical T-cell surface antigen; mT = mature T-cell surface antigen. The early replicating cells in the thymus and bone marrow are in the majority. Thymocytes are educated to recognize self-MHC haplotype (cf. p. 279). Tolerance to self-antigens is induced in the immature B- and T-cells within the primary lymphoid organs. Ia^+, μ^- pre-B cell precursors are Tdt^+; the Tdt enzyme may be involved as one of the mechanisms controlling the generation of diversity. In the mouse, the earliest thymocytes acquire surface Thy1; this then increases in surface density and is accompanied by the TL antigen (p. 258); cells ready to leave the thymus have lost TL and have a reduced Thy1.

culture with bone marrow cells *in vitro*. Of the four major candidates for the role of thymic hormone, 'thymosin', 'thymopoietin', 'thymic humoral factor' and 'facteur thymique serique' (FTS), only FTS (J.F. Bach) is a single molecular species. It is a nonapeptide of molecular weight 847 which can be detected in the cytoplasm of thymic epithelial cells by immuno-fluorescence and which binds to specific receptors on T-cells to cause an increase in cAMP formation. High doses are said to stimulate mature T-suppressor cells. Blood levels of FTS fall steadily with age as the thymus involutes (? and the cells wearily approach their Hayflick number), and precipitously in certain autoimmune disorders (SLE and NZB mice—chapter 10) at a time corresponding roughly with the onset of disease.

The microenvironment for the differentiation of B-cells is provided by the bursa of Fabricius in the chicken and the bone marrow itself in mammalian species (a nameless immunologist regularly slays his students by recalling that 'the bursa is strictly for the birds'). The early, rapidly dividing pre-B cells display cytoplasmic μ chains but no light chains (figure 4.16). It is likely that the genetic mechanisms responsible for the generation of receptor diversity (in T-cells as well) operate at this stage. In the immature B-cell, the receptor for which the cell is finally programmed is inserted into the plasma membrane as a specific IgM molecule. As immune competence emerges, the ability to mount an antibody response to each of a defined series of antigens appears sequentially and in the same order in different members of the same species, suggesting that the individual genes in the antibody V gene repertoire are recruited for receptor synthesis in a predetermined fashion. Immature B-cells have a lower density of surface immunoglobulins than primed lymphocytes and, unlike their mature counterparts, have difficulty in resynthesizing them after they have been stripped from the cell by treatment with anti-Ig which leads to 'shedding' or endocytosis. As discussed previously, this phenomenon could be related to the finding that bone marrow cells are easier to tolerize by exposure to thymus-dependent antigens than mature lymphocytes and that tolerance can be more readily induced in the new-born as compared with the adult. The relevance to the establishment of 'self-tolerance' to circulating body components at this stage hardly needs stressing; almost certainly, comparable events occur in the thymus.

At the next stage of differentiation, the cell develops a commitment to producing a particular antibody class and either bears surface IgM alone or in combination with IgA or IgG. The further addition of surface IgD now marks the readiness of the virgin B-cell for priming by antigen. Some cells, therefore, bear surface Ig of 3 different classes; M, G and D or M, A and D, but all Ig molecules on a single cell have the same idiotype and therefore are derived from the same V_H and V_L genes. IgD is lost on antigenic stimulation so that memory cells lack this Ig. At the terminal stages in the life of a fully mature plasma cell, virtually all surface Ig is shed. Injection of anti-μ (anti-IgM heavy chain) into chick embroyos prevents the subsequent maturation of IgM and IgG antibody producing cells, whereas anti-γ inhibits only IgG development. Whether the switch from

IgM production to other classes is partly antigen-driven (cf. p. 94) or occurs entirely as a result of microenvironmental factors is still unresolved. In the embryonic chicken bursa, a regular switch from IgM to IgG is observed and it seems possible that local influences in the gut will prove to be responsible for the predominant development of IgA bearing cells. These cells are generated in Peyer's patches, pass into the blood via the thoracic duct and return to populate the diffuse lymphoid tissue in the lamina propria of the gut.

Lymph node and spleen remain relatively underdeveloped in the human even at birth except where there has been intra-uterine exposure to antigens as in congenital infections with rubella or other organisms. The ability to reject grafts and to mount an antibody response is reasonably well developed by birth but the immunoglobulin levels with one exception are low particularly in the absence of intra-uterine infection. The exception is IgG which is acquired by placental transfer from the mother, a process dependent upon Fc structures specific to this Ig class. This material is catabolized with a half-life of approximately 30 days and

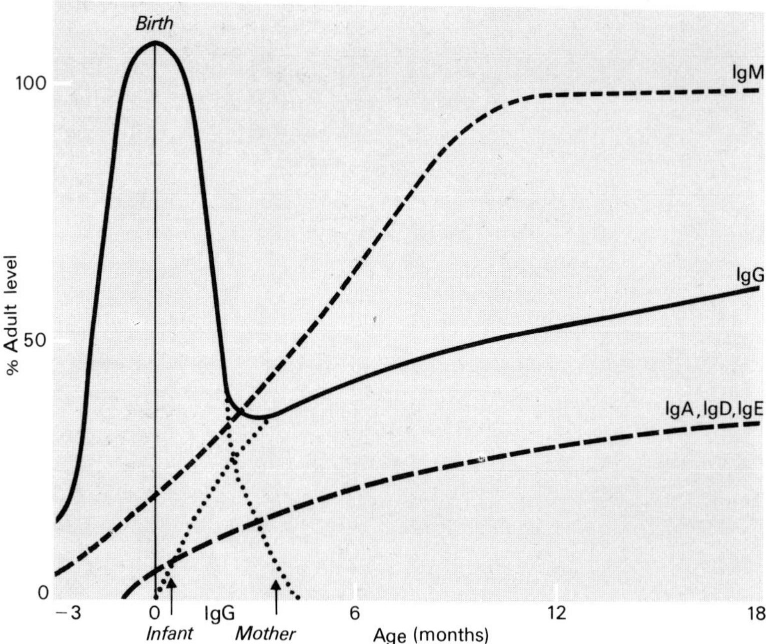

FIGURE 4.17. Development of serum immunoglobulin levels in the human (after Hobbs J. R. (1969) in *Immunology & Development*, ed. M. Adinolfi, p. 118. Heinemann, London).

there is a fall in IgG concentration over the first three months accentuated by the increase in blood volume of the growing infant. Thereafter the rate of synthesis overtakes the rate of breakdown of maternal IgG and the overall concentration increases steadily. The other immunoglobulins do not cross the placenta and the low but significant levels of IgM in cord blood are synthesized by the baby (figure 4.17). IgM reaches adult levels by nine months of age. Only trace levels of IgA, IgD and IgE are present in the circulation of the newborn.

Lymphoid malignancies

Lymphoid cells at almost any stage in their differentiation or maturation may become malignant and proliferate to form a clone of cells which are virtually 'frozen' in the developmental stage of the parent cell and bear the markers of the normal cell type from which they are derived. Thus, chronic lymphocytic leukaemia cells which originate from mature B-lymphocytes all stain for surface Ig and Ia and

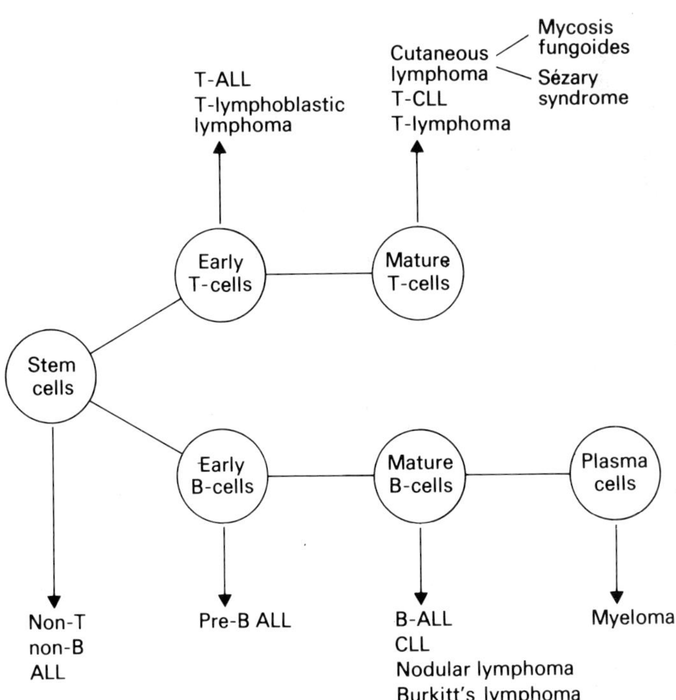

FIGURE 4.18. Cellular origin of human lymphoid malignancies. ALL, acute lymphoblastic leukaemia; CLL, chronic lymphocytic leukaemia. (After Greaves M.F. & Janossy G.)

bear identical idiotypes in a given patient. Using the Tdt enzyme and antisera directed against Ia, Ig and specific antigens on cortical thymocytes, mature T-cells and non-T, non-B acute lymphoblastic leukaemia cells, it has been possible to classify the lymphoid malignancies in terms of the phenotype of the equivalent normal cell (figure 4.18). This is proving to be of great value in the diagnosis, prognosis and treatment of many of these conditions. For example, whereas T-ALL and B-ALL cases have a poor prognosis, the non-T, non-B ALL patients who include most childhood leukaemias, belong to a prognostically favourable group many of whom are curable with current therapies.

Phylogeny of the immune response

It has long been known that natural defence mechanisms such as phagocytosis occur in invertebrates. More recently it has become clear that bactericidins may be induced in the haemolymph of species like the lobster by infection with different gram negative and positive bacteria. The bactericidins can reach a maximum in one to two days with peak titres of 1 : 100 or more. They show broad reactivity in that they can kill bacteria antigenically unrelated to the inducing organism; characterization of these molecules to see if they are related in any way to vertebrate immunoglobulins is awaited with interest. With respect to cell-mediated immune reactions, there are now reports that the earthworm can develop transplantation immunity to tissues of the same or other species while permanently accepting autografts (i.e. grafts of its own tissue). An understanding of the nature of these cellular and humoral responses will surely provide some insight into whether the cellular reaction is really the most primitive in evolutionary terms.

All vertebrates are capable of generating an immunological response on antigenic stimulation. Both B- and T-cell responses can be elicited even in the lowliest vertebrate studied, the California hagfish. This unpleasant cyclostome (which preys upon moribund fish by entering their mouths and eating the flesh from the inside) was originally considered 'the negative hero of the phylogeny of immunity' since unlike the lamprey, a more advanced cyclostome, it appeared incapable of reacting immunologically. It now transpires that hagfish can make antibodies to haemocyanin and reject allografts, provided they are maintained at temperatures approaching 20° (in general poikilotherms make antibodies better at higher temperatures). The antibodies were present in a 28*S* macroglobulin fraction, but further up the evolutionary scale in the cartilaginous fishes, well-defined 18*S* and 7*S* immunoglobulins with heavy and light chains have now been defined.

It is worthy of note that the thymus is lymphoid in the bony and cartilaginous fishes but in the lamprey there is no clear indication of a lymphoid thymus although a primitive epithelial organ has been recognized. So far there has been no definite evidence of thymus tissue in the hagfish although a small round cell with a thin rim of basophilic cytoplasm found in peripheral blood may be a candidate for an 'early lymphocyte'.

One could imagine the way in which immunoglobulins might have evolved from enzymes. Take for example an enzyme which has as its substrate a sugar common to the surface of many types of bacterium. The enzyme will bind to the substrate molecule on the bacterial surface using the same forces which are involved in antigen-antibody interactions. If mutation in the enzyme molecule were to produce a configuration capable of binding to a structure on the surface of a phagocyte (or if mutation changed the phagocyte so that it could bind the enzyme), we would have a bacterium-binding protein cytophilic for phagocytes which would thereby act as an opsonin to increase the rate of bacterial phagocytosis (cf. p. 181). Further mutations would lead to variations in the substrate (antigen)-recognizing portion and in the phagocyte-binding region giving molecules with different recognition specificities and a variety of biological functions.

Summary

Antibody-forming cells can be recognized by immunofluorescence or plaque techniques. Ig peptide chains are synthesized as a single unit starting at the N-terminal end. In myeloma, the monoclonal protein shows as a sharp 'M' band on paper electrophoresis or a 'bump' on the precipitin arc in immunoelectrophoresis; in some cases heavy chains with a central deletion are excreted in the urine. Myeloma light chain dimers appear as Bence-Jones protein in the urine and the variable regions can polymerize to form amyloid deposits. Immortal cell lines making monoclonal antibodies provide powerful new immunological reagents. IgM antibody responses reach an early peak and decline; IgG levels are quantitatively much higher and more persistent. Some Ig classes are particularly thymus dependent. Freund's adjuvant which stimulates T-cell activity only improves the response to thymus-dependent antigens.

Approximately 10 genes control the overall antibody response to complex antigens: some affect macrophage antigen handling and some the rate of proliferation of differentiating B-cells. Genes coding for antibodies of given specificities may be inherited together with (i.e. linked to) genetic markers for the heavy chain. Immune response genes linked to the major histocompatibility locus define products (with Ia specificities) on the T- and B-cells and macrophages which control the interactions required for T-B collaboration.

Regulation of the antibody response is strongly influenced by antigen concentration; since the response is antigen-driven, as effective antigen levels fall through catabolism and antibody feedback, the synthesis of antibody wanes. T-cells regulate B-lymphocyte responses not only through co-operative help but also by T-cell suppressor activity. Clonal proliferation is blocked by the development of an immune response to the antibody idiotype; an interlocking network based on recognition of idiotypes within the lymphocyte system provides a regulatory mechanism (Jerne).

Immunological tolerance can be induced by exposure to antigens in neonatal and (less readily) in adult life. T-cells are more readily tolerized than B-cells leaving T-dependent B-cells 'helpless'. Elimination of specific cells or generation of T-suppressors may occur.

Multipotent haemopoietic stem cells from the bone marrow differentiate within the thymus to become immunocompetent T-cells. In mammals the bone marrow itself provides the microenvironment for differentiation of B-cells. In man, maternal IgG is the only class to cross the placenta.

Lymphoid cells may become malignant and proliferate clonally, maintaining the developmental stage and specific markers of the parent cell.

Primitive lymphoid tissue and both B- and T-cell adaptive immune responses are associated phylogenetically with the appearance of the lowliest vertebrates.

Further reading

Beer A.E. & Billingham R.E. (1976) *The Immunobiology of Mammalian Reproduction.* Prentice-Hall.

Bevan M.J., Parkhouse R.M.R., Williamson A.R. & Askonas B.A. (1972) Biosynthesis of immunoglobulins. *Progress in Biophysics* & *Mol.Biol.*, **25**, 131.

Cantor H. & Gershon R.K. (1979) Immunological circuits: cellular composition. *Fed. Proc.*, **38**, 2058.

Cooper M. *et al.* (ed) (1979) *B Lymphocytes in the immune response.* Developments in Immunology, vol. 3. Elsevier/N. Holland, New York.

Dresser D.W. (ed) (1976) Immunological tolerance. *Brit.med.Bull.*, **32**, No. 2.

Fougereau M. & Dausset J. (eds) (1980) *Progress in Immunology IV.* Academic Press, London.

Greaves M.J. & Janossy G. (1978) Patterns of gene expression and the cellular origins of human leukaemias. *Biochim. biophys. Acta*, **516**, 193–230.

Hildemann W.H. & Reddy A.L. (1973) Phylogeny of immune responsiveness: marine invertebrates. *Fed.Proc.*, **32**, 2188.

Jerne N.K. (1973) The immune system (Network theory). *Scientific American*, p. 52.

Marchalonis J.J. (ed) (1976) *Comparative immunology.* Blackwell Scientific Publications, Oxford.

Melchers F. *et al.* (1978) *Lymphocyte hybridomas.* (Milstein's technique of fusion to establish monoclonal cell lines). *Current Topics in Microbiol. & Immunol.* **81**. Springer-Verlag, Berlin.

Milstein C. *et al.* (1979) Monoclonal antibodies and cell surface antigens. In *Human genetics, possibilities and realities.* p. 251 Ciba Foundation series 66 (Excerpta Medica).

Moller E. (ed) (1978) *Acquisition of the T cell repertoire. Immunol.Rev.* **42**.

Moller E. (ed) (1978) *Role of macrophages in the immune response. Immunol.Rev.* **40**.

Porter, Ruth & Knight, Julie (1972) *Ontogeny of Acquired Immunity.* Ciba Foundation Symposium. Elsevier, Amsterdam.

Quesenberry P. & Levitt L. (1979) Haemopoietic stem cells. *N. Engl. J. Med*, **301**, 755, 819 & 868.

Taniguchi M., Takei I & Tada T. (1980). Functional and molecular organization of an antigen-specific suppressor factor from a T-cell hybridoma. *Nature*, **283**, 227.

Uhr J.W. *et al.* (1979) Organization of the immune response genes. *Science*, **206**, 292.

Watson J., Trenkner E. & Cohn M. (1973) The use of bacterial lipopolysaccharides to show that two signals are required for the induction of antibody synthesis. *J.exp.Med.*, **138**, 699. (Note that these authors do not consider cross-linking of receptors to be a necessary condition for induction.)

Zucker–Franklin D., Greaves M.F., Grossi C.E. & Marmont A.M. (1980) *Atlas of blood cells. Function and pathology.* E.E., Milan.

5 The Immune Response III—Theoretical Aspects

Instructive theory

The ability of animals to synthesize antibodies directed against determinants such as dinitrobenzene and sulphanilic acid, which were so unlikely to occur in nature, made it difficult to accept the idea based on Ehrlich's earlier views that the body has preformed antibodies whose production is further stimulated by the entry of antigen. Instead attention turned to theories in which the antigen acted instructively as a template around which a standard unfolded γ-globulin chain could be moulded to provide the appropriate complementary shape. The molecule would be stabilized in this configuration by disulphide linkages, hydrogen bonds and so forth; on separation from the template the molecule would now have a specific combining site for antigen (figure 5.1).

Selective theory

An alternative view holds that the information required for the synthesis of the different antibodies is already present in the genetic apparatus. The gene which codes for a specific antibody is selected and 'switched on' by contact of antigen with the cell, and through transcription and translation of the appropriate messenger RNA, immunoglobulin peptide chains with corresponding individual primary amino acid sequences are synthesized; based on the sequence, these chains then fold spontaneously to a preferred globular configuration which possesses the specific antigen-combining sites (figure 5.1).

An analogy may help in the comparison of these two theories. If we consider the purchase of a suit, two courses of action are open. We may *instruct* the tailor to make the suit to measure, in which case we act as a template for the suit to be made on. Alternatively the tailor may be an enterprising fellow who has already made up 10^4

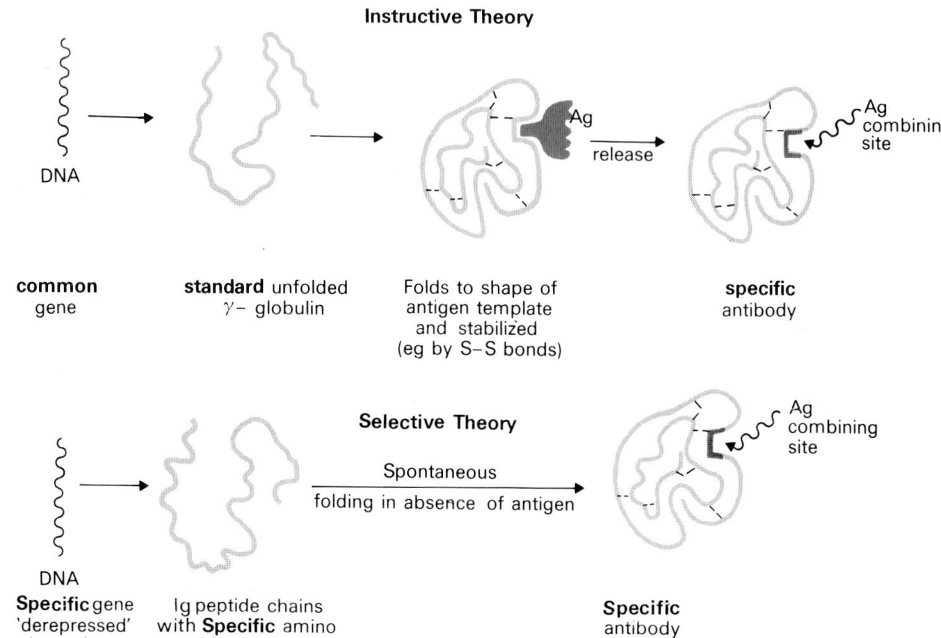

FIGURE 5.1. Comparison of instructive and selective theories for generating specific antigen-combining site.

different suits, one of which is almost certain to fit any intending purchaser; all we have to do is *select* the best fit for ourselves. Although in both cases the know-how of making suits (cf. protein synthesis) is there, in the first instance we provide essential information for the final shape (as the antigen does), whereas in the second situation the tailor himself had the foresight to make a whole variety of differently shaped suits (information already in the DNA) before seeing the customer (antigen).

Evidence for a selective theory

ABSENCE OF ANTIGEN FROM PLASMA CELLS

Using autoradiography to visualize highly radioactive antigens combined with immunofluorescence to identify cells making specific antibody, Nossall has shown that nearly all cells which contain intracellular antibody do not have demonstrable antigen molecules. This is clearly at variance with the idea of antigen acting as a template.

UNFOLDING EXPERIMENTS

Reduction of disulphide bonds in IgG or its Fab fragment followed by treatment with high concentrations of guanidine effectively destroys any organized secondary structure. However, removal of the guanidine from the unfolded molecules by dialysis and reoxidation restores significant specific antigen-binding activity. This is inconsistent with the instructive view (which requires the presence of antigen for the formation of a specific antibody) and indicates that the information held in the primary amino acid sequences is sufficient to allow the correct tertiary structure to be formed by spontaneous refolding. An analogous result has been obtained with ribonuclease; after unfolding, the molecule can spontaneously recover its enzymic activity.

AMINO ACID SEQUENCE OF ANTIBODIES

Purified antibodies show differences in amino acid sequence. As mentioned previously, myeloma proteins which represent individual immunoglobulin molecules show considerable variability in the sequences of the N-terminal part of both light and heavy chains. Indeed of the many human myeloma light chains so far sequenced, none have proved to have identical structures. These differences in amino acid sequence reflect differences in DNA nucleotide sequences strongly implicating genetic control of specificity.

GENETIC STUDIES

Immune responsiveness to certain defined antigens has indeed been associated with genetic constitution, not only with respect to MHC-linked genes controlling the synthesis of antigen specific Ia molecules concerned in T-cell regulation of the antibody response but in particular with the Ig-allotype linked genes encoding certain antibody clones and idiotypes which provides strong evidence for the view that the capacity to form particular antibodies is inherited through the possession of Ig *V*-region genes (p. 95).

Clonal selection model

The evidence clearly favours a genetic theory and we should now examine how this can be expressed in cellular terms. Clonal selection, based largely on the ideas elaborated by

Burnet, is generally regarded as an acceptable working model for antibody synthesis.

It is envisaged that each lymphocyte is genetically programmed to make one particular antibody and molecules of that antibody are built into the cell-surface membrane as receptors. Different lymphocytes make different antibodies so that all the body lymphocytes between them present antibodies with a wide spectrum of specificities. Antigen will combine with those lymphocytes carrying antibody on their surface which is a good fit, and these cells will be stimulated by the reaction on the plasma membrane to differentiate and divide to form a clone of cells synthesizing antibody with the same specificity as that on the surface of the parent lymphocyte (figure 5.2). Some of the progeny revert to small lymphocytes and become memory cells.

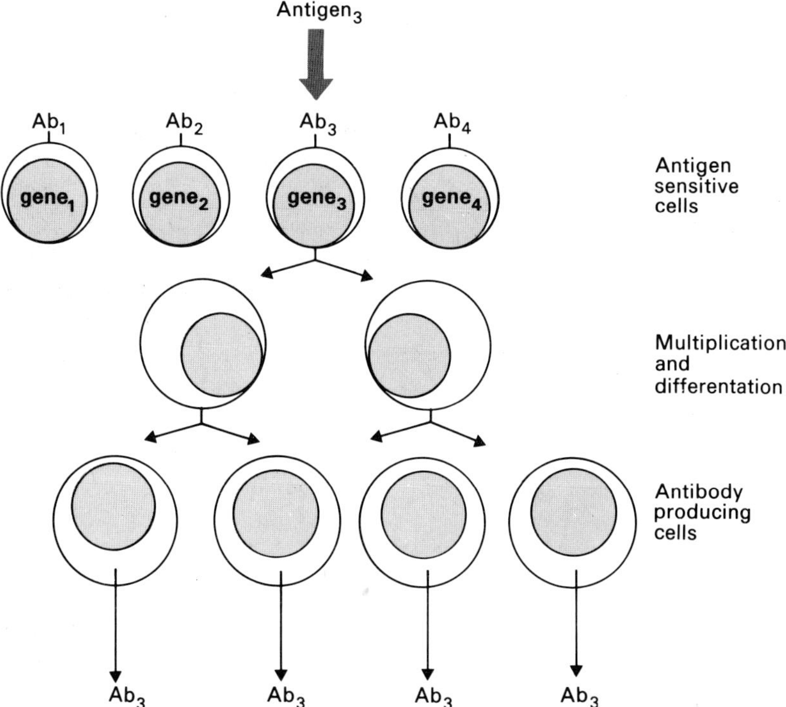

FIGURE 5.2. Clonal selection model. Each lymphocyte expresses the genes coding for one specific antibody, several molecules of which are built into the surface membrane to act as receptors. In the diagram, $antigen_3$ combines with the cell capable of making the complementary $antibody_3$ and this reaction at the cell surface leads to the formation of a clone of daughter cells making and exporting that specific antibody.

Evidence for clonal selection model

ONE CELL/ONE IMMUNOGLOBULIN

With immunofluorescent techniques, immunoglobulin-producing cells can be stained for either κ- or λ-chains but not both, and in the heterozygous rabbit, for the maternal allotypic marker or the paternal but never both together (*allelic exclusion*). Furthermore plasma cell tumours only produce one, and not more than one, myeloma protein. Similar restrictions apply to the staining of surface Ig on B-lymphocytes described in the previous chapter (p. 67).

That these surface immunoglobulins can behave as antibodies is suggested by the ability of a small percentage of lymphocytes to bind specific antigens such as sheep cells (forming 'rosettes') or radioactive salmonella flagellin. This binding can be blocked by anti-immunoglobulin sera. Humphrey has further shown that the percentage of cells binding antigen is increased in primed and decreased in tolerant animals.

When a soluble antigen like polymerized flagellin binds to a specific cell it causes patching and capping of the surface Ig in just the same way as an anti-Ig serum (cf. p. 67). If the antigen-capped cells are now stained with fluorescent anti-Ig, all the Ig is found in the cap, there being none on the remainder of the lymphocyte surface, i.e. when antigen reacts with a cell, all the Ig molecules on the cell surface combine with the antigen showing that they have similar specificity. In summary, the surface Ig of each B-lymphocyte represents the product of only one of the two chromosomes which code for each Ig chain and behaves as antibody of a single specificity.

RELATION OF SURFACE ANTIBODY TO FUTURE PERFORMANCE

When cells are taken from an animal which has given a primary response to both ovalbumin and bovine serum albumin (BSA) and are passed down a column of glass beads coated with BSA, they retain the ability to give a secondary antibody response to ovalbumin but are unresponsive to BSA. Thus the BSA-responsive cells have anti-BSA receptors on their surface which cause them to stick to the BSA-coated beads (figure 5.3).

Other investigations have shown that cells primed for

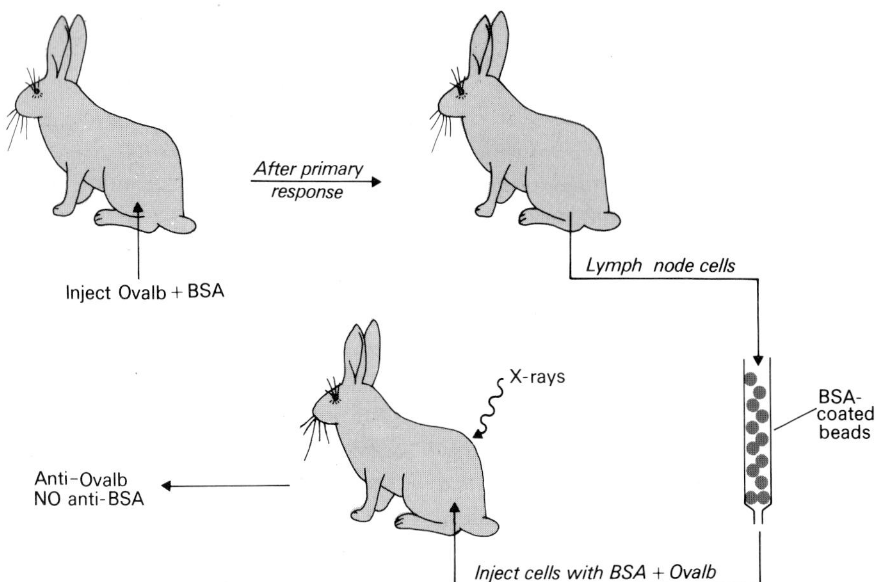

FIGURE 5.3. Absorption of antibody-forming cell precursors on antigen coated column. Lymph node cells primed to ovalbumin (ovalb) and bovine serum albumin (BSA) are run down a column of BSA-coated glass beads and injected into an irradiated recipient. On secondary challenge anti-ovalb but no anti-BSA is produced showing that the cells destined to make anti-BSA were bound to the column presumably through their specific anti-BSA receptors on the surface. (Based upon the work of Wigzell H. & Anderson B., *J.exp.Med.* 1969, **129**, 23.)

a humoral secondary response can be inhibited if treated with anti-immunoglobulin serum before the second contact with antigen. Furthermore, specific antibodies can be induced in mice by injection of a guinea pig IgG_1 anti-idiotype, the presumption being that this simulates antigen by activating cells bearing the idiotype marker through combination with the binding site of the antibody. One may conclude that the surface antibody plays a key role in the recognition of antigen for the triggering of the lymphocyte response.

Validity of the clonal selection model

Antibody affinity and antigen dosage

The combination of antigen and antibody is reversible and the complex may readily dissociate, depending upon the strength of binding. This can be defined broadly through the equilibrium constant of the reaction:

$$\mathrm{Ag} + \mathrm{Ab} \rightleftharpoons \mathrm{AgAb}$$

and the reactants will behave according to the laws of mass action (cf. chapter 1, p. 13). If the antigen and antibody fit together very closely, the equilibrium will lie well over to the right; we refer to such antibodies which bind strongly to the antigen as *high-affinity antibodies* (strictly *high avidity* in the case of multivalent antigens, cf. p. 15). Experimentally it is found that injection of *small* amounts of antigen leads to the production of *high*-affinity antibodies whereas *larger* amounts of antigen give more antibody of *lower* affinity. How can we account for this on the clonal selection model?

It may be supposed that when an appropriate number of antigen molecules are bound to the antibody receptors on the cell surface, the lymphocyte will be stimulated to develop into an antibody-producing clone. When only small amounts of antigen are present, only those lymphocytes with high-affinity antibody receptors will be able to bind sufficient antigen for stimulation to occur and their daughter cells will, of course, also produce high-affinity antibody. Consideration of the antigen–antibody equilibrium equation will show that as the concentration of antigen is increased, even antibodies with relatively low affinity will bind more antigen; therefore at high doses of antigen the lymphocytes with lower affinity antibody receptors will also be stimulated and, as may be seen from figure 5.4, these are more abundant than those with receptors of high affinity.

Feedback inhibition of antibody synthesis

It was mentioned earlier (p. 99) that the injection of preformed antibody could inhibit an immune response to antigen and that this suggests a possible negative feedback model for control of antibody synthesis *in vivo*. The higher the affinity of the injected IgG antibody used to inhibit the immune response, the more effective it is. On the basis of the clonal selection model it may be argued that there will be a competition between injected antibody and the lymphocyte receptors for antigen and only cells with receptors of higher affinity than the administered antibody will be triggered. The higher the affinity of the antibody, the smaller will be the percentage of the total cells available (cf. figure 5.4).

Increase of affinity during immunization

As immunization proceeds, only lymphocytes with higher and higher affinity receptors can be triggered because the

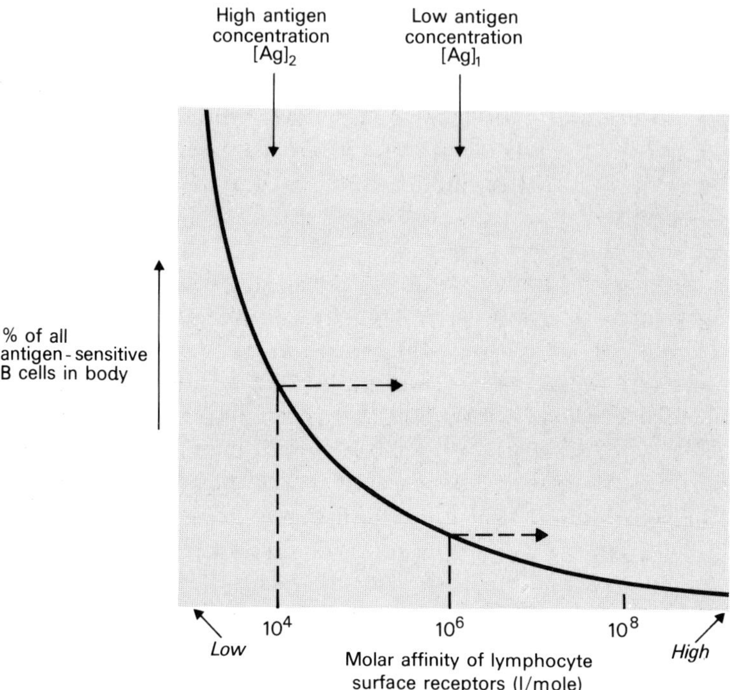

FIGURE 5.4. Antigen concentration in relation to affinity of surface antibody receptors on lymphocytes which are stimulated. A certain antigen concentration $[Ag]_1$ will lead to binding of sufficient antigen molecules to lymphocytes bearing receptors of affinity 10^6 litre/mole and higher to cause stimulation; assuming the cells will synthesize the same antibody as that present on their surface, the antibodies so produced will thus have affinity of 10^6 litre/mole and higher. At a much higher antigen concentration $[Ag]_2$, lower affinity receptors will now be capable of binding the requisite number of antigen molecules to be triggered. Thus the antibodies produced will now be of affinity 10^4 litre/mole and higher, but as the cell distribution curve shows that the number of cells capable of synthesizing the low-affinity antibodies is much greater, the resulting antiserum will consist predominantly of these low-affinity immunoglobulins.

concentration of available antigen steadily falls and feedback inhibition by synthesized antibody will 'turn off' cells with equal or lower affinity receptors.

Hapten inhibition of antibody synthesis

Mitchison has found that if lymphoid cells are taken from a mouse primed with a hapten-carrier complex, treated *in vitro* with excess of free hapten and then transferred to an irradiated recipient, they fail to give a secondary response to the hapten-carrier injected simultaneously. This inhibition by free hapten is ascribed to its binding to lymphocyte surface receptors so making them unavailable for reaction with the antigen hapten-carrier complex. When a cross-reacting hapten is used for the inhibition step, the final antiserum produced gives reasonably good binding with the homologous hapten but very poor cross-reaction, i.e. the hapten used for inhibition had selectively suppressed the reactivity of those cells with which it was best able to combine.

Effect of net charge of the antigen

Rabbit IgG antibodies can be separated by ion exchange chromatography into two major fractions, in one of which the proteins have a greater net positive charge than in the other. Antigens with a net negative charge favour the synthesis of the more positively charged antibodies and *vice versa* (Sela & Mozes). This would be fully consistent with the preferential binding of antigens to cells with surface receptors of opposite charge, other factors being equal.

Immunological tolerance

The clonal selection model readily provides a basis for the mechanism of tolerance induction. It has only to be postulated that under the conditions known to cause unresponsiveness, contact with antigen causes death or long-term inactivation of the antigen-sensitive cell rather than its

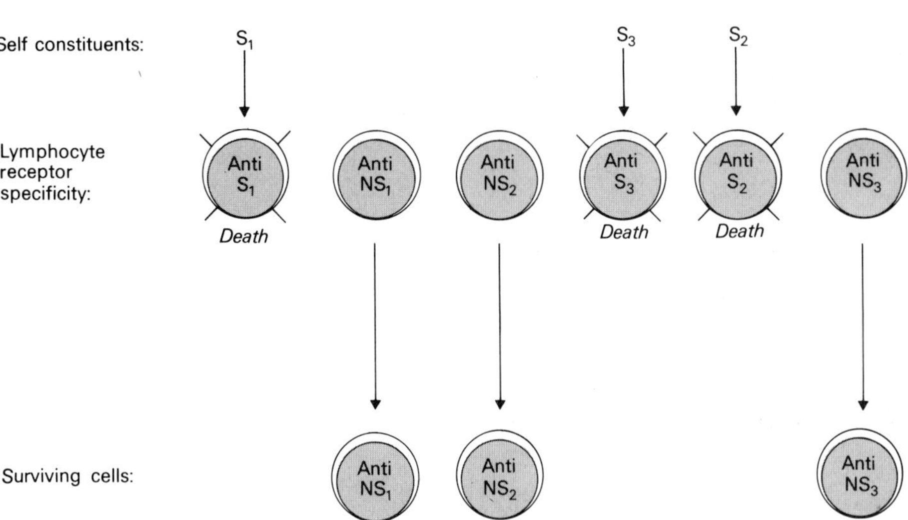

FIGURE 5.5. Induction of tolerance to self-constituents (S_1–S_3) by selective elimination of lymphocytes with self-reacting surface receptors. These cells are either killed or inactivated or inhibited by specific T suppressors. Surviving cells are able to react only with non-self (NS) foreign antigens of specificity NS_1, NS_2, NS_3 etc.

stimulation. Although we are uncertain of the mechanism, the idea that deletion or inactivation of specific clones is responsible for tolerance induction is attractive. For example, it can account for the development of self-tolerance since all lymphocytes having receptors capable of reäcting with circulating or accessible self-components would be eliminated or suppressed leaving only those cells with receptors for non-self determinants in the immunological armamentarium (figure 5.5).

Genetic theories of antibody variability

The variation in primary amino acid sequence of different antibodies, the differences between animal strains in their immunological responsiveness to selected synthetic and viral antigens and the plausibility of the clonal selection model all speak for a genetic basis underlying antibody variability. Similarities in amino acid sequence (homology) between the loops formed by intrachain disulphide bonds in the constant parts of heavy and light chains (figure 2.13) and to some extent between variable and constant parts, suggest that the existing genes controlling immunoglobulin structure are derived from a primitive smaller gene—perhaps coding for a peptide half the length of a light chain—by a process of duplication and translocation with early divergence of *V* genes.

Rough estimates place the total repertoire of different antibody molecules which can be synthesized by a given individual, at around 10^8 or perhaps even more. To help us understand the genetic basis for this quite remarkable diversity, we should first review the current status of our knowledge concerning the form and number of inherited (i.e. germ line) genes encoding antibody molecules.

GENES CODING FOR ANTIBODY

These fall into three clusters on three different chromosomes coding for κ, λ and heavy chains respectively. There appears to be only one variable region (V) gene for mouse λ chain and the genetic basis for the synthesis of this peptide is illustrated in figure 5.6. In common with other eukaryotic proteins, the chain is encoded in multiple distinct gene segments separated by intervening nucleotide sequences, *introns*, which are removed either by DNA translocation or

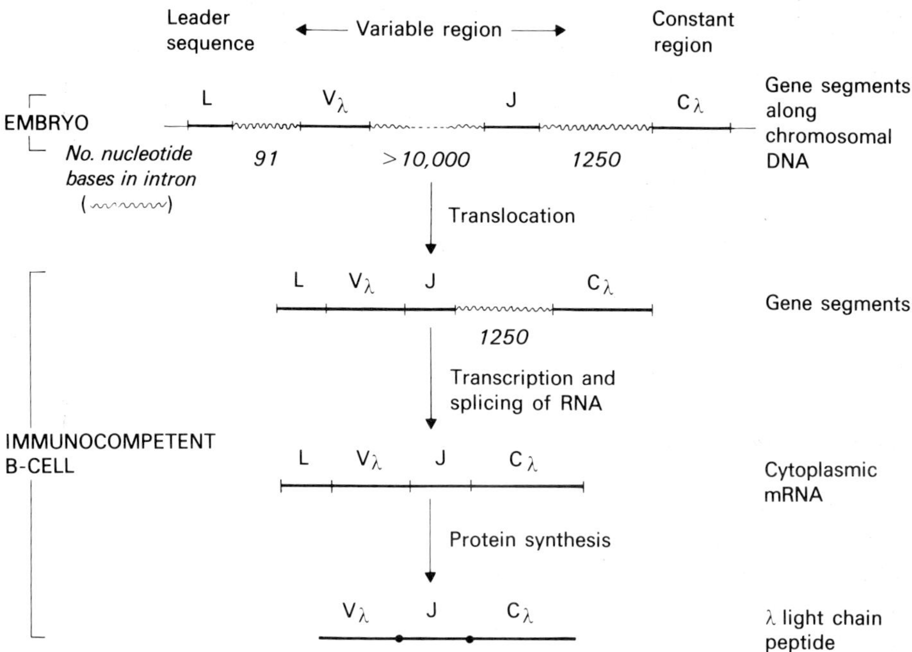

FIGURE 5.6. Genetic basis for synthesis of mouse λ chain. The variable region gene segment formed by the combination of V_λ with the joining segment J, is separate from the gene encoding the constant region as originally predicted by Dreyer and Bennett. In the human, the V_λ genes are more complex (cf. V_κ genes below).

by excision of the corresponding mRNA sequence. There is a leader sequence required for passage of the peptide through the endoplasmic reticulum, a V_λ segment coding for amino acid residues 1 to 98, a joining segment (J—not to be confused with the J peptide in IgM and IgA) encoding the remaining 11 amino acids of the variable region, and a C_λ gene segment giving rise to the constant region. As a lymphocyte undergoes differentiation to become an immunocompetent cell capable of synthesizing λ chains, there is a rearrangement or translocation of the DNA bringing the L, V_λ and J segments together but still separated from the C_λ by an intron of 1250 nucleotides. Splicing of the transcribed RNA in the nucleus produces an mRNA which can now be used for the synthesis of a continuous λ chain peptide.

The same general principles apply to the arrangement of κ and heavy chain genes although they exist in far greater variety (figure 5.7). The V_κ genes occur as a series of 50–100 clusters or sets each containing 6–8 closely related individual genes. Although the genes within a given set show some

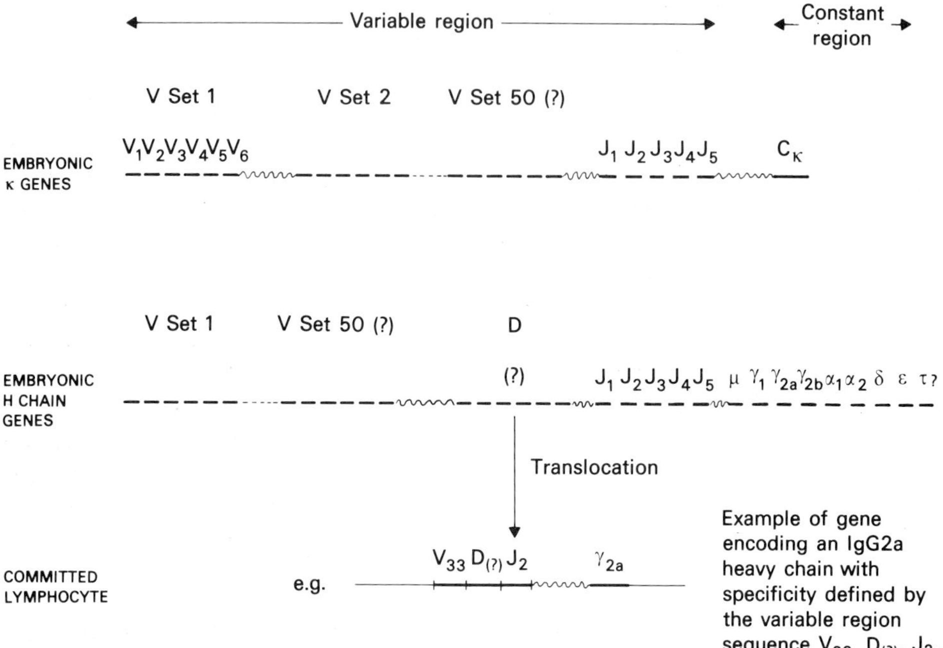

FIGURE 5.7. Genes coding for κ and heavy chain peptides in the mouse. The genetic basis for the highly variable D segment in the heavy chain which lies between the V and J segments is uncertain. The evidence suggests that a T-cell receptor heavy chain gene (τ) is likely to be included in the constant region group as shown.

framework and hypervariable diversity, they resemble each other far more than they do V genes in other sets. There are 5 different J segments but just a single constant region gene. The heavy chain constellation shows additional features: the subclass constant region genes form a single cluster and there is evidence for a highly variable sequence (D segment) inserted between the V and J regions. The D and J segments together encode almost the entire third hypervariable region which forms one side of the combining site groove (figure 2.10).

Since each cell has chromosome complements derived from each parent, the differentiating B-cell has 4 light and 2 heavy chain gene clusters to choose from. Once the V–J DNA rearrangement has occurred within one light and one heavy chain cluster, the V genes on the other 4 chromosomes are held by some mechanism in the embryonic state so that the cell is able to express *only one light and one heavy chain.* As we have discussed above, this is essential for clonal selection to work since the cell is then only programmed to make the one antibody it uses as a cell surface receptor to recognize antigen. Furthermore, this gene exclusion mechanism prevents the formation of molecules containing 2 different light or 2 different heavy chains which would have non-identical combining sites and therefore, be functionally monovalent with respect to the majority of antigens; such antibodies would be non-agglutinating and would tend to have low avidity because the bonus effect of multivalency could not operate.

The arrangement of heavy chain genes would clearly permit a given V–J variable region to associate sequentially with different constant region genes and account for class switch during the antibody response and for the presence of antibodies of different class (e.g. IgM and IgD) bearing the same idiotype on the surface of a given lymphocyte. Whether this occurs at the DNA or mRNA level is still unresolved.

THE GENERATION OF DIVERSITY

The problem of generating 10^8 or more different antibody molecules is now seen as a problem of generating 10^8 or more different combining sites since the V genes in any cluster can all link with the same constant region segment and it is therefore only necessary to have single C region genes. There are essentially two possibilities. Either: (a) we inherit *all* variable region genes—*the germ line theory*, or (b) we inherit just a few V genes from which diversity is generated by *somatic mutation* (figure 5.8).

Germ line concepts were initially criticized on the basis that 10^8 or so different V genes could not possibly be accommodated within the available genetic material. However, the finding through analysis of monoclonal proteins and DNA sequencing that light and heavy chain gene clusters each may have 5×10^2 or more V segments and around 5 separate J segments, leads to an explanation of diversity based upon random combinations of these genetic elements which may occur in the following ways:

(i) *Intra-chain amplification* of V and J segments by random DNA combination would lead to approximately 2.5×10^3 V–J regions (5×10^2V $\times$ 5J), and because the J chain may have an influence on the combining site, this would represent 2.5×10^3 different combining specificities. Variation in the N-terminal codon of the J segment caused by variation in the way a given V and J region are combined (at least in the κ chain) would increase this figure to around 10^4.

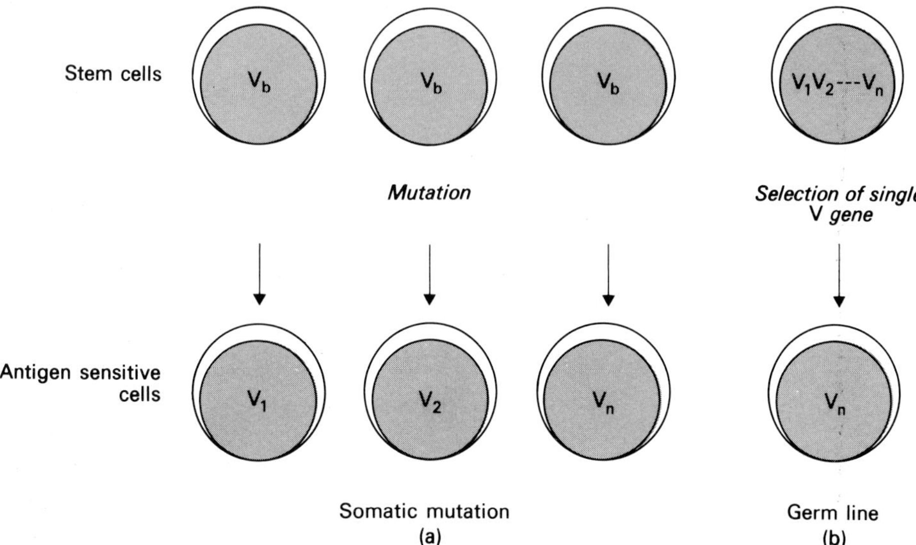

FIGURE 5.8. Somatic mutation and germ-line theories of antibody diversity: (a) a basic gene V_b undergoes somatic mutation during evolution from a stem cell to give different genes, one in each lymphocyte, coding for different antibodies with specificities from 1 to n; (b) each lymphocyte has the full range of genes coding for specificities 1 to n but only expresses one of these genes as it differentiates to immunocompetence.

(ii) *Inter-chain amplification* occurs by random association of heavy and light chains so that 10^4 heavy and 10^4 light chain V–J regions would code for 10^8 ($10^4 \times 10^4$) antibody specificities.

In other words, random interactions between 10^3 or so basic gene segments could allow the expression of around 10^8 different antibodies and it seems likely that diversity can be accounted for largely on the basis of germ line genes. Nonetheless, there is evidence that somatic mutation may play some role. Analysis of 18 murine λ myelomas revealed 12 with identical structure, 4 showing just one amino acid change, 1 with 2 changes and 1 with 4 changes, all within the hypervariable regions and indicative of somatic mutation of the single mouse λ germ line gene. Cunningham's work suggests that new specificities may appear in a small fraction of the progeny of a committed clone. The highly variable D segment between the heavy chain V and J regions which is a further important generator of diversity, might be encoded by multiple germ line 'minigenes' or arise through some new somatic mutation mechanism. To summarize, a body of germ line V and J genes may provide virtually the full diversity of antibody response needed but somatic mutation could increase this variation further.

Summary

Antigen does not act as a template for antibody production; the complete information for antibody synthesis is already in the genome. Folding of the antibody molecule and hence specificity, depends upon the primary amino acid structure and differences in amino acid sequence between different antibodies reflect differences in DNA nucleotide sequence. Immune responsiveness is genetically controlled.

The clonal selection model assumes that each immunocompetent lymphocyte is programmed to synthesize one immunoglobulin which is inserted into the plasma membrane as a surface receptor. An antigen which reacts strongly with this surface antibody will be bound selectively, trigger the cell and cause clonal amplification and differentiation to provide a large population of cells all making antibody of the required specificity plus an expanded population of memory cells. The model accounts for the inverse relation between antigen dose and antibody affinity, the greater effectiveness of high affinity antibody in feedback inhibition of the immune response and the increase in affinity with immunization; it envisages immunological tolerance in terms of deletion or inactivation of specific clones.

There are 3 distinct clusters of genes coding for κ, λ and heavy Ig peptide chains. In each cluster there are multiple V and J (joining) gene segments but only single genes encoding the constant region. Random joining of V and J segments occurs as the lymphocyte differentiates to a committed cell; since the V–J combined gene segment encodes the variable region, this mechanism provides for the generation of $V \times J$ specificities. Additional amplification occurs through random association of heavy and light chains; p heavy plus q light chain genes would produce $p \times q$ different antibodies. The 1000 or so different gene segments in the germ line could give rise to around 10^8 different antibodies by such mechanisms. Somatic mutation could increase this variation further. In the secreting cell, coupling between the V–J and the constant region is effected by splicing the nuclear mRNA; a switch to coupling with another C gene leads to production of antibody with the same specificity but different class or subclass.

Further reading

Cunningham A.J. (ed.) (1976) *The generation of antibody diversity. A new look.* Academic Press, London.

Edelman G. (ed.) (1974) Cellular Selection and Regulation in the Immune Response. *Soc.Gen.Physiol.Series*, **29**. Raven Press, New York.

Fudenberg H.H., Pink J.R.L., Stites D.P. & Wang A-C. (1977) *Basic Immunogenetics*, 2nd ed. Oxford University Press, New York.

Hofmann G.W. (1975) A theory of regulation and self-nonself discrimination in an immune network. *Eur.J.Immunol.*, **5**, 638.

Marx J.L. (1978) Antibodies: new information about gene structure. *Science*, **202**, 298 & 412.

Schilling J., Clevinger B., Davie J.M. & Hood L. (1980) Amino acid sequence of homogeneous antibodies to dextran and DNA rearrangements in heavy chain V-region gene segments. *Nature*, **283**, 35.

Siskind G.W. & Benacerraf B. (1969) Cell selection by antigen in the immune response. *Adv. Immunol.*, **10**, 1.

Williamson A.R. (1979) Control of antibody formation: certain uncertainties. *J.clin.Path.*, **32**, Suppl.(Roy. Coll. Path.) **13**, 76.

6 Interaction of antigen and antibody

The primary interaction between an antigenic determinant and the combining site of an antibody, governed by the affinity, gives rise to a number of secondary phenomena such as precipitation, agglutination, phagocytosis, cytolysis, neutralization and so on. In this chapter we consider the practical implications of this interaction and begin to explore its consequences.

Precipitation

Multivalent antigens mixed with bivalent antibodies in solution can combine to form complexes which aggregate and precipitate. As described in chapter 1 (p. 5) the amount of precipitate varies with the proportions of the reagents and, generally speaking, insoluble complexes are formed in *antibody excess* while the complexes generated in *antigen excess* tend to be soluble. A variety of techniques depend upon visualization of the precipitation reaction in gels.

PRECIPITATION IN GELS

In the double diffusion method of Ouchterlony, antigen and antibody placed in wells cut in agar gel, diffuse towards each other and precipitate to form an opaque line in the region where they meet in optimal proportions. A preparation containing several antigens will give rise to multiple lines. The immunological relationship between two antigens can be assessed by setting up the precipitation reactions in adjacent wells; the lines formed by each antigen may be completely confluent indicating immunological identity, they may show a 'spur' as in the case of partially related antigens, or they may cross, indicative of unrelated antigens (figure 6.1). The origins of these patterns are explained in figure 6.2. It should be emphasized that even in the case of confluent lines this can only indicate immunological identity in terms of the antiserum used, not necessarily molecular identity. For example, purified antibodies to

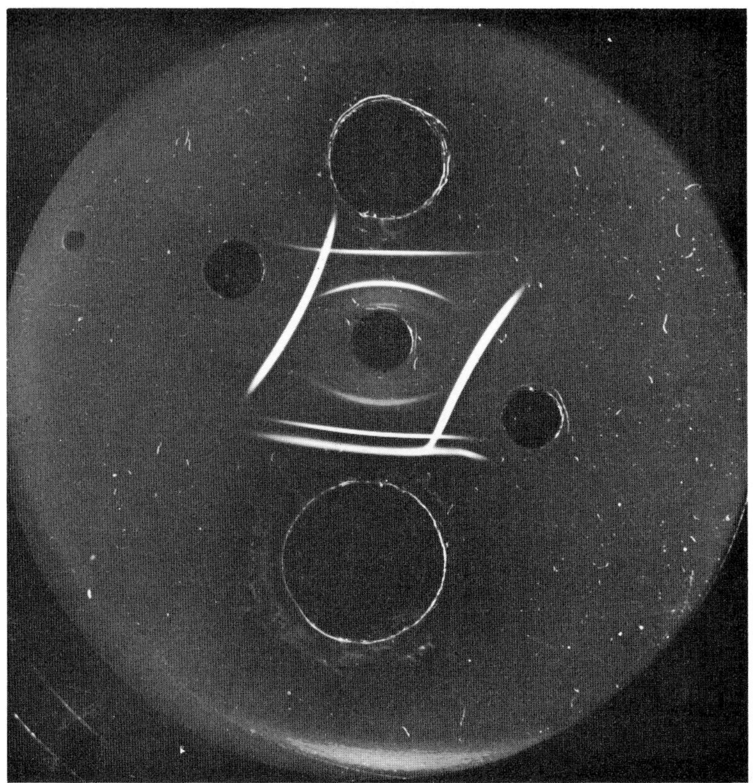

Antiserum in centre well

FIGURE 6.1. Multiple lines formed in the Ouchterlony test (double-diffusion precipitation) when rabbit antiserum (centre well) reacts in agar gel with 4 different antigen preparations (peripheral wells). Non-identity and partial identity of antigens are shown respectively by crossing over and spur formation between precipitin lines.

the dinitrobenzene hapten would give a line of confluence when set up against dinitrobenzene–ovalbumin and dinitrobenzene–serum albumin conjugates placed in adjacent wells.

Where reagents are present in balanced proportions, the line formed will generally be concave to the well containing the reactant of higher molecular weight, be it antigen or antibody. This is a consequence of the usually slower diffusion rate of larger sized molecules.

The gel precipitation method can be made more sensitive by incorporating the antiserum in the agar and allowing the antigen to diffuse into it; up to 90 per cent serum in agar may be employed (Feinberg). This method of single radial immuno-diffusion is used for the quantitative estimation of antigens.

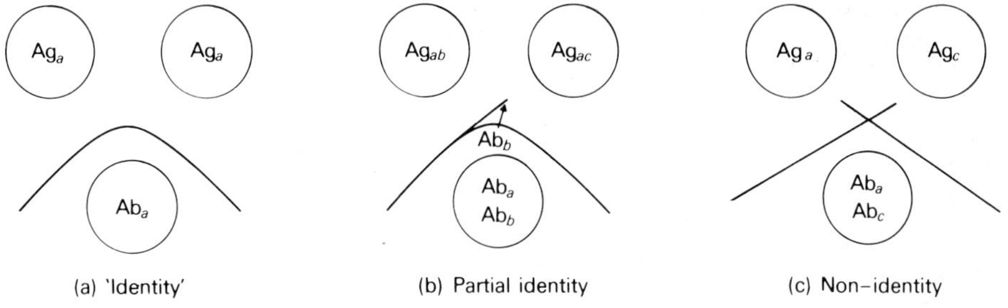

FIGURE 6.2. (a) Line of confluence obtained with two antigens which cannot be distinguished by the antiserum used.

(b) Spur formation by partially related antigens having a common determinant *a* but individual determinants *b* and *c* reacting with a mixture of antibodies directed against *a* and *b*. The antigen with determinants *a* and *c* can only precipitate antibodies directed to *a*. The remaining antibodies (Ab_b) cross the precipitin line to react with the antigen from the adjacent well which has determinant *b* giving rise to a 'spur' over the precipitin line.

(c) Crossing over of lines formed with unrelated antigens.

SINGLE RADIAL IMMUNODIFFUSION (SRID)

When antigen diffuses from a well into agar containing suitably diluted antiserum, initially it is present in a relatively high concentration and forms soluble complexes; as the antigen diffuses further the concentration continuously falls until the point is reached at which the reactants are nearer optimal proportions and a ring of precipitate is formed. The higher the concentration of antigen, the greater the diameter of this ring (figure 6.3). By incorporating, say, three standards of known antigen concentration in the plate, a calibration curve can be obtained and used to determine the amount of antigen in the unknown samples tested (figure 6.4). The method is used routinely in clinical immunology, particularly for immunoglobulin determinations, and also for substances such as the third component of complement, transferrin, C-reactive protein and the embryonic protein, α-foetoprotein, which is associated with certain liver tumours.

IMMUNOELECTROPHORESIS

The principle of this has been described earlier (p. 29). The method is of value for the identification of antigens by their electrophoretic mobility, particularly when other

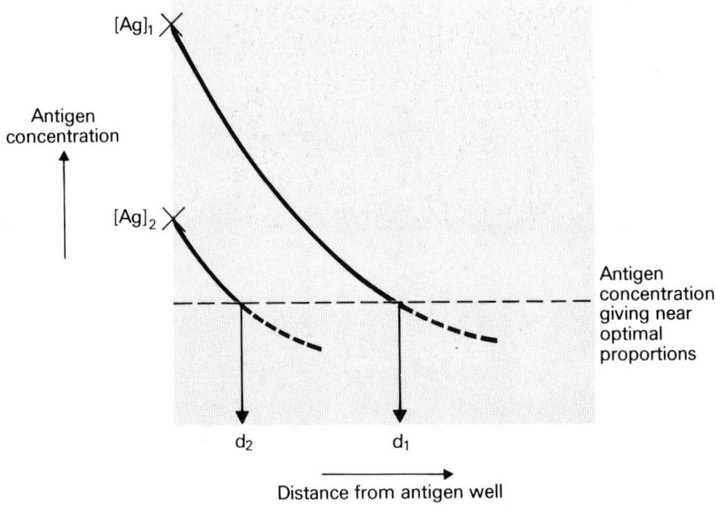

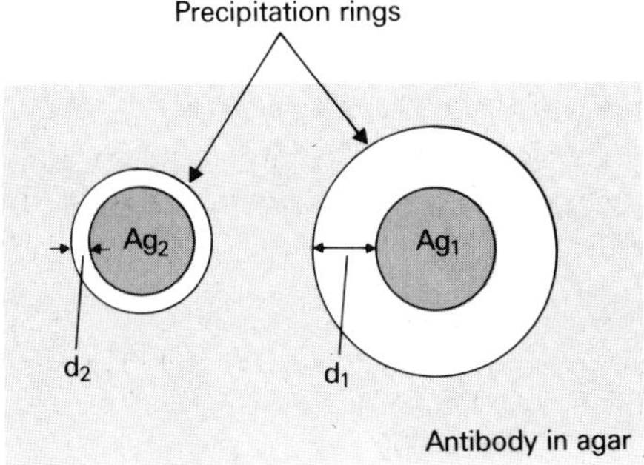

FIGURE 6.3. Single radial immunodiffusion: relation of antigen concentration to size of precipitation ring formed. Antigen at higher concentrations diffuses further from the well before it falls to the level giving precipitation with antibody near optimal proportions.

antigens are also present. In clinical immunology, semi-quantitative information regarding immunoglobulin concentrations and identification of myeloma proteins is provided by this technique.

There have been some felicitous developments of the principle combining electrophoresis with immunoprecipitation in which movement in an electric field drives the antigen directly into contact with antibody. *Countercurrent immunoelectrophoresis* may be applied to antigens which migrate towards the positive pole in agar (see figure 6.5).

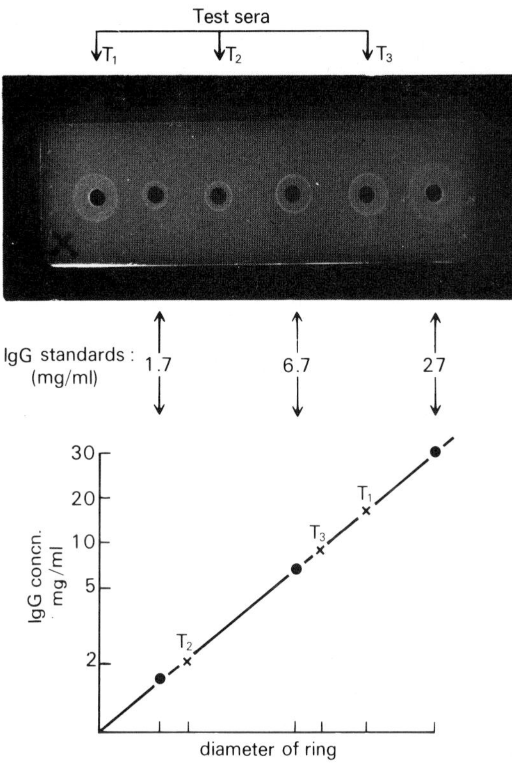

FIGURE 6.4. Measurement of IgG concentration in serum by single radial immuno-diffusion. The diameter of the standards (●) enables a calibration curve to be drawn and the concentration of IgG in the sera under test can be read off:

T_1—serum from patient with IgG myeloma; 15 mg/ml
T_2—serum from patient with hypogammaglobulinaemia; 2.6 mg/ml
T_3—normal serum; 9.6 mg/ml.

(Courtesy of Dr. F.C. Hay.)

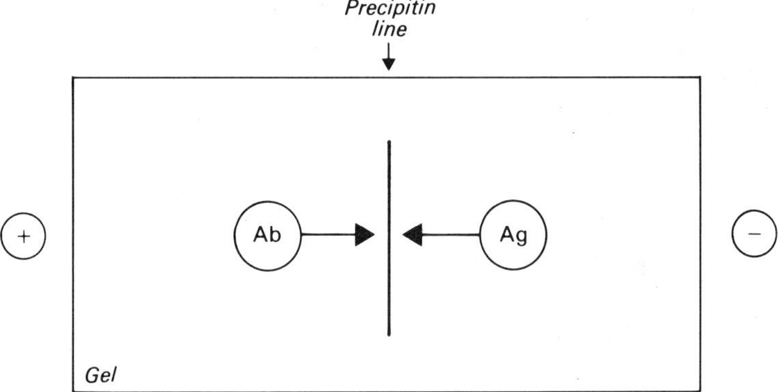

FIGURE 6.5. Countercurrent immunoelectrophoresis. Antibody moves 'backwards' in the gel on electrophoresis due to endosmosis; an antigen which is negatively charged at the pH employed will move towards the positive pole and precipitate on contact with antibody.

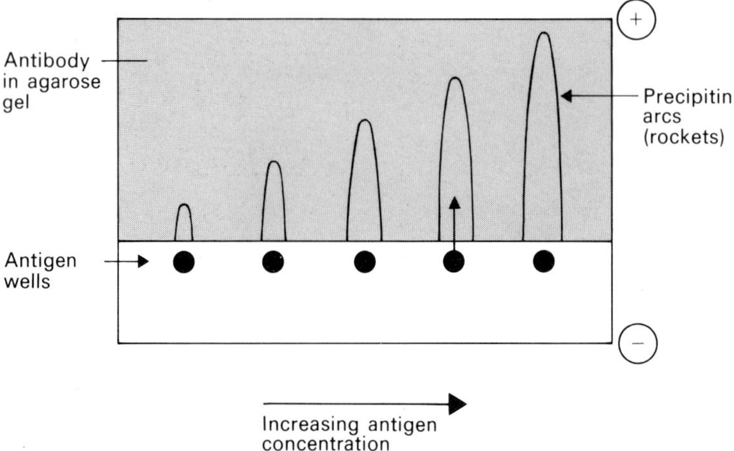

FIGURE 6.6. Rocket electrophoresis. Antigen is electrophoresed into gel containing antibody. The distance from the starting well to the front of the rocket shaped arc is related to antigen concentration.

This qualitative technique is much faster and considerably more sensitive than double diffusion (Ouchterlony) and is used for the detection of hepatitis B antigen or antibody, DNA antibodies in SLE (p. 296), autoantibodies to soluble nuclear antigens in mixed connective tissue disease, and *Aspergillus* precipitins in cases with allergic bronchopulmonary aspergillosis. *Rocket electrophoresis* is a quantitative method which involves electrophoresis of antigen into a gel containing antibody. The precipitation arc has the appearance of a rocket, the length of which is related to antigen concentration (figure 6.6). Like countercurrent electrophoresis this is a rapid method but again the antigen must move to the positive pole on electrophoresis; it is therefore suitable for proteins such as albumin, transferrin and caeruloplasmin but immunoglobulins are more conveniently quantitated by single radial immunodiffusion. One powerful variant of the rocket system, Laurell's *two-dimensional immunoelectrophoresis*, involves a preliminary electrophoretic separation of an antigen mixture in a direction perpendicular to that of the final 'rocket-stage' (figure 6.7a). In this way one can quantitate each of several antigens in a mixture. One straightforward example is the estimation of the degree of conversion of the third component of complement (C3) to the inactive form C3c (cf. pp. 162 and 240) which may occur in the serum of patients with

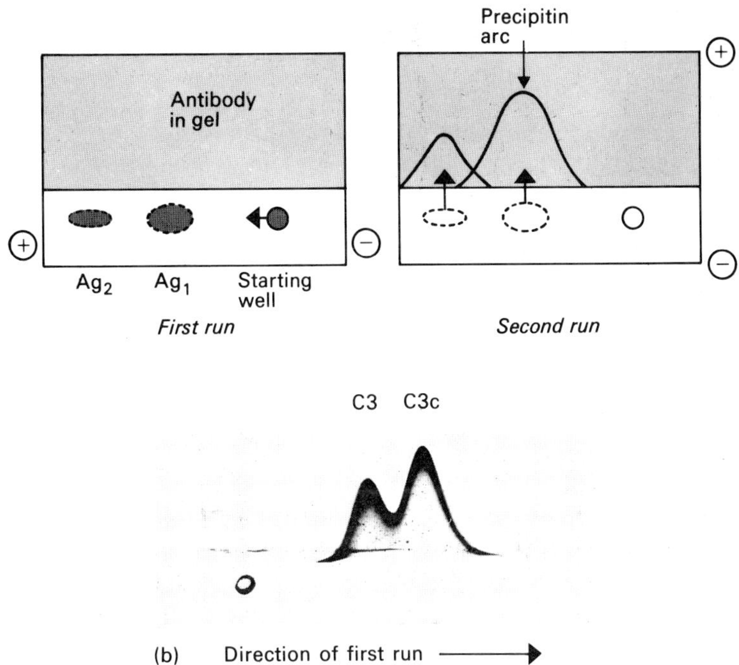

FIGURE 6.7. Two-dimensional immunoelectrophoresis. (a) Antigens are separated on the basis of electrophoretic mobility. The second run at right angles to the first drives the antigens into the antiserum-containing gel to form precipitin peaks; the area under the peak is related to the concentration of antigen. (b) Actual run showing C3 conversion (C3 → C3c) in serum. In this case the arcs interact because of common antigenic determinants. (Courtesy of Dr. C. Loveday.)

active SLE or the synovial fluid of affected joints in active rheumatoid arthritis, to give but two examples (figure 6.7b).

QUANTIFICATION BY NEPHELOMETRY

The small aggregates formed when dilute solutions of antigen and antibody are mixed creates a cloudiness or turbidity which can be measured by the scattering of an incident light source (nephelometry). Greater sensitivity can be obtained by using monochromatic light from a laser and by adding polyethylene glycol to the solution so that aggregate size is increased. In favoured laboratories which can sport the appropriate equipment, this method is replacing single radial immunodiffusion for the estimation of immunoglobulins, C3, C-reactive protein etc.

Radioactive binding techniques

MEASUREMENT OF ANTIBODY

These methods assess antibody level either by determining the capacity of an antiserum to complex with radioactive antigen or by measuring the amount of immunoglobulin binding to an insoluble antigen preparation. Perhaps the point should be made that it is not possible to define the *absolute* concentration of antibody in a given serum because each serum contains immunoglobulins with a range of binding affinities and the estimation of the amount of antigen bound to antibody depends upon the concentration and affinities of the antibodies as well as the nature and sensitivity of the test. With this proviso, the quantitative tests described do give a measure of the antibody content of a serum which is of practical value.

Using radioactive antigen

The two methods to be considered involve the addition of excess radio-labelled antigen to the antiserum followed by assessment of the amount of antigen which has been complexed with antibody (this being the antigen binding capacity). This is achieved either by:

(a) *the Farr technique* in which complexed antigen is separated from that in the free form by precipitation with 50 per cent ammonium sulphate (only applicable to those antigens soluble at this salt concentration), or

(b) *the antiglobulin coprecipitation technique* in which the antigen bound to antibody is precipitated together with the rest of the immunoglobulin by an antiglobulin serum, leaving free antigen in the supernatant (figure 6.8). By using antibodies to different immunoglobulin classes and subclasses as the antiglobulin reagent, it is possible to determine the distribution of antibody activity among the classes. For example, addition of a radioactive antigen to human serum followed by a precipitating rabbit antihuman IgA, would indicate how much antigen had been bound to the serum IgA. The data documented in figure 4.4 on p. 93 were obtained by similar methods.

Using insoluble antigen

The antibody content of a serum can be assessed by the ability to bind to antigen which has been insolubilized

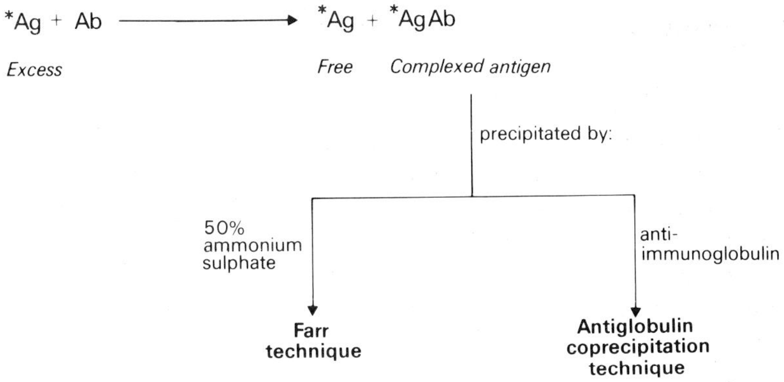

FIGURE 6.8. Determination of antigen-binding capacity. After addition of excess radioactive antigen (*Ag), that part bound to antibody as a complex is precipitated either by ammonium sulphate (Farr) or by an antiglobulin (antiglobulin coprecipitation).

either by coupling to an immunoadsorbent or by physical adsorption to a plastic tube; the bound immunoglobulin may then be estimated by addition of a radiolabelled anti-Ig raised in another species (figure 6.9). Consider, for example, the determination of DNA autoantibodies in systemic lupus erythematosus (cf. p. 296). When a patient's serum is added to a plastic tube coated with antigen (in this case DNA), the autoantibodies will bind to the tube and remaining serum proteins can be readily washed away. Bound antibody can now be estimated by addition of ^{125}I-labelled purified rabbit anti-human IgG; after rinsing out excess unbound reagent, the radioactivity of the tube will clearly be a

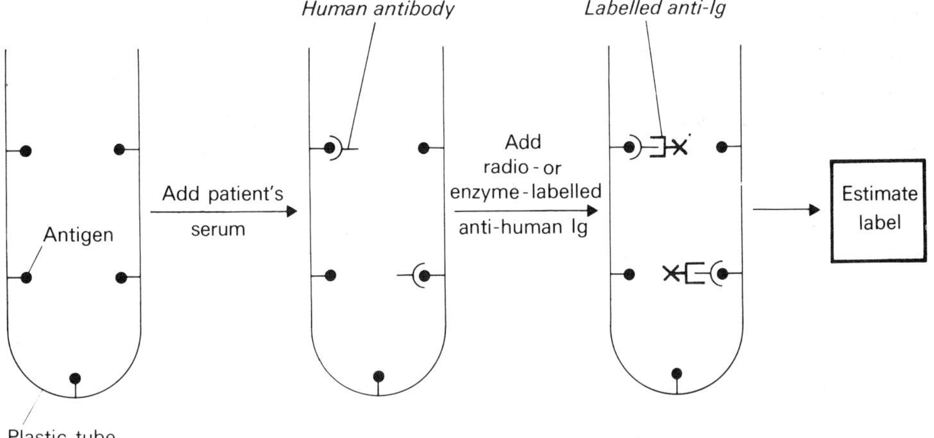

FIGURE 6.9 The 'tube test' for quantitative determination of antibody.

measure of the autoantibody content of the patient's serum. The distribution of antibody in different classes can obviously be determined by using specific antisera. Take the radio-allergosorbent test (RAST) for IgE antibodies in allergic patients. The allergen (e.g. pollen extract) is covalently coupled to a paper disc which is then treated with patient's serum. The amount of specific IgE bound to the paper is then estimated by addition of labelled anti-IgE.

MEASUREMENT OF ANTIGEN

Radioimmunoassay

The binding of radioactively labelled antigen to a limited fixed amount of antibody can be partially inhibited by addition of unlabelled antigen and the extent of this inhibition can be used as a measure of the unlabelled material added. The principle of this form of saturation analysis is explained in figure 6.10. Methods vary in the means used to separate free antigen from that bound to antibody: some use coprecipitation of the complex with anti-immunoglobulin sera, others adsorption of free antigen onto charcoal and so on.

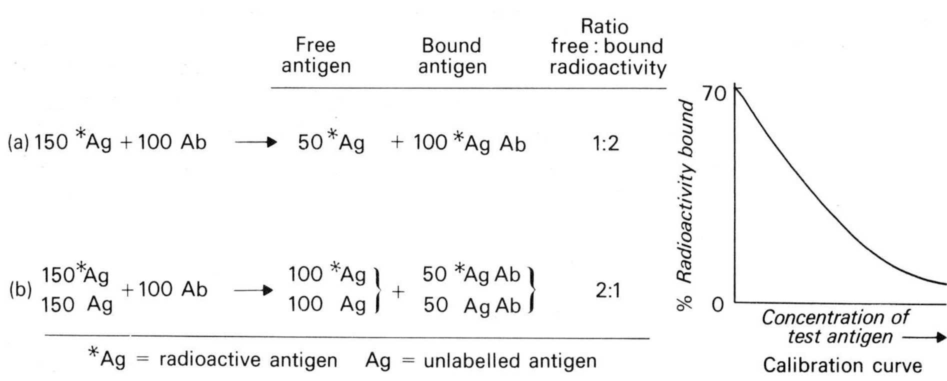

FIGURE 6.10. Principle of radioimmunoassay (simplified by assuming a very highly avid antibody and one combining site per antibody molecule).

(a) If we add 150 mol of radiolabelled Ag to 100 mol of Ab, 50 mol of Ag will be free and 100 bound to Ab. The ratio of the counts of free to bound will be 1:2.

(b) If we now add 150 mol of unlabelled Ag plus 150 mol radio Ag to the Ab, again only 100 mol of total Ag will be bound, but since the Ab cannot distinguish labelled from unlabelled Ag, half will be radioactive. The remaining antigen will be free and the ratio free: bound radioactivity changes to 2:1. This ratio will vary with the amount of unlabelled Ag added and this enables a calibration curve to be constructed.

With the development of methods for labelling antigens to a high specific activity, very low concentrations down to the 10^{-12} g/ml level can be detected and most of the protein hormones can now be assayed with this technique. One disadvantage is that these methods cannot distinguish active protein molecules from biologically inactive fragments which still retain antigenic determinants. Other applications include the assay of carcinoembryonic antigen, hepatitis B (Australia) antigen and smaller molecules such as steroids, prostaglandins and morphine-related drugs (appropriate antibodies are raised by coupling to an immunogenic carrier).

Immunoradiometric assay

This differs from radioimmunoassay in the sense that the labelled reagent is used in excess. For the estimation of antigen, antibodies are coated onto a solid surface such as plastic and the test antigen solution added; after washing, the amount of antigen bound to the plastic can be estimated by adding an excess of radiolabelled antibody. The specificity of the method can be improved by using solid phase and labelled antibodies with specificities for different parts of the antigen:

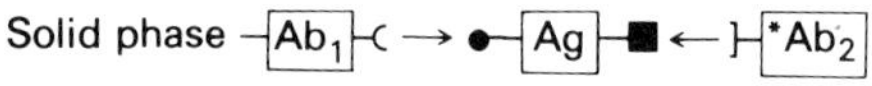

Solid phase —[Ab_1]—(→ ●—[Ag]—■ ← —)—[$^*Ab_2$]

One widely used application is the radioimmunosorbent test (RIST) for IgE. Rabbit anti-IgE is coupled by cyanogen bromide to microcrystalline cellulose and reacted with dilutions of an IgE-containing standard serum or the patient's serum under test. Bound IgE is then measured by addition of labelled anti-IgE.

NON-RADIOACTIVE LABELS

Because of health hazards, the expense of counting equipment and the deterioration of labelled reagents through radiation damage, other types of label have been sought. Enzymes such as peroxidase and phosphatase which give a coloured reaction product have been successfully employed particularly in the ELISA (enzyme-linked immunosorbent assay), an immunometric assay for antibody (figure 6.9) or antigen. Chemiluminescent and new fluorescent tags are under active scrutiny but almost the ultimate in sensitivity (around 10^3 molecules of antigen) is claimed for a method combining enzyme label with radioactive substrate.

Immunohistochemistry

IMMUNOFLUORESCENCE

Fluorescent dyes such as fluorescein and rhodamine can be coupled to antibodies without destroying their specificity. Coons showed that such conjugates would combine with antigen present in a tissue section and that the bound antibody could be visualized in the fluorescence microscope. In this way the distribution of antigen throughout a tissue and within cells can be demonstrated. Looked at another way, the method can also be used for the detection of antibodies directed against antigens already known to be present in a given tissue section or cell preparation. There are three general ways in which the test is carried out.

1. *Direct test*

The antibody to the tissue substrate is itself conjugated with the fluorochrome and applied directly (figure 6.11a). For example, suppose we wished to show the tissue distribution of a gastric autoantigen reacting with the autoantibodies

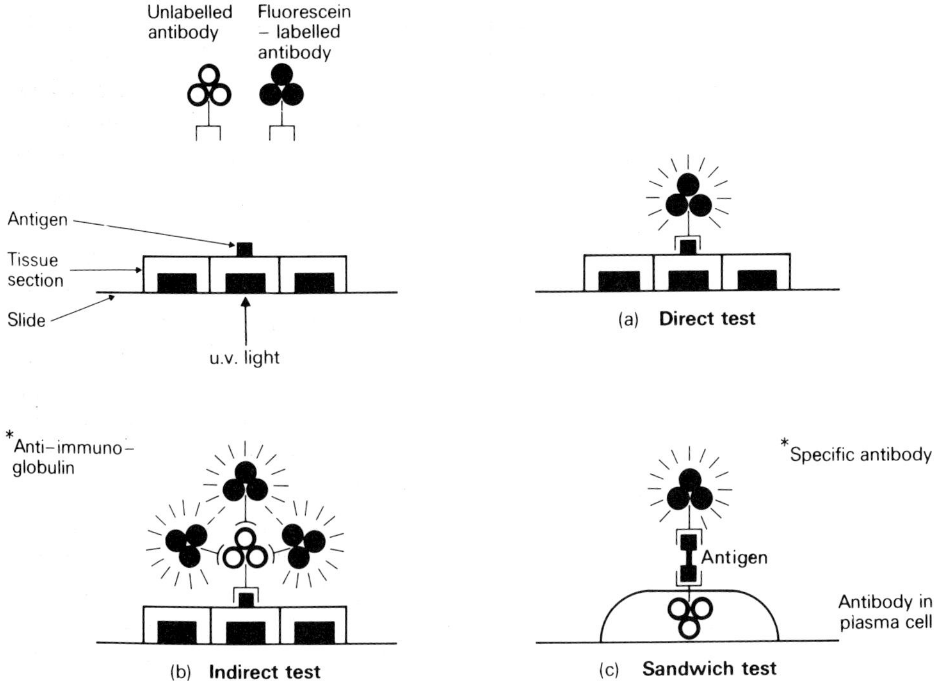

FIGURE 6.11. Fluorescent antibody tests. * = fluorescein labelled.

present in the serum of a patient with pernicious anaemia. We would isolate IgG from the patient's serum, conjugate it with fluorescein, and apply it to a section of human gastric mucosa on a slide. When viewed in the fluorescence microscope we would see that the cytoplasm of the parietal cells was brightly stained. By using antisera conjugated to dyes which emit fluorescence at different wavelengths, two different antigens can be identified simultaneously in the same preparation. In figure 3.6h (p. 60), direct staining of fixed plasma cells with a mixture of rhodamine-labelled anti-IgG and fluorescein-conjugated anti-IgM craftily demonstrates that these two classes of antibody are produced by different cells.

2. *Indirect test*

In this double layer technique, the unlabelled antibody is applied directly to the tissue substrate and visualized by treatment with a fluorochrome-conjugated anti-immunoglobulin serum (figure 6.11b). In this case, in order to find out whether the serum of a patient has antibodies to gastric parietal cells, we would first treat a gastric section with the serum, wash well and then apply a fluorescein-labelled rabbit anti-human immunoglobulin; if antibodies were present, there would be staining of the parietal cells (figure 6.12a).

This technique has several advantages. In the first place the fluorescence is brighter than with the direct test since several fluorescent anti-immunoglobulins bind onto each of the antibody molecules present in the first layer (figure 6.11b). Secondly, since the conjugation process is lengthy, much time can be saved when many sera have to be screened for antibody because it is only necessary to prepare a single labelled reagent, viz. the anti-immunoglobulin. Furthermore, the method has great flexibility. For example, by using conjugates of antisera to individual immunoglobulin heavy chains, the distribution of antibodies among the various classes and subclasses can be assessed at least semi-quantitatively. One can also test for complement fixation on the tissue section by adding a mixture of the first antibody plus a source of complement, followed by a fluorescent anti-complement reagent as the second layer. Even greater sensitivity can be attained by using a third layer. Thus, in the example quoted of antibodies to parietal cells, we could treat the stomach section sequentially with the following: patient's serum containing antibodies to parietal cells,

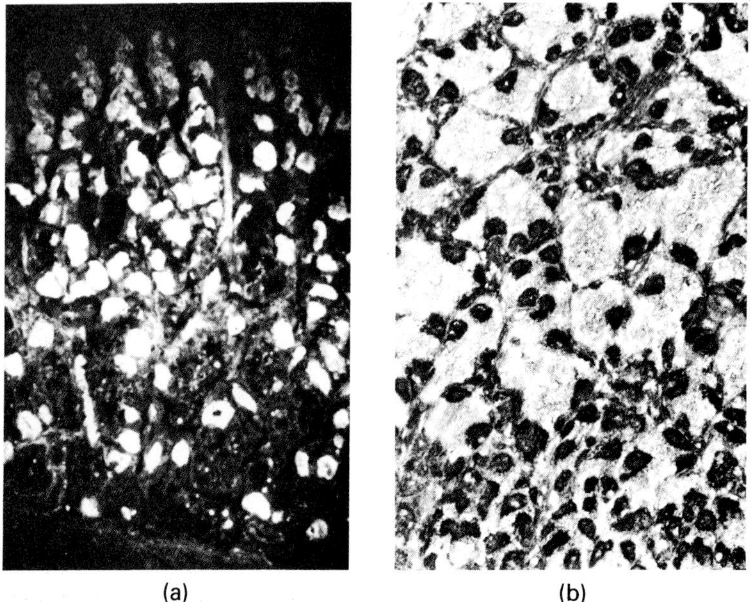

FIGURE 6.12. Staining of gastric parietal cells by (a) fluorescein and (b) peroxidase linked antibody. The sections were sequentially treated with human parietal cell autoantibodies and then with the conjugated rabbit anti-human IgG. The enzyme was visualized by the peroxidase reaction. (Courtesy of Miss V. Petts.)

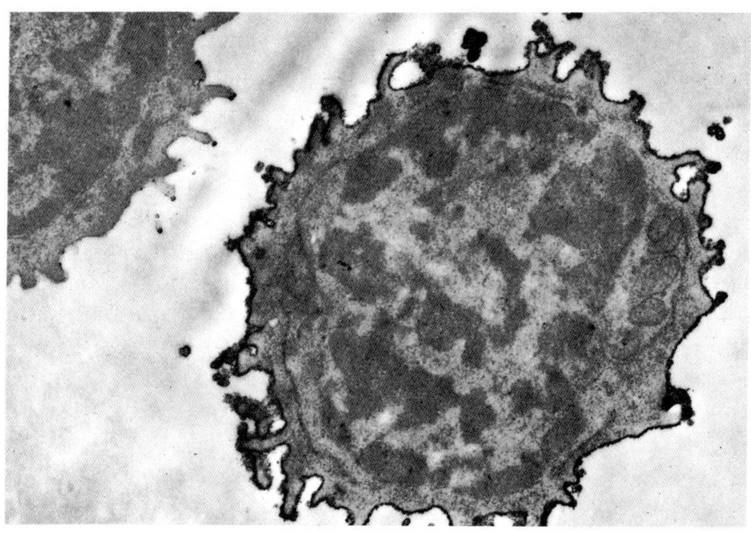

FIGURE 6.13. Electron microscopic visualization of human IgG on the surface of a B-lymphocyte by treatment of viable cell suspensions with peroxidase coupled anti-IgG. Note the adjacent unstained lymphocyte. (Courtesy of Miss V. Petts.)

then a rabbit anti-human IgG, and finally a fluorescein-conjugated goat anti-rabbit IgG. However, as with most immunological techniques as *sensitivity* is increased, *specificity* becomes progressively reduced and careful controls are essential.

Applications of the indirect test may be seen in figure 6.12a and in chapter 10 (e.g. figure 10.2, pp. 298–9).

3. *Sandwich test*

This is a double layer procedure designed to visualize specific antibody. If, for example, we wished to see how many cells in a preparation of lymphoid tissue were synthesizing antibody to pneumococcus polysaccharide, we would first fix the cells with ethanol to prevent the antibody being washed away during the test, and then treat with a solution of the polysaccharide antigen. After washing, a fluorescein labelled antibody to the polysaccharide would then be added to locate those cells which had specifically bound the antigen (figure 6.11c). The name of the test derives from the fact that antigen is sandwiched between the antibody present in the cell substrate and that added as the second layer.

OTHER LABELLED ANTIBODY METHODS

In place of fluorescent markers, other workers have evolved methods in which enzymes such as peroxidase or phosphatase are coupled to antibodies and these can be visualized by conventional histochemical methods at both light microscope (figure 6.12b) and electron microscope (figure 6.13) level. Intracytoplasmic antigens pose certain problems since the cells must be damaged to allow penetration by the labelled antibody and in order to avoid morphological degeneration of cellular structures it is necessary to fix the tissue; however the greater the degree of fixation, the more difficult it is for the antibody to diffuse through the cytoplasm. Technological improvements in this area would not be amiss.

Reactions with cell surface antigens

BINDING OF ANTIBODY

Surface antigens can be detected and localized by the use of labelled antibodies. Because antibodies cannot readily

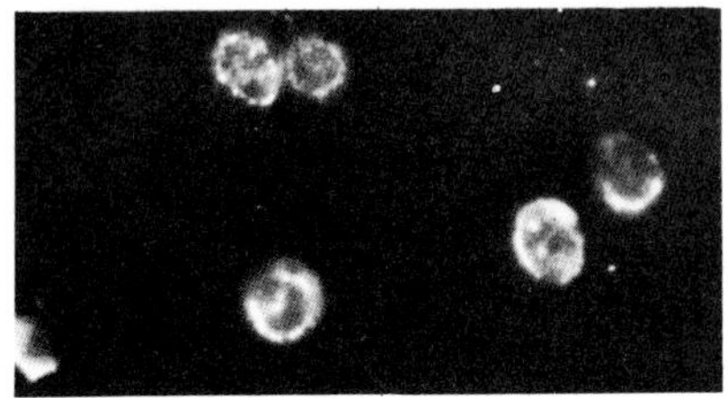

FIGURE 6.14. Antigens on the surface of viable human thyroid cells as demonstrated with thyroid autoantibodies in the indirect test. Note the patchy distribution. (Courtesy of Mrs. H. Lindqvist; after Fagreus A. & Jonsson J.)

penetrate living cells except by endocytosis, treatment of cells with labelled antibody in the cold (to minimize endocytosis) should lead to staining only of antigens on the surface. Such studies have been carried out using antibodies labelled with peroxidase (figure 6.13) and with fluorescein (figures 3.9 and 6.14). The amount of fluorescent antibody bound to the cell can be quantified by flow cytofluorography as described earlier (p. 67) and an example of the data which can be generated by these machines is given in figure 6.15.

After combination with antibody, many antigens are removed from the cell surface either through capping and endocytosis, or shedding into the extracellular medium as complexes. This 'stripping' process may have deleterious consequences for the host if it makes virally infected cells or tumours refractory to immunological attack.

Immunochemical analysis of surface antigens is possible if they are radiolabelled either by lactoperoxidase iodination of viable cells, by sequential oxidation of the surface glycoproteins and reduction with tritiated sodium borohydride or by metabolic incorporation of radioactive precursors. The membrane antigens can then be solubilized in a detergent which does not influence antigen-antibody interactions, and precipitated through combination with a specific antibody. The molecular weight of the antigen and its constituent peptides can be determined by running the precipitate in SDS-polyacrylamide gel electrophoresis and looking for the distribution of radioactivity (figure 6.16).

AGGLUTINATION

Whereas the cross-linking of multivalent protein antigens by antibody leads to precipitation, cross-linking of cells or large particles by antibody directed against surface

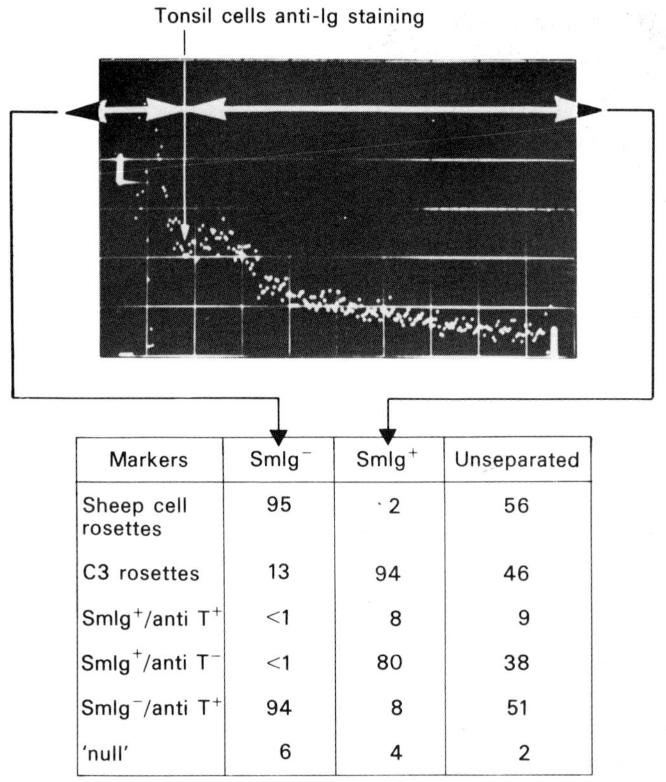

Markers	SmIg$^-$	SmIg$^+$	Unseparated
Sheep cell rosettes	95	2	56
C3 rosettes	13	94	46
SmIg$^+$/anti T$^+$	<1	8	9
SmIg$^+$/anti T$^-$	<1	80	38
SmIg$^-$/anti T$^+$	94	8	51
'null'	6	4	2

FIGURE 6.15. Separation of B- and T-cells from human tonsil lymphocytes by the fluorescence activated cell sorter (cf. p. 67). After staining with fluorescein-conjugated anti-Ig, the viable cells were analysed by flow cytofluorimetry to give the histogram shown (vertical axis = number of cells; horizontal axis, increasing relative fluorescence intensity). The lymphocytes were separated into a surface membrane Ig positive (SmIg$^+$) and a negative (SmIg$^-$) population depending upon the fluorescence intensity being either above or below the arbitrary cut-off point. Analysis of the % of cells positive for each marker (cf. p. 59) is shown. The anti-T serum was a fluorescent rabbit anti-monkey thymus made specific by absorption with B lymphoblastoid cell lines. 'Null' cells were negative with both anti-Ig and anti-T reagents. (Data kindly provided by Dr. M.F. Greaves.)

antigens leads to agglutination. Since most cells are electrically charged, a reasonable number of antibody links between two cells is required before the mutual repulsion is overcome. Thus agglutination of cells bearing only a small number of determinants may be difficult to achieve unless special methods such as further treatment with an antiglobulin reagent are used. Similarly, the higher avidity of multivalent IgM antibody relative to IgG (cf. p. 42)

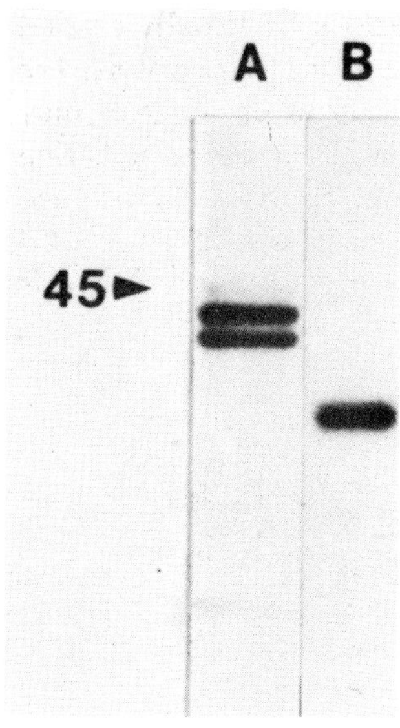

FIGURE 6.16. Analysis of membrane-bound classical transplantation antigens (cf. p. 257). The membranes from human cells pulsed with ^{35}S-methionine were solubilized and immunoprecipitated with a monoclonal antibody to HLA-A and B molecules. An autoradiograph (A) of the precipitate run in SDS-polyacrylamide gel electrophoresis shows the HLA-A and B chains as a 43,000 molecular weight doublet (the position of a 45,000 marker is arrowed). If membrane vesicles were first digested with Proteinase K before solubilization, a labelled band of molecular weight 39,000 can be detected (B) consistent with a transmembrane orientation of the HLA chain: the 4,000 hydrophilic C-terminal fragment extends into the cytoplasm and the major portion, recognized by the monoclonal antibody and by tissue typing reagents, is present on the cell surface (cf. figure 9.8). (From data and autoradiographs kindly supplied by Dr. M.J. Owen.)

makes the former more effective as an agglutinating agent, molecule for molecule.

Agglutination reactions are used to identify bacteria and to type red cells; they have been observed with leucocytes and platelets and even with spermatozoa in certain cases of male infertility due to sperm agglutinins. Because of its sensitivity and convenience, the test has been extended to the identification of antibodies to soluble antigens which have been artificially coated onto various types of particle. Red cells have been popular and they can be coated with proteins after first modifying their surface with tannic acid or chromium chloride, or by direct use of bifunctional cross-linking agents such as bisdiazobenzidine. The large rapidly sedimenting red cells of the turkey are finding increasing favour for this purpose. The tests are usually carried out in the wells of plastic agglutination trays where the settling pattern of the cells on the bottom of the cup may be observed (figure 6.17); this provides a more sensitive indicator than macroscopic clumping. Inert particles such as bentonite and polystyrene latex have also been coated with antigens for agglutination reactions particularly those used to detect the rheumatoid factors (figure 6.18).

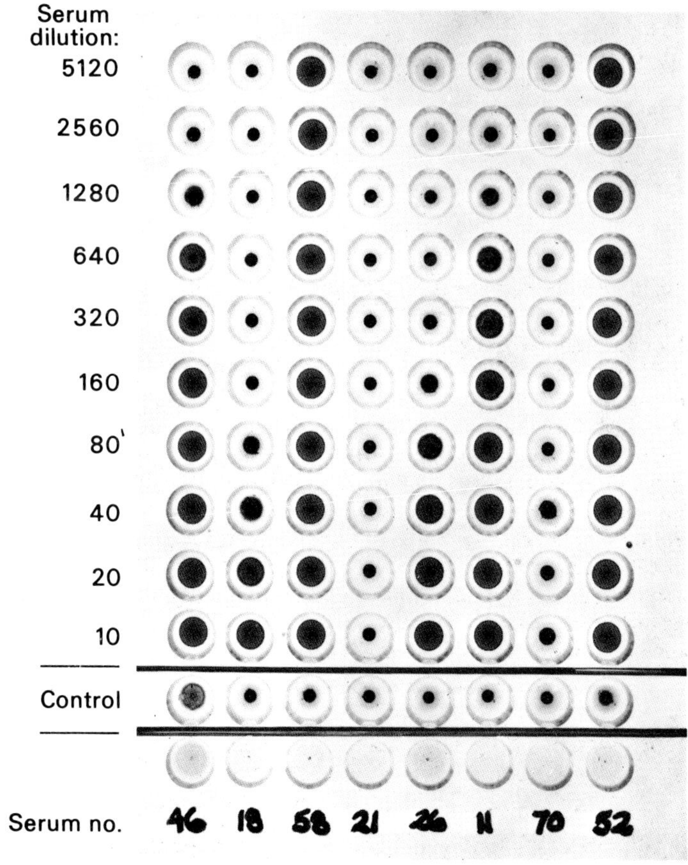

FIGURE 6.17. Tanned red cell haemagglutination test for thyroglobulin autoantibodies. Thyroglobulin-coated cells were added to dilutions of patients' sera. Uncoated cells were added to a 1:10 dilution of serum as a control. In a positive reaction, the cells settle as a carpet over the bottom of the cup. Because of the 'V'-shaped cross-section of these cups, in negative reactions the cells fall into the base of the 'V' forming a small easily recognizable button. The reciprocal of the highest serum dilution giving an unequivocally positive reaction is termed the *titre*. The titres reading from left to right are: 640, 20, >5,120, neg, 40, 320, neg, >5,120. The control for serum No. 46 was slightly positive and this serum should be tested again after absorption with uncoated cells.

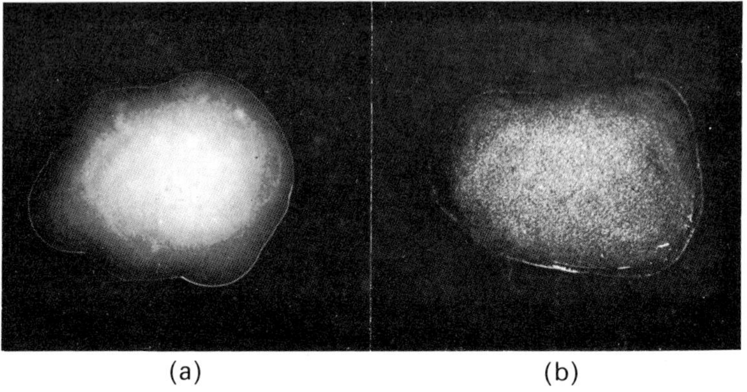

FIGURE 6.18. Macroscopic agglutination of latex coated with human IgG by serum from a patient with rheumatoid arthritis. This contains rheumatoid factor, an autoantibody directed against determinants on IgG. (a) normal serum, (b) patient's serum.

OPSONIC (FC) ADHERENCE

On combination with IgG antibodies, antigens develop an increased adherence to polymorphonuclear leucocytes and macrophages through the specific IgG Fc binding sites on the surface of these cells. To take one example, bacteria coated with antibody become '*opsonized*'—i.e. 'ready for the table' or 'tasty for the phagocytes'—and will adhere to phagocytic cells; this in turn facilitates the engulfment and subsequent digestion of the micro-organisms. Opsonic adherence and the related *immune adherence* reactions which involve binding through complement components (see below) are of major importance in the defence against infection. They may also be concerned in the removal of lymphocytes from the circulation by anti-lymphocyte serum and of red cells by the autoantibodies in autoimmune haemolytic anaemia. The *extracellular killing* of antibody-coated target cells (cf. p. 226) depends upon adherence to Fc receptors on the effector cell surface. IgE-mediated degranulation of mast cells by antigen which triggers acute inflammatory responses and sometimes anaphylaxis, provides an interesting contrast, since in this case the Ig molecules are already firmly bound to their Fc receptors before the reaction with antigen.

STIMULATION

A quite unexpected phenomenon has been observed in that antibodies to cell-surface components may sometimes lead not to cytotoxic reactions as discussed below, but to actual stimulation of the cell. This probably occurs if the antibodies are directed against receptors on the surface which can generate a stimulatory signal when triggered by combination with the antibody. Examples are:

(i) The transformation and mitosis induced in small lymphocytes by anti-lymphocyte serum and anti-immunoglobulin sera *in vitro*. The latter combine with the immunoglobulin antigen receptors on the cell surface and mimic the configurational changes produced by antigen which activate the cell.

(ii) Degranulation of human mast cells by anti-IgE serum. The anti-IgE brings about the same sequence of changes as would specific antigen combining with the surface bound IgE molecules.

(iii) Stimulation of thyroid cells by autoantibodies present in the serum of patients with thyrotoxicosis.

(iv) Parthenogenetic division of sea-urchin eggs by antibody.

Stimulation may also be observed at the molecular level as in the increase in enzymic activity of certain penicillinase and β-galactosidase variants caused by addition of the appropriate antibodies which induce allosteric changes in the enzyme conformation.

CYTOTOXIC REACTIONS

If antibodies directed against the surface of cells are able to fix certain components present in the extracellular fluids, collectively termed *complement*, a cytotoxic reaction may occur. Historically, complement activity was recognized by Bordet who showed that the lytic activity against red cells of freshly drawn rabbit anti-sheep erythrocyte serum was lost on ageing or heating to 56°C for half-an-hour but could be restored by addition of fresh serum from an unimmunized rabbit. Thus, for haemolysis one requires a relatively heat stable factor, the antibody, plus a heat labile factor, complement, present in all fresh sera.

Complement

NATURE OF COMPLEMENT

The classical activity ascribed to complement (C′) depends upon the operation of nine protein components (C1–C9)

TABLE 6.1.

	C1q	C4	C3
Serum concn., μg/ml	100–200	400	1,200
Molecular weight	400,000	230,000	185,000
Thermolability	+	–	–
Immunoelectrophoresis	γ	β_{1E}	β_{1C}

acting in sequence of which the first consists of three major subfractions termed C1q, C1r and C1s. Some of the characteristics of the three most abundant components are given in table 6.1.

When the first component is activated by an immune complex (e.g. antibody bound to a red cell), it acquires the ability to activate several molecules of the next component in the sequence; each of these is then able to act upon the next component and so on producing a cascade effect with amplification. In this way, the triggering of one molecule of C1 can lead to the activation of thousands of the later components. At each stage, activation is accompanied by the appearance of a new enzymic activity and since one enzyme molecule can process several substrate molecules, so each complement factor can cause the processing or activation of many molecules of the next component in the sequence (figure 6.19). The terminal components of the complement cascade have the ability to punch a 'functional hole' through the cell membrane on which they are fixed, presumably by some perturbation of phospholipid

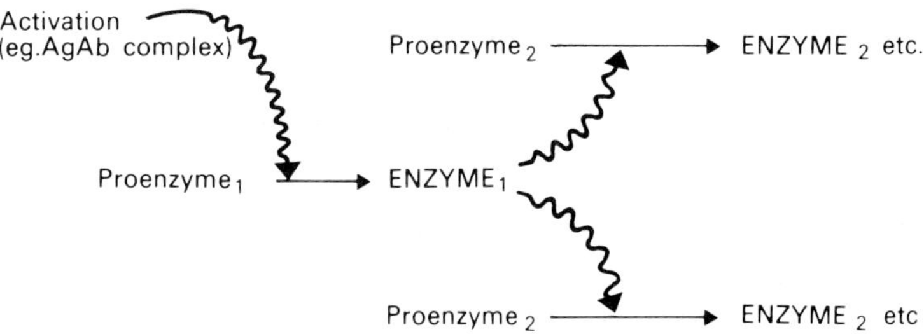

FIGURE 6.19. Enzymic basis of the amplifying complement cascade. The activated *enzyme*$_1$ splits a peptide fragment from several molecules of *proenzyme*$_2$ which all become active *enzyme*$_2$ molecules capable of splitting *proenzyme*$_3$ and so on.

structure, and this leads to cell death. Thus, through this sequential amplification process, the activation of one C1 molecule can lead to a macroscopic event, namely the lysis of a cell. As will be seen later, the intermediate stages in the complement sequence also give rise to other biological activities which are of importance in health and disease. Like the blood clotting, kallikrein and fibrinolytic systems which also involve enzyme cascades, the complement components have a complex system of inhibitors to regulate activation.

Complement is measured as an activity as are other enzyme systems and is expressed in terms of the degree of lysis of a standard suspension of antibody coated sheep red cells produced within a fixed time (figure 6.20).

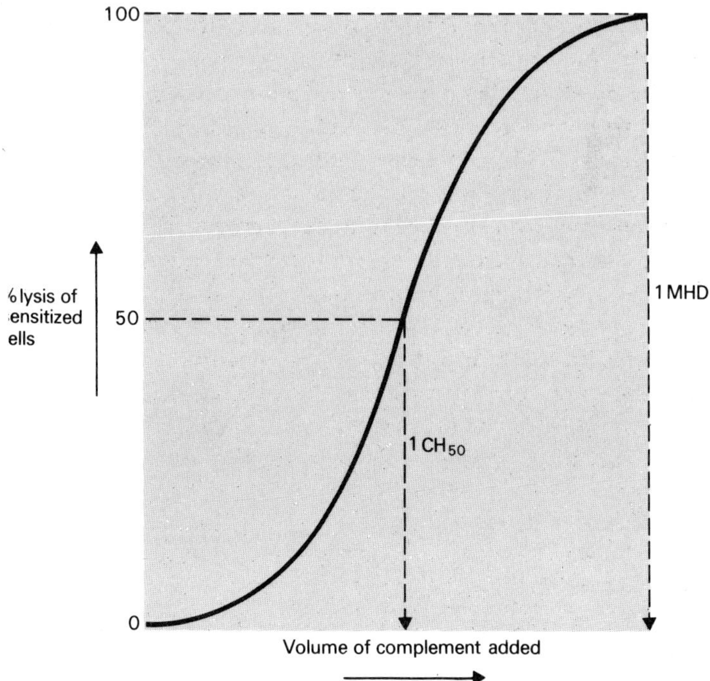

FIGURE 6.20. Relationship of added complement to percentage lysis of standard suspension of sensitized red cells. At the 50 per cent lysis point, the curve is steep and the amount of C′ giving 50 per cent lysis (1 CH_{50}) can be accurately determined. The curve only gradually reaches 100 per cent lysis and the amount of C′ giving 100 per cent lysis (1 Minimum Haemolytic Dose: 1 MHD) is less precisely assessed. The MHD is nonetheless adequate for routine serological purposes but for more accurate work the CH_{50} unit is preferred.

ACTIVATION OF COMPLEMENT

The activation of C1 is initiated by binding through C1q to C_H2 sites on the immunoglobulins forming a complex with antigen. Aggregation of immunoglobulin as by heating to 60°C for 20 minutes also leads to the changes in structure which allow complement activation. Different immunoglobulin classes have different Fc structures and only IgG and IgM can bind C1. There are differences even within the IgG subclasses: IgG1 and IgG3 fix complement well, IgG2 modestly and IgG4 poorly, if at all. C1q is polyvalent with respect to Ig binding and consists of a central collagen-like stem branching into 6 peptide chains each tipped by an Ig binding subunit (resernbling the blooms on a bunch of flowers). At least two of these subunits must bind to immunoglobulin C_H2 sites for activation of C1q. With IgM this is less of a problem since several Fc regions are available within a single molecule, although these only become readily accessible when the $F(ab')_2$ arms bend out of the plane of the inner Fc region on combination with antigen (cf. figure 2.17). On the other hand, IgG antibodies will only fix complement when two or more molecules are bound to closely adjacent sites on the antigen. It is for this reason that IgM antibodies to red cells have a high haemolytic efficiency since a 'single hit' will produce full complement activation and cell death. With IgG antibodies, a far larger number of 'hits' will be required before, by chance, two IgG antibodies are bound at adjacent sites and are then able to initiate the complement sequence.

Complement can be activated by another route, the so-called *alternative pathway* (see below). This can be stimulated by certain cell wall polysaccharides such as bacterial endotoxin and yeast zymosan, by some aggregated immunoglobulins such as human IgA and guinea pig IgG1 known to be ineffective for C1q binding, and, as we shall see later, by a feedback mechanism from the classical pathway.

THE COMPLEMENT SEQUENCE

Classical pathway (figure 6.21)

Let us analyse the sequence of events which take place when IgM or IgG antibodies combine with the surface membrane of a cell in the presence of complement. C1q is linked in a trimolecular complex through calcium to

C1r and C1s. After the binding of C1q to the Fc regions of the immune complex, C1s acquires esterase activity and brings about the activation and transfer to sites on the membrane (or immune complex) of first C4 and then C2 (unfortunately components were numbered before the sequence was established). This complex has 'C3-convertase' activity and splits C3 in solution to produce a small peptide fragment (C3a) and a residual molecule (C3b) which have quite distinct functions:

1. C3a is chemotactic for polymorphonuclear leucocytes and has *anaphylatoxin* activity in that it causes histamine release from mast cells.

2. C3b, like C2 and C4, displays a very short-lived hydrophobic site immediately after proteolytic cleavage of the parent C3 which enables it to stick readily to adjacent regions on the membrane. By this means a large number of C3b molecules may be transferred to the surface membrane through the action of the convertase. There are specific receptors for this membrane-bound C3b on polymorphs and macrophages (all mammalian species studied), platelets (rabbits) and red cells (primates) which allow *immune adherence* of the antigen–antibody-C3b complex to these cells so facilitating subsequent phagocytosis (figure 6.21). The

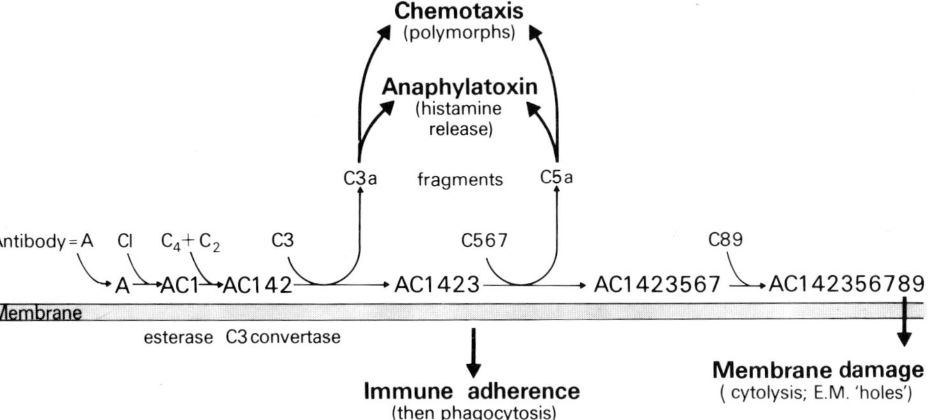

FIGURE 6.21. Sequence of classical complement activation by membrane-bound antibody showing formation of C3a and C5a fragments chemotactic for polymorphs and with anaphylatoxin activity causing histamine release. Immune adherence through C3 to macrophages, platelets or red cells facilitates phagocytosis. Fixation of C8 and 9 generates cytolytic activity. Fragments released during the activation of C4 and C2 are thought to have chemotactic and kinin-like activity respectively.

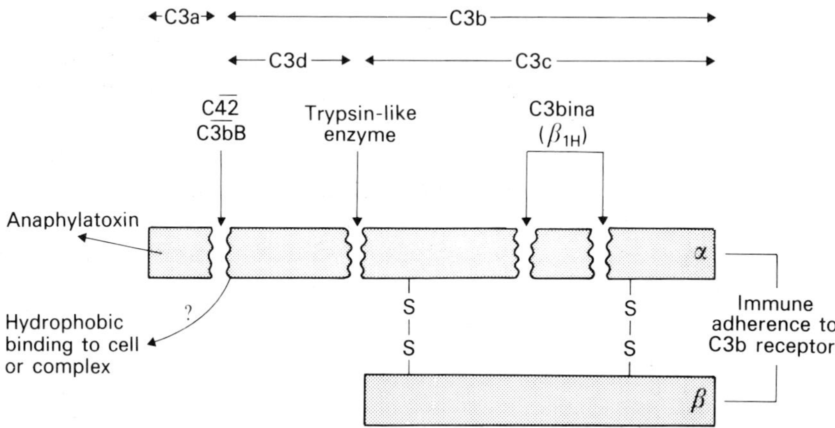

FIGURE 6.22. The structural basis for the cleavage of C3 by C3 convertases and the inactivation of C3b by successive action of C3b inactivator and a protease.

bound C3 presents a new structural configuration not present on the native molecule which can provoke the formation of the autoantibody *immunoconglutinin*. Control of C3b levels is maintained through the action of a C3b inactivator (C3bina; previously termed KAF). C3b readily combines with β_{1H} to form a complex which is broken down by C3bina and loses its haemolytic and immune adherence properties; it then becomes highly susceptible to attack by trypsin-like enzymes present in the body fluids and splits to form the fragments C3c and C3d (figure 6.22).

Alternative pathway

In the classical pathway we have just discussed, the active C3b fragment is formed by the action of C142 convertase. Another C3 convertase, C$\overline{3bB}$ can be generated by a distinct series of reactions collectively termed the alternative pathway (figure 6.23) which can be triggered by extrinsic agents, in particular microbial polysaccharides such as endotoxin, acting independently of antibody. The convertase is formed by the action of factor D on C3b and factor B. This creates an interesting positive feedback loop in which the product of C3 breakdown helps to form more of the cleavage enzyme.

The present view is that the low concentrations of C3b in plasma can give rise to C$\overline{3bB}$ convertase under normal conditions; however, the lability of C$\overline{3bB}$ and the action of C3b inactivator prevent the system from getting out of hand and allow the feedback loop to 'tick over' quietly. Microbial polysaccharides and other initiators of the alternative pathway boost the levels of $\overline{\text{C3bB}}$ convertase by providing a surface upon which the enzyme is stabilized (perhaps with the help of properdin).

The alternative pathway can be studied independently of the classical sequence under circumstances where the latter is inoperative as, for example, in C4-deficient serum or in a serum treated with Mg-EGTA to complex Ca^{2+} and inactivate C1.

The solubilization of immune complexes by coating with C3b appears to be due to activation of the alternative pathway perhaps through stabilization of convertase on the surface of the complex. An unexpected finding was the observation that factor B can be detected on the surface of B-lymphocytes. Is this connected with a role for C3b as a second signal for lymphocyte induction?

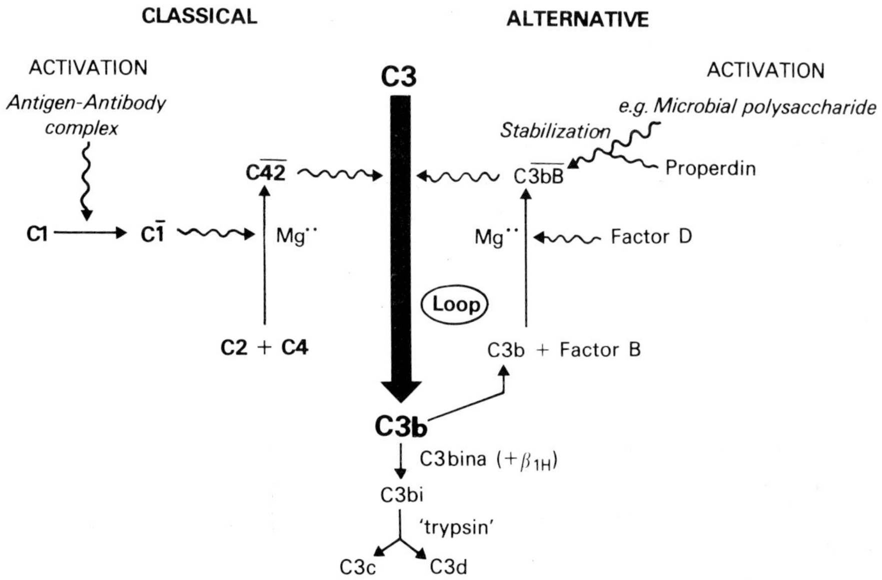

CLASSICAL
ALTERNATIVE
ACTIVATION
Antigen-Antibody complex
C3
ACTIVATION
e.g. Microbial polysaccharide
Stabilization
Properdin
$\overline{\text{C42}}$
$\overline{\text{C3bB}}$
C1
$\overline{\text{C1}}$
Mg··
Mg··
Factor D
Loop
C2 + C4
C3b + Factor B
C3b
C3bina (+β_{1H})
C3bi
'trypsin'
C3c
C3d

FIGURE 6.23. The alternative complement pathway showing points of similarity with the classical sequence. Both pathways generate a C3 convertase, $\overline{\text{C42}}$ in one case and $\overline{\text{C3bB}}$ in the other, which activates C3 to provide the central event in the complement system. The C3b inactivator may split C4b in the same manner as it does C3b. C3 and C4 resemble each other structurally as do C2 and Factor B. The alternative pathway is probably the older of the two in phylogenetic terms. ⟿ represents an activation process. The convention of using a horizontal bar above a complement component to designate its activation is used. The activated components are usually fragments of the original molecules e.g. the alternative pathway convertase is actually $\overline{\text{C3bBb}}$, but in the interests of simplicity in a complicated system, such details have been omitted.

Post C3 pathway

The sequence reaches its full amplitude at the C3 stage which represents the essential heart of the complement system. Thereafter C5 is split by C3b to give C5a and C5b fragments. C5a degranulates mast cells and is the dominant polymorph chemotactic agent in the complement system; it also brings about the extracellular secretion of leucocyte lysosomal enzymes. Both C3a and C5a are inactivated by a carboxypeptidase which removes the terminal arginine. Meanwhile, the C5b binds as a complex with C6 and 7 to form a thermostable site on the membrane which recruits the final components C8 and C9 and these administer the coup de grâce by generating *membrane damage*. The cytolytic component is C8 but C9 enhances its activity (figure 6.21); incredibly just one molecule of C8 is sufficient to lyse a red cell.

Yet more complexity is introduced by the phenomenon of *reactive lysis* (Lachmann & Thomson); a proportion of the activated C5b67 complexes formed remain free and not only are they chemotactic for neutrophils but are also able to bind to 'innocent' cells in the vicinity. Once fixed to the cell surface they can complete the complement sequence by binding C8, 9 with resultant cell lysis.

ROLE IN DEFENCE

Cytolysis

The full complement system leading to membrane damage can cause bacteriolysis in Gram-negative organisms by allowing lysozyme to reach the plasma membrane where it destroys the mucopeptide layer (p. 181). Negatively stained preparations in the electron microscope show the 'pits' on the surface (figure 6.24) which correspond with individual sites of complement activation and which resemble those seen on the red cell.

Immune (C3b) adherence

This plays a major role in facilitating the phagocytosis of micro-organisms after coating with antibody and C′ or after activation of the alternative complement pathway. Since many C3 molecules are bound onto the surface at each site of C′ activation, adherence to macrophages and polymorphs may operate largely through C3 binding

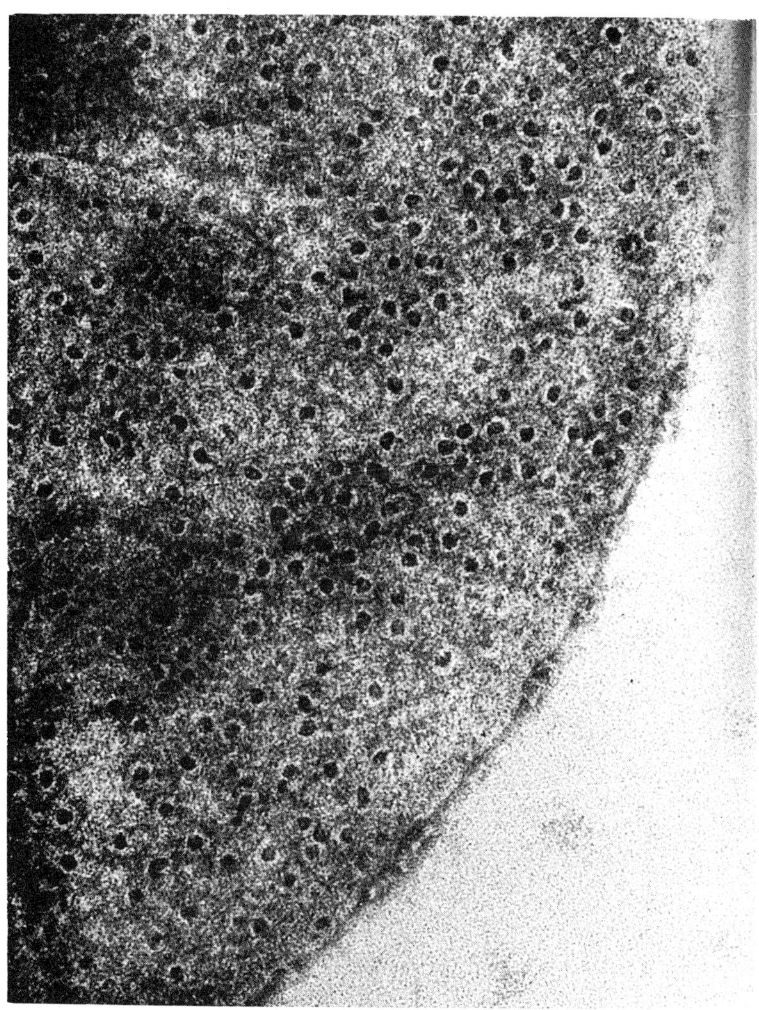

FIGURE 6.24. Multiple lesions in cell wall of *Escherichia coli* bacterium caused by interaction with IgM antibody and complement. Each lesion is caused by a single IgM molecule and shows as a 'dark pit' due to penetration by the 'negative stain'. This is somewhat of an illusion since in reality these 'pits' are like volcano craters standing proud of the surface, and are each single complexes containing one each of the terminal C5-8 components plus 6 molecules of C9. C8 opens and shuts a transmembrane channel which eventually causes lysis, and C9 acts to jam this channel open. Comparable results may be obtained in the absence of antibody since the cell wall endotoxin can activate the alternative pathway. Magnification ×400,000. (Courtesy of Drs. R. Dourmashkin and J.H. Humphrey.)

although it should be noted that subsequent phagocytosis is provoked to a greater extent by IgG rather than C3b. Purified C3b has been shown to trigger extracellular release of lysosomal enzymes from macrophages and it is possible, but not yet established, that this could damage adhering micro-organisms.

Immunoconglutinin

This may play a role by agglutinating relatively small complexes containing bound C3 thereby making them more susceptible to phagocytosis.

Acute inflammation

The fragments produced during complement consumption stimulate two helpful features of the acute inflammatory response. First, the chemotactic factors attract phagocytic neutrophil polymorphs to the site of C′ activation, and secondly anaphylatoxin, through histamine release, increases vascular permeability and hence the flow of serum antibody and more C′ to the infected area.

ROLE IN DISEASE

Complement is implicated in disease processes involving cytotoxic and immune-complex mediated hypersensitivities which will be discussed in more detail in chapter 8. Cytotoxic reactions are seen in nephrotoxic nephritis and autoimmune haemolytic anaemia. Complexes formed in antibody excess giving rise to immune vasculitis of the Arthus type are seen, for example, in Farmer's lung and cryoglobulinaemia with cutaneous vasculitis; soluble complexes formed in antigen excess give 'serum sickness' type reactions with considerable deposition in the kidney glomeruli as found in many forms of chronic glomerulonephritis. Some patients with mesangiocapillary glomerulonephritis and partial lipodystrophy have low complement levels due to the presence in serum of the so-called C3 nephritic factor which appears to be an autoantibody capable of activating the alternative pathway by combining with and stabilizing the $\mathrm{C3\overline{bB}}$ convertase.

In paroxysmal nocturnal haemoglobinuria (PNH) the erythrocytes are particularly susceptible to reactive lysis as a result of an unusual, as yet unexplained ability to fix the activated trimolecular complex, C567. Massive complement activation can lead to disseminated intravascular coagulation. A good model for this is the Shwartzmann reaction produced in rabbits by intravascular endotoxin. This activates the alternative pathway so that the endotoxin becomes coated with C3b and sticks to platelets by immune adherence; the C567 complexes generated cause platelet destruction by reactive lysis with release of clotting factors. Although in man, C3b adherence reactions involve red cells and leucocytes rather than platelets, somewhat similar mechanisms associated with intense complement consumption underly the disseminated intravascular coagulation seen in human patients with Gram-negative septicaemia or dengue haemorrhagic shock produced by a substantial viraemia occurring in the second infection of individuals with high titre antibodies.

COMPLEMENT DEFICIENCIES

A transient fall in C′ can be induced by injection of aggregated IgG or of a cobra venom factor which contains the reptilian equivalent of C3b. This fires the alternative pathway but because of its insensitivity to the mammalian C3b inactivator it persists long enough to cause C3 exhaustion. The importance of C′ in defence against infections is emphasized by the occurrence of repeated infections in a patient lacking C3b inactivator. Because of his inability to destroy C3b there is continual activation of the alternative pathway through the feedback loop leading to very low C3 and Factor B levels with normal C1, 4 and 2. On the other hand, permanent deficiencies in C5, C6 and C7 have all been described in man yet in virtually every case the individuals are healthy and not particularly prone to infection. Thus full operation of the C′ system up to C8,9 does not appear to be essential for survival and adequate protection must be afforded by opsonizing antibodies and the immune adherence mechanism.

Failure to generate the classical C3-convertase through deficiencies in C1r, C4 and C2 have been reported in a small number of cases associated with an unusually high incidence of SLE-like syndromes (cf. p. 294) perhaps due to a decreased ability to eliminate antigen–antibody complexes (cf. p. 238). An inhibitor of active C1 is grossly lacking in hereditary angioneurotic oedema and this can lead to recurring episodes of acute circumscribed noninflammatory oedema. The patients are heterozygotes and synthesize small amounts of the inhibitor which can be raised to useful levels by administration of testosterone or, in critical cases, of the purified inhibitor itself.

GENETICS

Multiple allotypic (polymorphic) forms of human C3, C6 and Factor B have been described, the latter showing genetic linkage to HLA (the major histocompatibility locus). Genes responsible for C4 and C2 deficiencies are present in the same region.

In the mouse, control of C3 levels is linked to H-2 while regulation of C4 maps in the Ss region (figure 4.5).

Neutralization of biological activity

To continue our discussion on the interaction of antigen and antibody we may focus attention on a number of biological reactions which can be inhibited by addition of specific antibody. Thus the agglutination of red cells by interaction of influenza virus with receptors on the erythrocyte surface can be blocked by antiviral antibodies and this forms the basis for their serological detection. Neutralization of the growth of hapten-conjugated bacteriophage provides an exquisitely sensitive assay for anti-hapten antibodies. A test for antibodies to salmonella H antigen present on the flagella depends upon their ability to inhibit the motility of the bacteria *in vitro*. Likewise, mycoplasma antibodies can be demonstrated by their inhibitory effect on the metabolism of the organisms in culture. The successful treatment of cases of drug overdose with the Fab fragment of specific antibodies has been described and may become a practical proposition if a range of hybridomas can be assembled. Antibodies to hormones such as insulin and TSH can be used to probe the specificity of biological reactions *in vitro*; for example the specificity of the insulin-like activity of a serum sample on rat epididymal fat pad can be checked by the neutralizing effect of an antiserum. Such antibodies can be effective *in vitro* and as part of the world-wide effort to prevent disastrous over-population, attempts are in progress to immunize against chorionic gonadotropin using fragments of the β-chain coupled to appropriate carriers, since this hormone is needed to sustain the implanted ovum.

Summary

The formation of single bands of precipitate when antigen and antibody react in gels can be used qualitatively to study the number of reacting components and the immunological relationship between different antigens (Ouchterlony double diffusion system) and the electrophoretic mobility of the antigens (immunoelectrophoresis). Quantitative measurement of antigen concentration is made by single radial immunodiffusion, 'rocket' electrophoresis and two-dimensional electrophoresis. Laser nephelometry provides a sensitive method for the quantification of antigens in solution.

Radioisotopic techniques for assessing the antibody content of serum include: (a) addition of radiolabelled antigen and determination of the amount bound to antibody by ammonium sulphate or a second antibody precipitation (antigen-binding capacity) and (b) determination of the amount of antibody binding to insoluble antigen by addition of a labelled anti-Ig (e.g. 'tube test'). Radioimmunoassay of antigen is a form of saturation analysis in which the test material competes with labelled antigen for a limited amount of antibody, the amount of label displaced being a measure of the antigen in the test sample. Immunoradiometric tests involve the binding of antigen to solid phase antibody and its estimation by excess labelled antibody.

The localization of antigens in tissues, within cells or on the cell surface can be achieved microscopically using antibodies tagged with fluorescent dyes or enzymes such as peroxidase whose reaction product can be readily visualized. In the direct test, the labelled antibody is applied directly to the tissue; in the indirect test the label is conjugated to an anti-Ig used as a second amplifying antibody. Fluorescent antibody bound to the surface of single cells e.g. lymphocytes, can be quantified by flow cytofluorography. For ultrastructural studies, antibodies are usually tagged with peroxidase.

Antibodies can be used for the immunochemical analysis of detergent solubilized antigens of the plasma membrane. Reaction of antibody with a cell surface antigen can lead to agglutination, enhancement of phagocytosis or extracellular killing, metabolic stimulation and mitosis, and complement-mediated cytotoxicity.

Complement, like the blood coagulation, fibrinolytic and kallikrein systems, involves a multicomponent enzymic cascade in which the first component, on activation, splits a small peptide from several molecules of the second component each of which is now an active enzyme able to act on the third component, etc.; a small number of initiating events leads to a large effect through this amplification method. The most abundant component, C3, is split by a convertase enzyme generated either by the *classical pathway* (C1,4,2) which is initiated by antibody, or by the alternative pathway (properdin, factors B and D) which is initiated in the absence of antibody by material such as bacterial polysaccharides. One split product, C3a, is chemotactic for polymorphonuclear leucocytes and increases vascular permeability through histamine release from mast cells and basophils. The other product, C3b, binds non-specifically to the antigen surface and increases the efficiency of binding to the polymorphs (attracted by C3a) because of C3b receptors on the surface of these phagocytic cells. C3b also activates C5 to release C5a (with similar properties to C3a) and generates C5b which fires the remainder of the sequence to C8 and 9 thereby leading to cell death through membrane damage. Through these effects complement plays an important role in the defence against infection. It is also concerned in certain hypersensitivity reactions involving combination of antibody with surfaces (e.g. nephrotoxic nephritis) and immune complexes (e.g. Farmer's lung, chronic glomerulonephritis). Massive activation of complement by microbial products can lead to disseminated intravascular coagulation. Deficiency in complement components predisposes to the development of SLE. Like the blood clotting system, inhibitors play a crucial role and if they are defective, disease may result, e.g. hereditary angioneurotic oedema (C1 inhibitor) or repeated infection (C3b inactivator).

Antigens with biological activity, e.g. hormones such as human chorionic gonadotropin, may be neutralized *in vivo* by antibody.

Further reading

Clausen J. (1969) *Immunochemical techniques for the identification and estimation of macromolecules*. North-Holland, Amsterdam.

Hudson L. & Hay F.C. (1980) *Practical Immunology*, 2nd ed. Blackwell Scientific Publications, Oxford.

Lachmann P.J. (1980) Complement. In *Clinical Aspects of Immunology*, 4th ed. Lachmann P.J. & Peters K. (eds). Blackwell Scientific Publications, Oxford.

Nairn R.C. (1976) *Fluorescent protein tracing*, 4th ed. Churchill Livingstone, Edinburgh.

Rose N.R. & Friedman H. (eds) (1976) *Manual of Clinical Immunology*. Amer. Soc. Microbiology, Washington, D.C.

Thompson R.A. (1974) *The Practice of Clinical Immunology*, Arnold, London.

Weir D.M. (ed.) (1973) *Handbook of Experimental Immunology*, 2nd ed. Blackwell Scientific Publications, Oxford.

Williams C.A. & Chase M.W. (1967–71) *Methods in Immunology and Immunochemistry*, Vols. I–IV. Academic Press, London.

7 Immunity to infection

Aside from ill-understood constitutional factors which make one species innately susceptible and another resistant to certain infections, a number of non-specific anti-microbial systems (e.g. phagocytosis) have been recognized which are '*innate*' in the sense that they are not intrinsically affected by prior contact with the infectious agent. We shall discuss these systems and examine how, in the state of *specific acquired immunity*, their effectiveness can be greatly increased by both B- and T-cell activity.

Innate immunity

PREVENTING ENTRY

The simplest way to avoid infection is to prevent the micro-organisms from gaining access to the body (figure 7.1). The major line of defence of course is the skin which, when intact, is impermeable to most infectious agents. Furthermore most bacteria fail to survive for long on the skin because of the direct inhibitory effects of lactic acid and fatty acids in sweat and sebaceous secretions and the low pH which they generate. An exception is *Staphylococcus aureus* which often infects the relatively vulnerable hair follicles and glands.

Mucus, secreted by the membranes lining the inner surfaces of the body, acts as a protective barrier and can inhibit the penetration of cells by viruses through competition with cell surface receptors for the viral neuraminidase. Microbial and other foreign particles trapped within the adhesive mucus are removed by mechanical stratagems such as ciliary movement, coughing and sneezing. Among other mechanical factors which help protect the epithelial surfaces, one should also include the washing action of tears, saliva and urine. Many of the secreted body fluids contain bactericidal components, e.g. acid in gastric juice, spermine in semen and lysozyme in tears, nasal secretions and saliva.

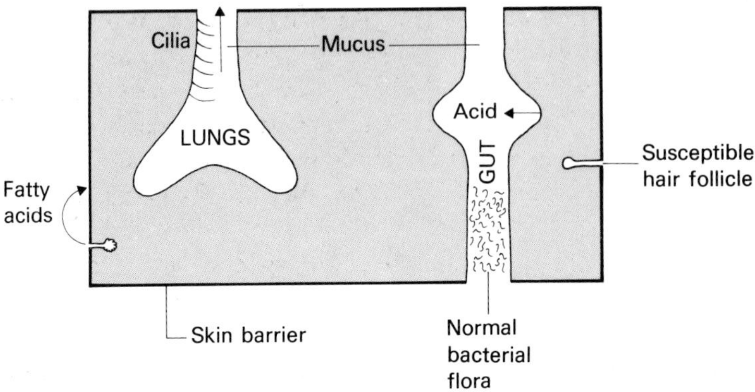

FIGURE 7.1. The first lines of defence against infection: protection at the external body surfaces.

A totally different mechanism is that of microbial antagonism associated with the normal bacterial flora of the body. These suppress the growth of many potentially pathogenic bacteria and fungi at superficial sites by competition for essential nutrients or by production of inhibitory substances such as colicins or acid.

COUNTER-ATTACK AGAINST THE INVADERS

When micro-organisms do penetrate the body, two main defensive operations come into play, the destructive effect of soluble chemical factors such as bactericidal enzymes and the mechanism of phagocytosis—literally 'eating' by the cell.

Humoral factors

Of the soluble bactericidal substances elaborated by the body, perhaps the most abundant and widespread is the enzyme lysozyme, a muramidase which splits the mucopeptide wall of susceptible bacteria. A number of plasma components, C-reactive protein (CRP), α_1 anti-trypsin, α_2-macroglobulin, fibrinogen, caeruloplasmin, C9 and factor B, collectively termed *acute phase proteins*, show a dramatic increase in concentration in response to infection or tissue injury. For example, CRP is released from the liver in response to endogenous pyrogen derived from endotoxin stimulated macrophages, and its concentration can rise 1000-fold. CRP shows a Ca-dependent binding to a number of micro-organisms which contain phosphoryl choline in their membranes, the complex having the useful property of activating complement by the classical pathway. We remember of course that many microbes activate the alternative pathway directly and we will explore the consequences in more detail below; suffice it to say under this head that such activation can result in damage to the outer membrane of the infective agent mediated by the terminal components C8 and C9.

Lastly we should include the non-specific antiviral agent *interferon I* which inhibits intracellular viral replication and is itself synthesized by cells in response to viral infection. Viral interference, the resistance of an animal or cell infected with one virus to superinfection with a second unrelated virus, may be attributed to interferon. In children given live measles vaccine, smallpox vaccine will not take if inoculated at the height of interferon production. It must be presumed that interferon plays a significant role in the recovery from, as distinct from the prevention of viral infections. The finding that interferon heightens the activity of non-specific killer cells (NK; p. 285) could have considerable significance if these are shown to be generally cytotoxic for virally infected cells since this would constitute a nicely integrated system.

Phagocytosis

The engulfment and digestion of micro-organisms is assigned to two major cell types recognized by Metchnikoff at the turn of the century as *micro-* and *macrophages*. The smaller polymorphonuclear neutrophil (cf. figure 3.6f) is a non-dividing short-lived cell with granules containing a wide range of bactericidal factors and glycogen stores which can be utilized by glycolysis under anaerobic conditions. It is the dominant white cell in the blood stream. Macrophages derive from bone marrow promonocytes which, after differentiation to blood monocytes, finally settle in the tissues as mature macrophages where they constitute the so-called *reticuloendothelial system*. They are present throughout the connective tissue and around the basement membrane of small blood vessels and are particularly concentrated in the lung (alveolar macrophages), liver (Kupffer cells), and lining of spleen sinusoids and lymph node medullary sinuses where they are strategically placed to filter off foreign material. Other examples are mesangial cells in the kidney glomerulus, brain microglia and osteoclasts in bone. Unlike the polymorphs, they are long-lived cells with significant rough-surfaced endoplasmic reticulum and mitochondria and whereas the polymorphs provide the major defence against pyogenic (pus-forming) bacteria, as a rough generalization it may be said that macrophages are at their best in combating those bacteria, viruses and protozoa which are capable of living within the cells of the host.

Before phagocytosis can occur, the microbe must first adhere to the surface of the polymorph or macrophage, an event mediated by some rather primitive recognition mechanism on the part of the phagocytic cells. Depending upon its nature, a particle attached to the membrane may initiate the ingestion phase in which it becomes engulfed by cytoplasmic processes and comes to lie within a vacuole termed a phagosome (figures 7.2 & 3.7g–j). A lysosomal granule then fuses with the vacuole to form a phagolysosome in which the ingested microbe is slaughtered by a battery of mechanisms (table 7.1). Dominant among these are the oxygen-dependent systems. Phagocytosis is associated with a dramatic increase in activity of the hexose monophosphate shunt providing NADPH and a burst of oxygen consumption as this is metabolized by a plasma membrane NADPH oxidase which is activated on contact with the microbe during ingestion and continues to function on the inner surface of the phagolysosome. The oxygen is converted to superoxide anion, hydrogen peroxide, singlet oxygen and hydroxyl radicals, all powerful microbicidal agents. The combination

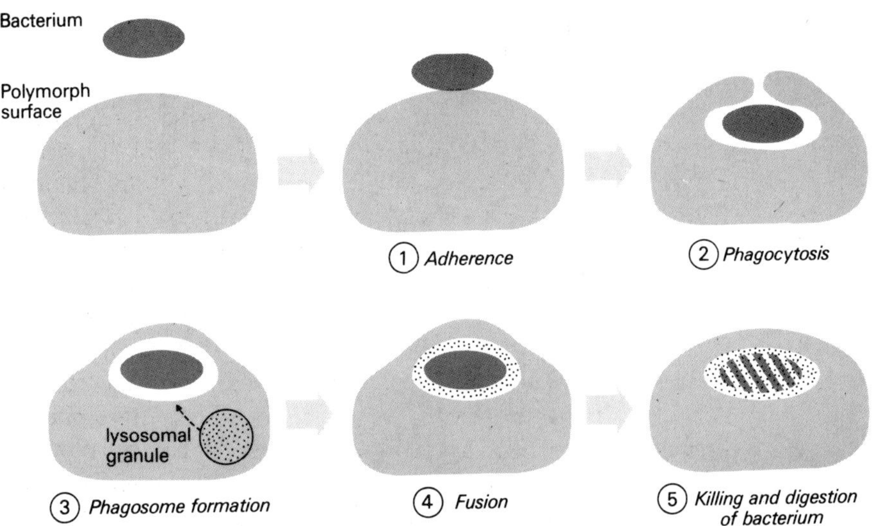

FIGURE 7.2. Phagocytosis of bacterium by neutrophil leucocyte (see also figure 3.7g–j).

TABLE 7.1. Antimicrobial systems in phagocytic vacuoles

**Oxygen dependent mechanisms:*			
Glucose + $NADP^+$	hexose monophosphate shunt $\longrightarrow$	pentose phosphate + NADPH	O_2 burst + generation of superoxide anion
NADPH + O_2	oxidase $\longrightarrow$	$NADP^+$ + $\mathbf{O_2^-}$	
$2O_2^-$ + $2H^+$	spontaneous dismutation $\longrightarrow$	$\mathbf{H_2O_2}$ + $\mathbf{^1O_2}$	Spontaneous formation of further microbicidal agents
O_2^- + H_2O_2	$\longrightarrow$	$\mathbf{\cdot OH}$ + OH^- + $\mathbf{^1O_2}$	
H_2O_2 + Cl^-	myeloperoxidase $\longrightarrow$	$\mathbf{OCl^-}$ + H_2O	Myeloperoxidase generation of microbicidal molecules
OCl^- + H_2O	$\longrightarrow$	$\mathbf{^1O_2}$ + Cl^- + H_2O	
$2O_2^-$ + $2H^+$	superoxide dismutase $\longrightarrow$	O_2 + H_2O_2	Protective mechanisms used by host + many microbes
$2H_2O_2$	catalase $\longrightarrow$	$2H_2O$ + O_2	
Oxygen independent mechanisms:			
Low pH (lactic acid formation)			Not a microbial paradise
Lysozyme			Splits mucopeptide in bacterial cell wall
Lactoferrin			Deprives bacteria of iron
Cationic proteins (leukin, phagocytin)			Damage to microbial membranes
Proteolytic enzymes (including elastase) Variety of other hydrolytic enzymes			Digestion of killed organisms

*Microbicidal species in bold type.
O_2^-, superoxide anion; $^1O_2$, singlet (activated) oxygen; $\cdot OH$, hydroxyl free radical.

of peroxide, myeloperoxidase and halide ions constitutes a potent halogenating system capable of killing both bacteria and viruses. Low pH, lysozyme, lactoferrin and the cationic proteins constitute a series of bacteriostatic and bactericidal factors which are oxygen-independent and can therefore function under anaerobic circumstances. The rich variety of proteolytic and other hydrolytic enzymes present are concerned in the digestion of the killed organisms.

To some extent there is an extracellular release of lysosomal constituents during phagocytosis which may play an amplifying role. The basic polypeptides, for example, stimulate an acute inflammatory reaction with increased vascular permeability, transudation of serum proteins and egress of leucocytes from blood vessels by diapedesis. The release of an endogenous pyrogen from the polymorphs may explain, in part at least, the fever which often accompanies an infection and the output of acute phase proteins from liver.

It is clear then, that the phagocytic cells possess an impressive anti-microbial potential, but when an infectious agent gains access to the body, this formidable array of weaponry is useless until some way is found to enable the phagocyte to 'home onto' the micro-organism. The body has solved this problem with the effortless ease that comes with a few million years of evolution by developing the complement system.

THE ROLE OF COMPLEMENT

As we argued in chapter 6, the surface carbohydrates of many microbial species are able to activate the alternative pathway thereby generating C3 convertase activity. The convertase now splits C3 to give C3b which binds to the surface of the microbe, and the small peptide C3a which provides the microbe, and the small peptide C3a which provides the answer we need through its ability to attract polymorphs (a later product of the sequence, C5a has similar powers cf. p. 164). The polymorphs move up the chemotactic C3a gradient until suddenly they come face to face with the C3b-coated micro-organisms to which they become attached by virtue of their surface C3b receptors so thoughtfully placed there by the subtle processes of evolution.

The formation of C3a and C5a (the anaphylatoxins) has further ramifications through their action on the mast cell which releases histamine and causes transudation of complement components and movement of polymorphs from the local blood vessels into the surrounding tissue providing the ingredients of an acute inflammatory reaction (figure 7.3).

Adherence to the surface of the phagocyte having been achieved, it remains only for the cell to be stimulated by its contact with the micro-organism for the ingestion phase to be initiated. How splendid—but what happens if the micro-organism should be of such physical and chemical constitution that it lacks the decency either (a) to activate the alternative complement pathway or (b) to be able to stimulate phagocytic ingestion? Once again the body has produced an ingenious solution: it has devised a variable adaptor molecule.

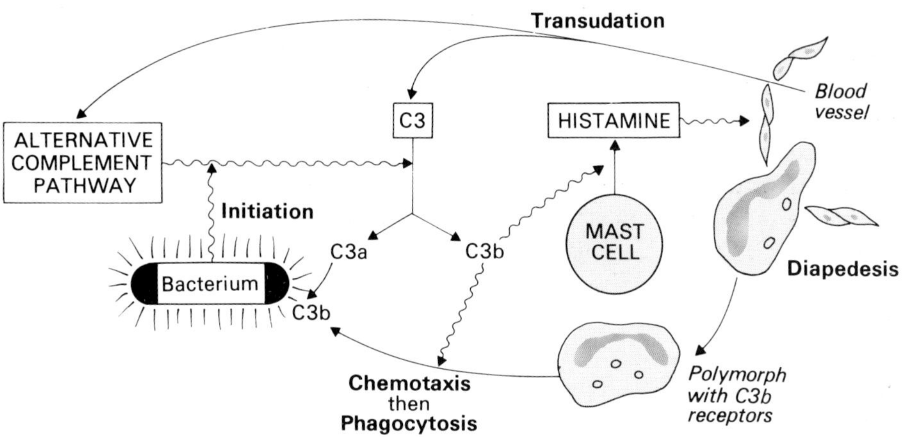

FIGURE 7.3. The role of complement in the defence against infection showing the consequences of activation of the alternative pathway by a bacterium with generation of an *acute inflammatory reaction* involving increased vascular permeability through separation of capillary endothelial cells and an influx of polymorphs. C5a is also chemotactic and the terminal components C8 and C9 may be lytic.

Acquired immunity

Looking at the problem teleologically (which usually gives the right answer for the wrong reasons), the body had to develop a molecule with the intrinsic ability to activate complement and phagocytosis but which could be adapted to stick onto any one of a host of different micro-organisms so that each would then become susceptible to the combined complement—phagocyte defence system. And lo and behold, it came to pass, and we marvelled and called it—ANTIBODY! An immunoglobulin of the appropriate class, e.g. human IgG1, activates complement by a separate pathway (classical) through binding C1q to its C_H2 domain thereby generating a C3 convertase; the C_H3 domain binds to specific Fc receptors on the phagocyte and presumably initiates ingestion (cf. figure 2.13, p. 36). The whole molecule is attached to the foreign invader through the antigen binding region of the variable domains, the body making sure of its defences by manufacturing antibody molecules with a wide range of combining specificities.

The B-lymphocyte system developed in order to produce antibodies, and by allowing each lymphocyte to synthesize only one type of antibody great flexibility could be introduced. Although there are sufficient lymphocytes to produce a wide range of different antibodies, it would be wasteful to maintain large numbers of lymphocytes capable of reacting with antigens which the body did not encounter. The system of clonal triggering and formation of memory cells ensures that the body only concentrates its main energies on antigens which it actually meets while retaining the potential to react against some obscure microbe which might infect the body at any time in the future. The ability to generate memory cells in response to a particular infection is, of course, the basis of *acquired* as distinct from *innate* immunity but it should be perfectly plain that antibody, as one agent of acquired immunity acts to enhance the mechanisms of innate immunity.

Immunity to bacterial infection

ROLE OF HUMORAL ANTIBODY

Enhancing phagocytosis

Many virulent forms of bacteria resist engulfment by phagocytic cells: for example, encapsulated forms of pneumococci do not stick readily to these cells and virulent strains of staphylococci and streptococci elaborate antiphagocytic substances including certain toxins. In accord with our previous discussion, antibody has a dramatic effect on phagocytosis and the rate of clearance of such organisms from the blood stream is strikingly enhanced when they are coated with specific Ig (figure 7.4). The less effective removal of coated bacteria in complement-depleted animals emphasizes the synergism between antibody and complement for 'opsonization' (cf. pp. 156 & 161) which is mediated through specific high affinity receptors for IgG and C3b on the phagocyte surface (figure 7.5). It is clearly advantageous that the subclasses which bind strongly to these Fc receptors (e.g. IgG1 and 3 in the human) also fix complement well.

Bacteria may also be captured by antibody already fixed to the Fc receptor site (cytophilic antibody) but it is probable that adherence is mediated more through opsonization than through the prior binding of cytophilic antibody to the phagocyte. Complexes containing C3 may show immune adherence to primate red cells and rabbit platelets to provide phagocytosable aggregates.

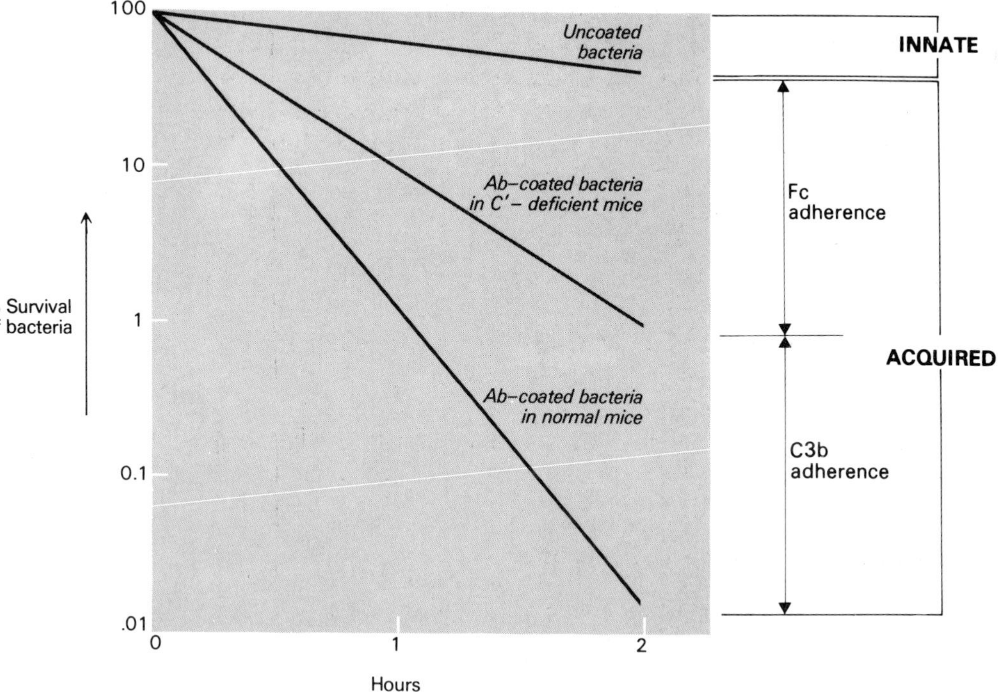

FIGURE 7.4. Effect of opsonizing antibody and complement on rate of clearance of virulent bacteria from the blood. The uncoated bacteria are phagocytosed rather slowly (INNATE IMMUNITY) but on coating with antibody, adherence to phagocytes is increased many-fold (ACQUIRED IMMUNITY). The adherence is somewhat less effective in animals temporarily depleted of complement.

Some strains of Gram-negative bacteria which have a lipoprotein outer wall resembling mammalian surface membranes in structure are susceptible to the bactericidal action of fresh serum containing antibody. The antibody initiates the development of a complement-mediated lesion producing similar 'holes' to those caused by complement in mammalian cells (cf. figure 6.24); this allows access of serum lysozyme to the inner wall of the bacterium with resulting cell death. Activation of complement through union of antibody and bacterium will also generate the C3a and C5a anaphylatoxins leading to extensive transudation of serum components including more antibody, and to the chemotactic attraction of polymorphs to aid in phagocytosis. In other words the series of events described in figure 7.3 can be entirely recreated by substituting the antibody-initiated classical complement sequence in place of the alternative pathway.

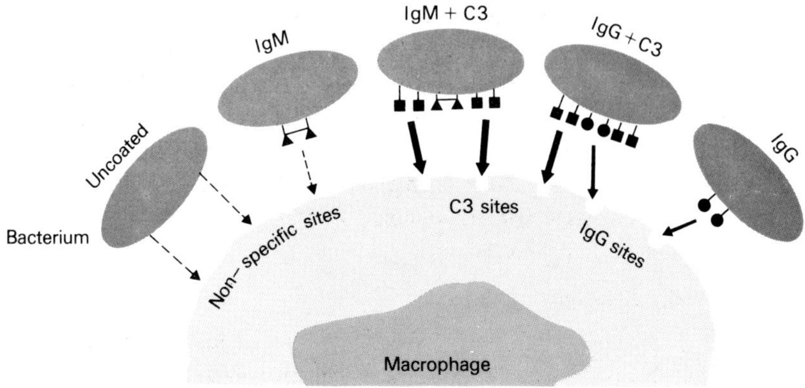

FIGURE 7.5. Immunoglobulin and complement coats greatly increase the adherence of bacteria (and other antigens) to macrophages and polymorphs. Uncoated or IgM ( ) coated bacteria adhere relatively weakly to non-specific sites but there are specific receptors for IgG (Fc) ( ) and C3 ( ) on the macrophage surface which considerably enhance the strength of binding. The augmenting effect of complement is due to the fact that two adjacent IgG molecules can fix many C3 molecules thereby increasing the number of links to the macrophage (cf. 'bonus' effect of multivalency; p. 15). Although IgM does not bind specifically to the macrophage, it promotes adherence through complement fixation.

Protecting external surfaces

IgA antibodies afford protection in the external body fluids, tears, saliva, nasal secretions and those bathing the surfaces of the intestine (so-called 'coproantibodies') and lung, by coating bacteria and viruses and preventing their adherence to mucosal surfaces. It might be anticipated that in order to fulfil this function, secretory IgA molecules would themselves have very little innate adhesiveness for cells and certainly no high affinity Fc receptors for this Ig class have yet been described. If an infectious agent succeeds in penetrating the IgA barrier, it comes up against the next line of defence of the MALT system (p. 84) which is manned by IgE. Although present in low concentration, IgE is bound very firmly to the Fc receptors of the mast cell (p. 218) and contact with antigen leads to the release of mediators which effectively recruit agents of the immune response. Thus histamine, by increasing vascular permeability, causes the transudation of IgG and complement into the area while chemotactic factors for neutrophils and eosinophils attract the effector cells needed to dispose of the infectious organism coated with specific IgG and C3b (figure 7.6). Where the opsonized organism is too large for phagocytosis, these cells can kill by an extracellular mechanism after attachment by their Fcγ receptors. This phenomenon, termed antibody-dependent cell-mediated cytotoxicity (ADCC) is discussed further in the following chapter but there is evidence for its involvement in parasitic infections (p. 195). There are obvious parallels between the ways in which complement-derived anaphylatoxins and IgE utilize the mast cell to cause local amplification of the immune defences.

Toxin neutralization

In addition to their role in removal of microbes, circulating antibodies act to neutralize the soluble exotoxins (e.g. phospholipase C of *Clostridium welchii*) released by bacteria. Combination near the biologically active site of the toxin would stereochemically block reaction with the substrate, particularly if it were macromolecular; combination distant from the active site may also cause inhibition through allosteric conformational changes. In its complex with antibody, the toxin may be unable to diffuse away rapidly and will be susceptible to phagocytosis, especially if the complex

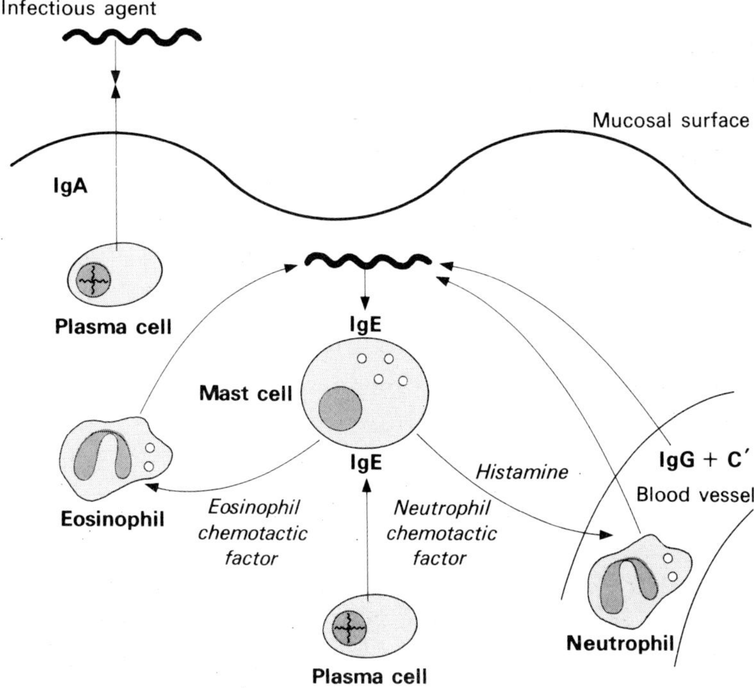

FIGURE 7.6. Defence of the mucosal surfaces. IgA prevents adherence of organisms to the mucosa. IgE recruits agents of the immune response by firing the release of mediators from mast cells.

can be increased in size by the action of naturally occurring antibodies to altered IgG (antiglobulin factors) and altered C3 (immunoconglutinin).

Specific organisms

Let us see how these considerations apply to the defence against infection by common organisms such as streptococci and staphylococci. β-Haemolytic streptococci were classified by Lancefield according to their carbohydrate antigen and the most important from the standpoint of human disease are those belonging to group A. However the most immunogenic surface component is the M-protein (variants of which form the basis of the Griffith typing). This protein inhibits phagocytosis and the protection afforded by antibodies to the M-component is attributable to the striking increase in phagocytosis which they induce. High titred antibodies to the streptolysin O exotoxin (ASO) are indicative of recent streptococcal infection. The erythrogenic toxin elaborated by strains which give rise to scarlet fever is neutralized by antibody and the erythematous intradermal reaction to the injected toxin is only seen in individuals lacking antibody (Dick reaction).

Virulent forms of staphylococci, of which *S. aureus* is perhaps the most common, resist phagocytosis. This may be due partly to capsule formation *in vivo* and partly to the elaboration of factors such as protein A which combines with the Fc portion of IgG (except for subclass IgG3) and inhibits binding to the polymorph Fc receptor. *S. aureus* is readily phagocytosed in the presence of adequate amounts of antibody but a small proportion of the ingested bacteria survive and they are difficult organisms to eliminate completely. Where the infection is inadequately controlled, severe lesions may occur in the immunized host as a consequence of type IV delayed hypersensitivity reactions. Thus, staphylococci were found to be avirulent when injected into mice passively immunized with antibody but caused extensive tissue damage in animals previously given sensitized T-cells (Glynn).

Other examples where antibodies are required to overcome the inherently anti-phagocytic properties of bacterial capsules are seen in immunity to infection by pneumococci, meningococci and *Haemophilus influenzae*. *Bacillus anthrax* possesses an anti-phagocytic capsule composed of a gamma polypeptide of D-glutamic acid but although anti-capsular antibodies effectively promote uptake by polymorphs, the exotoxin is so potent that vaccines are inadequate unless they also stimulate anti-toxin immunity.

IgA produced in genital secretions in response to gonococcal infection appears to be capable of inhibiting the attachment of the organisms, through their pili, to mucosal cells. Nonetheless, such antibody does not protect against reinfection, perhaps due to the ability of gonococcal protease to split IgA dimers, or to the existence of multiple non-cross-reacting serotypes.

ROLE OF CELL-MEDIATED IMMUNITY (CMI)

Some strains of bacteria such as the tubercle and leprosy bacilli, and listeria and brucella organisms, are able to live and continue their growth within the cytoplasm of macrophages after their uptake by phagocytosis. In an elegant series of experiments, Mackaness has demonstrated the importance of CMI reactions for the killing of these intracellular facultative parasites and the establishment of an immune state. Animals infected with moderate doses of *M. tuberculosis* overcome the infection and are immune to subsequent challenge with the bacillus. Surprisingly, if they are given an unrelated organism such as *Listeria monocytogenes* at *the same time* as the second infection with tubercle bacillus, they are resistant and can kill the listeria which have been engulfed by macrophages. Without the prior immunity to *M. tuberculosis* or the second challenge with this organism, the animal would have succumbed to listeria infection. In the same way, an animal immune to listeria can rapidly kill tubercle bacilli given at the same time as a second infection with listeria (table 7.2). Thus the triggering of a specific secondary immune response to one organism may endow the animal with a simultaneous but transient non-specific resistance to unrelated microbes of similar growth habits.

Immunity—both specific and non-specific—can be transferred to a normal recipient with lymphocytes but not macrophages or serum from an immune animal (figure 7.7). This strongly suggests that the specific immunity is mediated by T-cells. In support of this view is the greater susceptibility to infection with tubercle and leprosy bacilli of mice in which the T-lymphocytes have been depressed by thymectomy plus antilymphocyte serum. In human leprosy,

TABLE 7.2. Induction of non-specific immunity by a CMI reaction

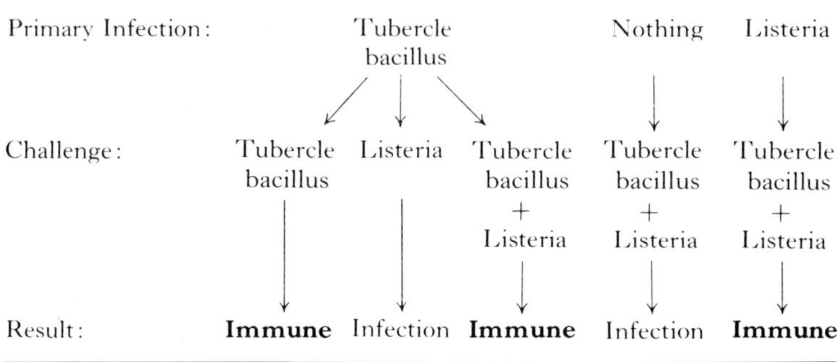

Primary Infection:	Tubercle bacillus	Tubercle bacillus	Tubercle bacillus	Nothing	Listeria
Challenge:	Tubercle bacillus	Listeria	Tubercle bacillus + Listeria	Tubercle bacillus + Listeria	Tubercle bacillus + Listeria
Result:	**Immune**	Infection	**Immune**	Infection	**Immune**

the disease presents as a spectrum ranging from the *tuberculoid* form with few viable organisms, to the *lepromatous* form characterized by an abundance of *Mycobacterium leprae* within the macrophages. As Turk has emphasized, the tuberculoid state is associated with an active T-lymphocyte system giving good PHA transformation of lymphocytes and cell-mediated dermal hypersensitivity responses, although still not good enough to completely eradicate the bacilli. In the lepromatous form, there is poor T-cell reactivity and the paracortical areas in the lymph nodes are depleted of lymphocytes although there are numerous plasma cells which contribute to a high level of circulating antibody. Clearly CMI rather than humoral immunity is important for the control of the leprosy bacillus.

The non-specific immunity to intracellular facultative bacteria described above can be induced by any cell-mediated hypersensitivity reaction. For example, guinea-pigs previously sensitized with bovine γ-globulin (BGG) in complete Freund's adjuvant, are resistant to challenge with brucella given at the same time as BGG. Animals also show non-specific immunity to such organisms during a graft vs. host reaction (cf. p. 260).

The intracellular organisms survive because they are able to thwart the killing mechanisms of the host macrophage. During a CMI reaction when sensitized T-lymphocytes are stimulated by contact with specific antigen, one of the many soluble factors released (e.g. MAF—p. 78) confers on these macrophages the power to kill the ingested organisms and it may be relevant to note that the oxygen-dependent microbicidal systems of such cells are enhanced. Thus the specificity lies at the level of the initial reaction of T-cell with its antigen; the non-specific immunity arises from the newly

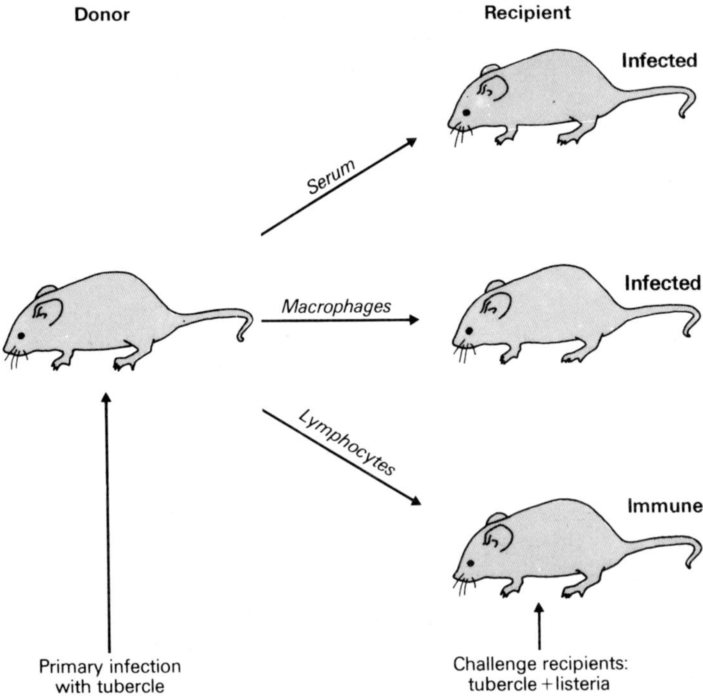

FIGURE 7.7. Transfer of specific and non-specific immunity by lymphocytes from an immune animal. The syngeneic recipient of the lymphocytes resisted simultaneous challenge with tubercle and listeria organisms. The recipients were not immune to listeria given without the tubercle. The lymphocytes lost their power to confer passive immunity on the recipients if treated with a cytotoxic anti-T cell serum plus complement prior to injection. Serum or macrophages were ineffective in transferring immunity (after Mackaness).

acquired ability of the macrophage to kill almost *any* organism it has phagocytosed (figure 7.8). Macrophages taken from animals with graft vs. host reactions where the grafted T-lymphocytes react against the host appear to be very active when examined *in vitro;* these 'angry' macrophages have very motile cytoplasmic processes and show well-developed intracellular granules. Similar changes have been induced in ordinary macrophage cultures treated with lymphokine preparations obtained by incubating sensitized T-cells with antigen.

Where the host has difficulty in effectively eliminating such organisms, the chronic CMI response to locally released antigen leads to the accumulation of densely packed macrophages which release fibrogenic factors and stimulate the formation of granulation tissue and ultimately fibrosis. The

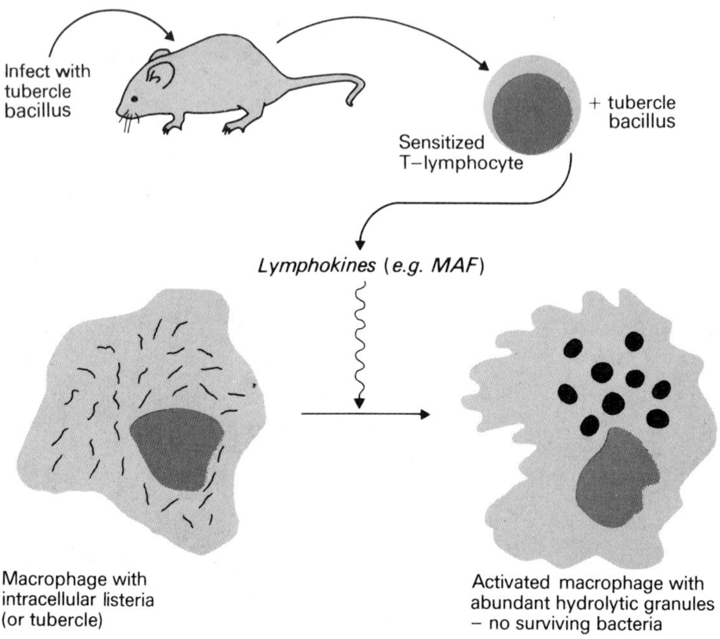

FIGURE 7.8. Macrophage killing of intracellular bacteria triggered by specific cell-mediated immunity reaction.

resulting structure, termed a granuloma, represents an attempt by the body to isolate a site of persistent infection.

Immunity to viral infection

Genetically controlled constitutional factors which render a host or certain of his cells non-permissive (i.e. resistant to takeover of their replicative machinery by virus) play a dominant role in influencing the vulnerability of a given individual to infection. Macrophages may readily take up viruses non-specifically and kill them. However, in some instances the macrophages allow replication and if the virus is capable of producing cytopathic effects in various organs, the infection may be lethal; with non-cytopathic agents such as lymphocytic choriomeningitis, Aleutian mink disease and equine infectious anaemia viruses, a persistent infection will result.

PROTECTION BY SERUM ANTIBODY

The antibody molecule can neutralize viruses by a variety of means. It may stereochemically inhibit combination with the receptor site on cells thereby preventing penetration and subsequent intracellular multiplication, the protective effect of antibodies to influenza viral neuraminidase providing a good example. It may lyse a virus particle directly through activation of the classical complement pathway or lead to aggregation, enhanced phagocytosis and intracellular death by mechanisms already discussed.

Relatively low concentrations of circulating antibody can be effective and one is familiar with the protection afforded by poliomyelitis antibodies, and by human γ-globulin given prophylactically to individuals exposed to measles. The most clear-cut protection is seen in diseases with long incubation times where the virus has to travel through the blood stream before it reaches the tissue which it finally infects. For example, in poliomyelitis the virus gains access to the body via the gastrointestinal tract and eventually passes through the circulation to reach the brain cells which become infected. Within the blood, the virus is neutralized by quite low levels of specific antibody while the prolonged period before the virus infects the brain allows time for a secondary immune response in a primed host.

LOCAL FACTORS

With other viral diseases, such as influenza and the common cold, there is a short incubation time related to the fact that the final target organ for the virus is the same as the portal of entry and no intermediate stage involving passage through the body occurs. There is little time for a primary antibody response to be mounted and in all likelihood the rapid production of interferon is the most significant mechanism used to counter the viral infection. Experimental studies certainly indicate that after an early peak of interferon production, there is a rapid fall in the titre of live virus in the lungs of mice infected with influenza (figure 7.9). Antibody, as assessed by the *serum* titre, seems to arrive on the scene much too late to be of value in aiding recovery. However, recent investigations have shown that antibody levels may be elevated in the *local* fluids bathing the infected surfaces, e.g. nasal mucosa and lung, despite low serum titres and it is the production of antiviral antibody (most prominently IgA) by locally deployed immunologically primed cells which may prove to be of great importance for the *prevention* of subsequent infection. Unfortunately, in so far as the common cold is concerned,

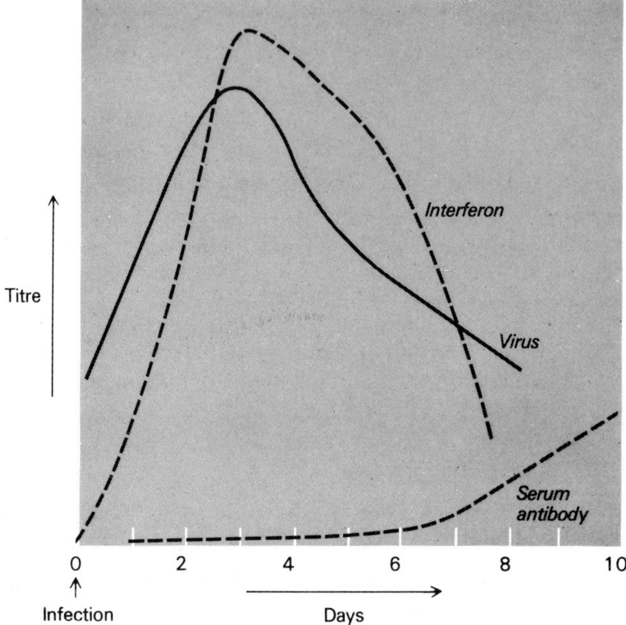

FIGURE 7.9. Appearance of inteferon and serum antibody in relation to recovery from influenza virus infection of the lungs of mice (from Isaacs A., *New Scientist* 1961, **11**, 81).

a subsequent infection is likely to involve an antigenically unrelated virus so that general immunity to colds is difficult to achieve.

CELL-MEDIATED IMMUNITY

Local or systemic antibodies can block the spread of cytolytic viruses but alone they are usually inadequate to control those viruses which modify the antigens of the cell membrane and bud off from the surface as infectious particles. Included in this group are: oncorna (=oncogenic RNA virus, e.g. murine leukaemogenic), orthomyxo (influenza), paramyxo (mumps, measles), toga (dengue), rhabdo (rabies), arena (lymphocytic choriomeningitis), adeno, herpes (simplex, varicella zoster, cytomegalo, Epstein-Barr, Marek's disease), pox (vaccinia), papova (SV40, polyoma) and rubella viruses. The importance of cell-mediated immunity for recovery from infection with these agents is underlined by the inability of children with primary T-cell immunodeficiency to cope with such viruses whereas patients with Ig deficiency but intact cell-mediated immunity are not troubled in this way.

T-lymphocytes from a sensitized host are directly cytotoxic to cells infected with viruses from this group, the new surface antigens on the target cells being recognized by specific receptors on the aggressor lymphocytes. Strikingly, these lymphocytes are not cytotoxic for cells infected with the same virus but carrying different major histocompatibility antigens (cf. figure 9.16, p. 280). The sensitized T-cells must therefore recognize (a) virally modified histocompatibility antigen, (b) a complex of histocompatibility antigen with virally associated antigen, or (c) *both* virally associated *and* self-histocompatibility antigens.

This direct attack on the cell will effectively limit the infection if the surface antigen changes appear before full replication of the virus, otherwise the organism will spread by two major routes. The first, involving free infectious viral particles released by budding from the surface can normally be checked by humoral antibody. The second, which depends upon the passage of virus from one cell to another across intercellular junctions, cannot be influenced by antibody but is countered by cell-mediated immunity. Macrophages, attracted to the site by chemotactic factors released by the interaction of T-cells with virally-associated antigen, appear to discourage the formation of these intercellular bridges, a capability which may be enhanced by other T-cell lymphokines such as macrophage-activating factor. Furthermore, interferon II, produced either by the reacting T-cell itself or by the lymphokine-stimulated macrophage will render the contiguous cells non-permissive for the replication of any virus acquired by intercellular transfer (figure 7.10). It may also increase the non-specific cytotoxicity of NK cells (p. 285) for infected cells. The generation of 'immune interferon' in response to non-nucleic acid viral components provides a valuable back-up mechanism when dealing with viruses which are intrinsically poor stimulators of interferon synthesis.

The neutralization of free virus particles by antibody is relatively straightforward but the interaction with infected cells is rather more complex. Access to the surface antigens by T-cells would be denied were they blocked by coating with antibody. Nonetheless, these antibodies should be able to initiate type II hypersensitivity reactions. Antibody-dependent cell mediated cytotoxicity (ADCC; p. 226) has

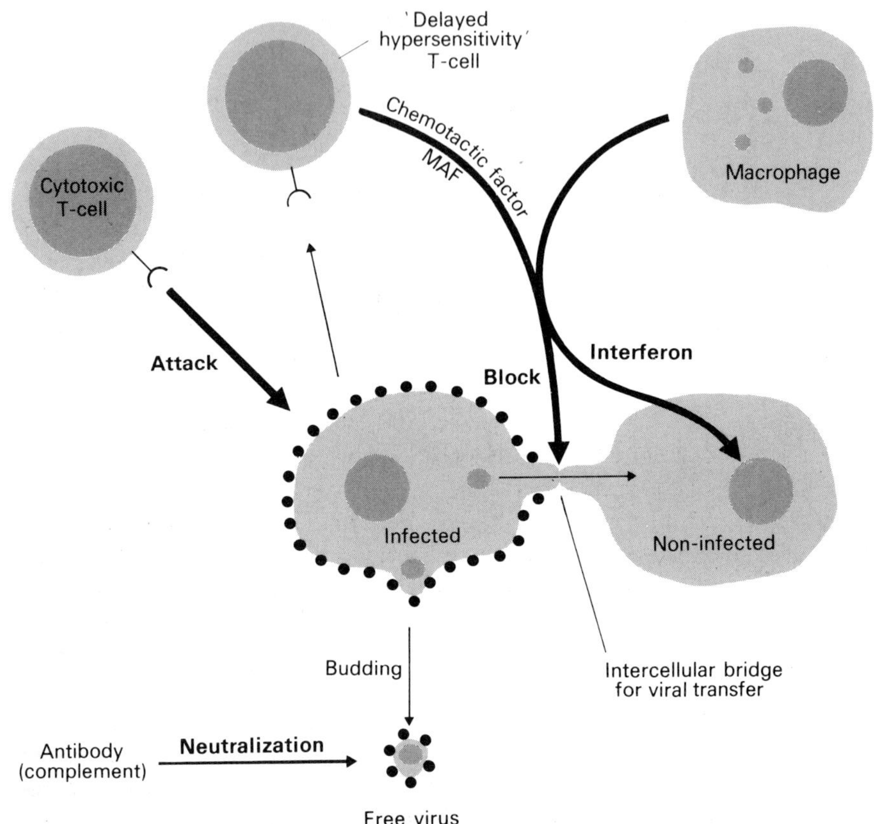

FIGURE 7.10. Control of infection by 'budding', viruses. Cytotoxic T-cells kill virally infected targets directly after recognition of new surface antigen (—●●●—). Interaction with a separate subpopulation of T-cells releases lymphokines which attract macrophages to inhibit intercellular virus transfer and prime contiguous uninfected cells with interferon. Free virus released by budding from the cell surface is neutralized by antibody (which if thymus-dependent points to yet another contribution by the T-cell to viral immunity).

been reported with herpes and mumps-infected target cells while Oldstone has described the complement-mediated killing of measles infected cells by $F(ab')_2$ antibody fragments via the alternative pathway (? suggesting a role for the C_{H1} domain as an initiator of this sequence). Antibody may play a different tune, however, since in the case of measles-infected cells, although 10^6 antibody molecules per cell permit complement-mediated cytotoxicity, 10^5 molecules do not kill but cause capping and shedding of surface antigen (cf. p. 68) leaving the cell resistant to attack by any immunological mechanism.

Immunity to parasitic infections

PROTOZOA

After recovery from parasitic infection, the organisms may be completely eradicated and the host remains solidly immune to reinfection: we speak of a *sterile immunity*. Often the parasites are not completely eliminated but small numbers continue to be harboured even though the host is able to resist superinfection; this state is referred to by parasitologists as *premunition*. The precise immunological mechanisms which operate in premunition are still not completely understood. Neither have the relative roles of humoral antibody or cell-mediated immunity been clearly established in relation to the defence against protozoal parasites. Perhaps the generalization may be made that a humoral response develops when the organisms invade the bloodstream (malaria, trypanosomiasis) whereas CMI is usually elicited by parasites which develop in the tissues (e.g. cutaneous leishmaniasis).

Circulating antibodies have often been shown to offer protection against the blood-borne forms but the parasites can be wily. Thus in toxoplasmosis, although antibody is protective it cannot eliminate the cystic stage; as a result the overt clinical disease is rare but subclinical infection is relatively frequent. In trypanosomiasis and malaria, the parasites escape from the cytocidal action of humoral antibody on their cycling blood forms by the ingenious trick of altering their antigenic constitution. Figure 7.11 illustrates how the trypanosome continues to infect the host, even after fully protective antibodies appear, by *antigenic variation* to a form which these antibodies cannot inactivate; as antibodies to the new antigens are synthesized, the parasite escapes again by changing to yet a further variant and so on. This may explain why in hyperendemic areas, children are subjected to repeated attacks of malaria for their first few years and are then solidly immune to further infection. Immunity must presumably be developed against all the antigenic variants before full protection can be attained, and indeed it is known that IgG from individuals with solid immunity can effectively terminate malaria infections in young children. Despite this problem of antigenic variation, recent experiments with monkeys have raised hopes that a human malaria vaccine may be a real possibility.

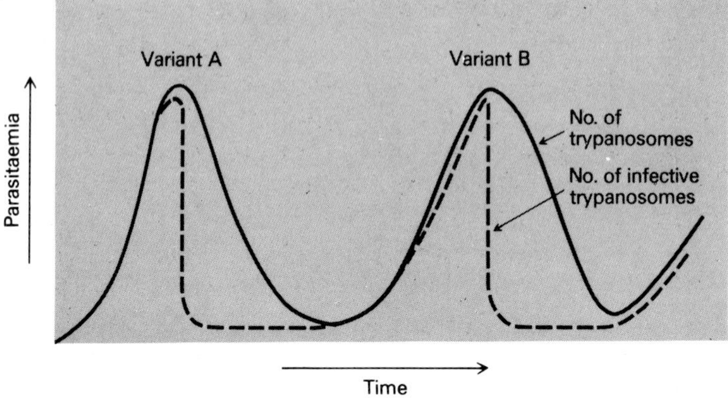

FIGURE 7.11. Antigenic variation during chronic trypanosome infection. As antibody to the initial variant A is formed, the blood trypanosomes become complexed prior to phagocytosis and are no longer infective leaving a small number of viable parasites which have acquired a new antigenic constitution. This new variant (B) now multiplies until it, too, is neutralized by the primary antibody response and is succeeded by variant C (after Gray A.R., see further reading list).

Trypanosoma cruzi, the organism producing Chagas' disease, may survive after ingestion by macrophages; activation of the macrophages by lymphokines stimulates the formation of hydrogen peroxide and leads to intracellular execution within 48 hours. Cell-mediated immunity is directly concerned in the recovery from certain forms of leishmaniasis but studies on laboratory models have not so far defined all the factors involved. For example, cultured guinea pig macrophages activated by the Mackaness phenomenon so that they non-specifically kill ingested listeria (cf. p. 185), take up *Leishmania enrietti* and allow the organisms to grow. Similarly, activated mouse macrophages which have ingested *Toxoplasma gondii* allow growth through a failure to effect lysosome fusion with the phagosome containing the organism. Almost certainly a further antigen-specific factor, probably antibody, is required to help the macrophage deal with the parasite; in other words the simple idea that a non-specifically activated macrophage will always kill *any* organism growing within its cytoplasm is going to need some amendment.

HELMINTHS

A marked feature of the immune reaction to helminthic infections such as *Trichinella spiralis* in man and *Nippostrongylus brasiliensis* in the rat is the high level of homocytotropic (reaginic) antibody produced. In man serum levels of IgE can rise from normal values of around 100 ng/ml to as high as 10,000 ng/ml. This exceptional increase has encouraged the view that IgE represents an important line of defence. One suggestion is that histamine released by contact of antigen with IgE-coated mast cells can aid the expulsion of the worm from the gut. Another view is that such a local anaphylactic reaction may lead to exudation of serum proteins known to contain high concentrations of protective antibodies in all the major immunoglobulin classes. Certainly IgE-mediated release of eosinophil chemotactic factor (cf. figure 7.6) would attract these cells which are known to bind to antibody coated nematodes. Transfer studies in rats (Ogilvie) have shown that although antibody produces some damage to the worms, cells lacking surface Ig from *immune* donors are required for vigorous expulsion. It is of interest that schistosomules have been killed in cultures containing both specific IgG and eosinophils, which are acting as effectors in a form of antibody-dependent cell-mediated cytotoxicity (figure 7.12); after 12 hours or so, the granules release the major basic protein forming its electron-dense core onto the parasite and this presumably is the agent of destruction. Further evidence for an involvement of this

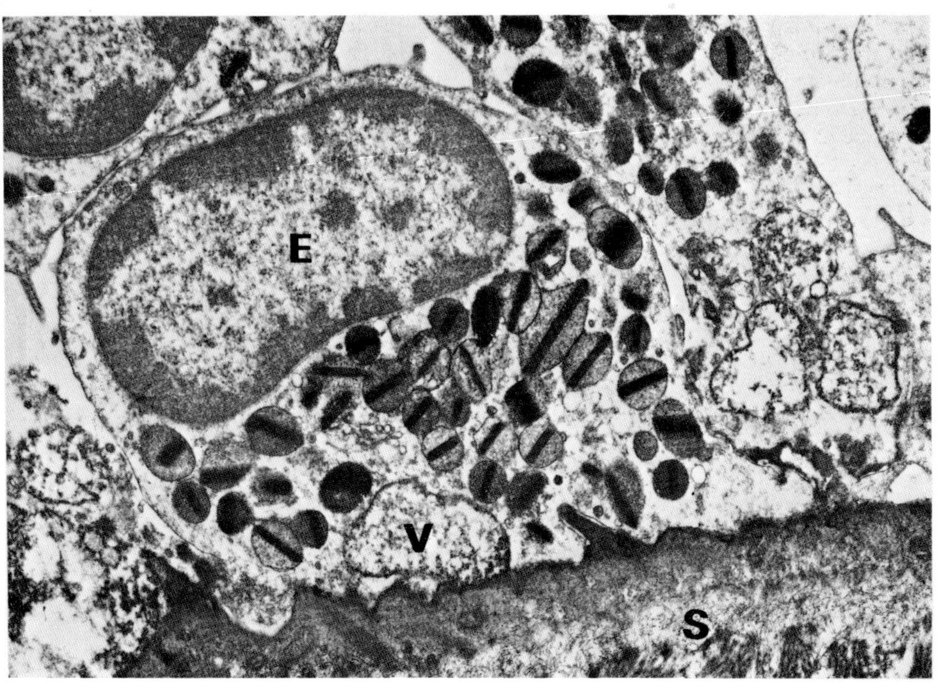

FIGURE 7.12. Electron micrograph showing an eosinophil (E) attached to the surface of a schistosomulum (S) in the presence of specific antibody. The cell develops large vacuoles (V) which appear to release their contents onto the parasite (x 16,500). (Courtesy of Drs. D.J. McLaren & C.D. Mackenzie.)

cell comes from the experiment in which the protection afforded by passive transfer of antiserum *in vivo* was blocked by pretreatment of the recipient with an antieosinophil serum.

Schistosomiasis presents another intriguing feature. The adult worm lives permanently within the mesenteric vessels of the host, despite the fact that the blood which bathes it contains antibodies which can prevent a second infection. Smithers and Terry have shown that the parasites make themselves resistant to these immune processes by disguising themselves with an outer coat of the host's antigens, either by direct acquisition or possibly through synthesis by the parasite itself as a form of antigenic 'mimicry'.

Prophylaxis

The control of infection is approached from several directions. One method of breaking the chain of infection has been achieved in the U.K. with rabies and psittacosis by controlling the importation of dogs and parrots respectively. Improvements in public health—water supply, sewerage systems, education in personal hygiene—prevent the spread of cholera and many other diseases. And of course when other measures fail we can fall back on the induction of immunity.

PASSIVELY ACQUIRED IMMUNITY

Temporary protection against infection can be established by giving preformed antibody from another individual of the same or a different species. As the acquired antibodies are utilized by combination with antigen or catabolized in the normal way, this protection is gradually lost.

Homologous antibodies

Maternal. In the first few months of life while the baby's own lymphoid system is slowly getting under way, protection is afforded by maternally derived antibodies acquired by placental transfer and by intestinal absorption of colostral immunoglobulins.

γ-Globulin. Preparations of pooled human adult γ-globulin are of value to modify the effects of chicken pox or measles, particularly in individuals with defective immune responses such as premature infants, children with primary immunodeficiency or protein malnutrition or patients on steroid treatment. Contacts with cases of infectious hepatitis and smallpox may also be afforded protection by γ-globulin, especially when in the latter case the material is derived from the serum of individuals vaccinated some weeks previously. Human anti-tetanus immunoglobulin is preferable to horse antitoxin which can cause serum reactions.

Isolated γ-globulin preparations tend to form small aggregates spontaneously and these can lead to severe anaphylactic reactions when administered intravenously on account of their ability to aggregate platelets and to activate complement and generate C3a and C5a anaphylatoxins. For this reason the material is always injected intramuscularly. Preparations free of aggregates would be welcome as would separate pools with raised antibody titres to selected organisms such as vaccinia, *Herpes zoster*, tetanus and perhaps rubella. This need will ultimately be satisfied when it becomes possible to produce human monoclonal antibodies on demand.

Heterologous antibodies

Horse globulins containing anti-tetanus and anti-diphtheria toxins have been extensively employed prophylactically, but at the present time the practice is more restricted because of the complication of serum sickness developing in response to the foreign protein. This is more likely to occur in subjects already sensitized by previous contact with horse globulin; thus individuals who have been given horse anti-tetanus (e.g. for immediate protection after receiving a wound out in the open) are later advised to undergo a course of active immunization to obviate the need for further injections of horse protein in any subsequent emergency.

ACTIVE IMMUNIZATION

In the case of tetanus, immunization is of benefit to the individual but not to the community since it will not eliminate the organism which is formed in the faeces of domestic animals and persists in the soil as highly resistant spores. Where a disease depends on human transmission, immunity in just a proportion of the population can help the whole community if it leads to a fall in the reproduction rate (i.e. the number of further cases produced by each infected individual) to less than one; under these circumstances the disease will die out, witness for example the disappearance of diphtheria from communities in which around 75% of the children have been immunized.

The objective of vaccination is to provide effective immunity by establishing adequate levels of antibody and a primed population of cells which can rapidly expand on renewed contact with antigen. The first contact with antigen during vaccination obviously should not be injurious and the manoeuvre is to modify the pathogenic effect without losing important antigens:

(a) *Toxoids.* Bacterial exotoxins such as those produced by diphtheria and tetanus bacilli can be successfully detoxified by formaldehyde treatment without destroying the major immunogenic determinants (figure 7.13). Immunization with the *toxoid* will therefore provoke the formation of protective antibodies which neutralize the toxin by stereochemically blocking the active site and encourage removal by phagocytic cells. The toxoid is generally given after adsorption to aluminium hydroxide which acts as an adjuvant and produces higher antibody titres.

(b) *Killed organisms.* Dead bacteria and viruses which have been inactivated provide a safe antigen for immunization. Examples are typhoid (in combination with the relatively ineffective paratyphoid A and B), cholera and killed poliomyelitis (Salk) vaccines. The success of the Salk vaccine was slightly marred by a small rise in the incidence and deaths from poliomyelitis in 1960–1 (figure 7.14) but this has now been attributed to poor antigenicity of one of the three different strains of virus used and present-day vaccines are

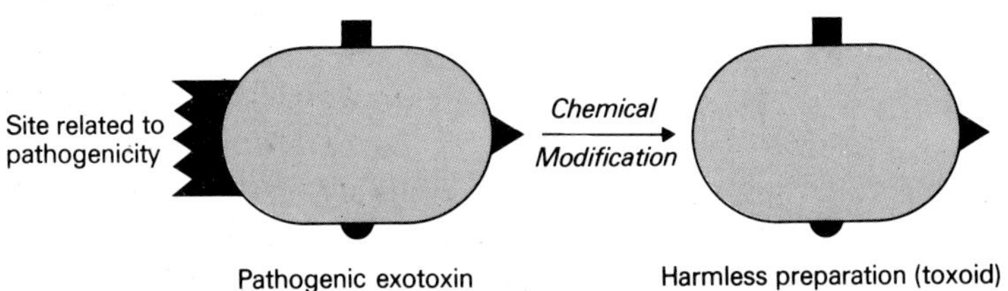

FIGURE 7.13. Modification of toxin to harmless toxoid without losing many of the antigenic determinants (■▲▲). Thus antibodies to the toxoid will react well with the original toxin. Utilizing a similar principle, micro-organisms can be rendered harmless by killing or attenuating to non-virulent but still living forms.

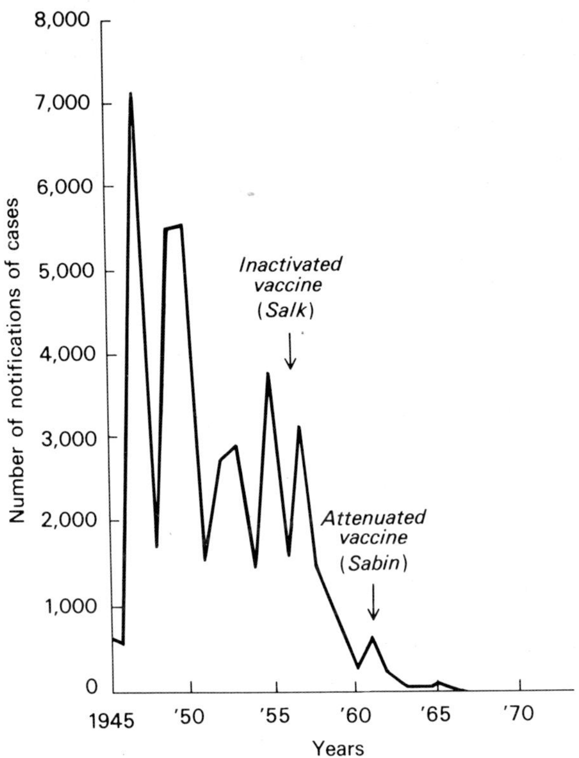

FIGURE 7.14. Notifications of paralytic poliomyelitis in England and Wales showing the beneficial effects of community immunization with killed and live vaccines. (Reproduced from 'Immunisation' by G. Dick, 1978, Update Books; with kind permission of author and publishers.)

far more potent. In other instances, the immunity conferred by killed vaccines, even when given with adjuvant (see below), is often inferior to that resulting from infection with live organisms. This must be partly because the replication of the living microbes confronts the host with a larger and more sustained dose of antigen and that with budding viruses, infected cells are required for the establishment of good cytotoxic T-cell memory. Another significant advantage is that the immune response takes place largely at the site of the natural infection. As an example cholera infection will be most efficiently dealt with by antibodies produced locally by the gut wall ('copro-antibodies') yet injected *killed* vaccine may stimulate antibody synthesis in the spleen and perhaps many lymph nodes without initiating an adequate response in the intestinal lymphoid system. Ideally immunity would be best established by infection with a modified but live (attenuated) form of cholera bacillus which would multiply at the site of the natural infection without producing disease. This is well illustrated by the nasopharyngeal IgA response to immunization with polio vaccine. In contrast with the ineffectiveness of parenteral injection of killed vaccine, intranasal administration evoked a good local antibody response; but whereas this declined over a period of 2 months or so, per oral immunization with *live attenuated* virus established a persistently high IgA antibody level (figure 7.15).

(c) *Attenuated organisms.* Pasteur first achieved the production of live but non-virulent forms of chicken cholera bacillus and anthrax by such artifices as culture at higher temperatures and under anaerobic conditions, and was able to confer immunity by infection with the attenuated organisms. A virulent strain of *Mycobacterium tuberculosis* became attenuated by chance in 1908 when Calmette and Guérin at the Institut Pasteur, Lille, added bile to the culture medium in an attempt to achieve dispersed growth. After 13 years of culture in bile-containing medium, the strain remained attenuated and was used successfully to vaccinate children against tuberculosis. The same organism, BCG (Bacille, Calmette, Guérin), is widely used today for immunization of tuberculin negative individuals; it may

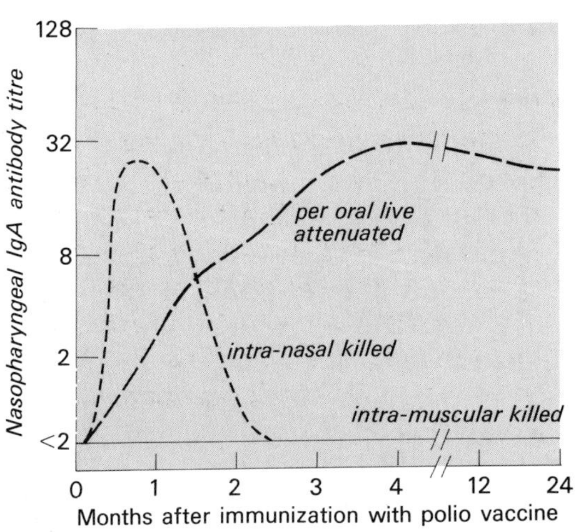

FIGURE 7.15. Local IgA response to polio vaccine. Local secretory antibody synthesis is confined to the specific anatomical sites which have been directly stimulated by contact with antigen. (Data from Ogra *et al.* in 'Viral Immunology & Immunopathology', p. 67. Ed: Notkins. Acad. Press 1975).

also bestow a reasonable degree of protection against *Mycobacterium leprae.*

Attenuated vaccines for poliomyelitis (Sabin), measles and rubella have gained general acceptance. The earlier inactivated measles vaccines produced an incomplete immunity which left the individual susceptible to the development of immunopathological complications on subsequent natural infection, but this is no longer the case with the more effective attenuated live strains currently employed. The technique of genetic recombination is being used to generate various attenuated strains of influenza virus with lower virulence for man, with temperature sensitivity (e.g. no replication at 37° in the lower respiratory tract and impaired growth at 32–34° in the upper respiratory tract) and with an increased multiplication rate in eggs (enabling newly endemic strains of influenza to be adapted for rapid vaccine production). A new approach termed 'infection permissive immunization' utilizes parenteral administration of a recombinant virus which bears the relevant neuraminidase (which has to bind to the cell before infection is possible) but an irrelevant haemagglutinin (the antigen which binds to red cells): the partial immunity so produced still permits natural infection but prevents the development of disease, and it is anticipated that this process will establish an effective resistance to subsequent contact with the virus.

Adjuvants

For practical and economic reasons prophylactic immunization should involve the minimum number of injections and the least amount of antigen. We have referred to the undoubted advantages of replicating attenuated organisms in this respect but non-living organisms frequently require an adjuvant which by definition is a substance incorporated into or injected simultaneously with antigen which potentiates the immune response (*L* adjuvare—to help). The mode of action of adjuvants may be considered under several headings:

(i) *Depot effects.* Free antigen usually disperses rapidly from the local tissues draining the injection site and an important function of the so-called repository adjuvants is to counteract this by providing a long-lived reservoir of antigen, either at an extracellular location or within macrophages. The most common adjuvants of this type used in man are aluminium compounds (phosphate and hydroxide) and Freund's incomplete adjuvant (in which the antigen is incorporated in the aqueous phase of a stabilized water in paraffin oil emulsion). Both types increase the antibody response but the emulsions tend to produce higher and far more sustained antibody levels with a broadening of the response to include more of the epitopes in the antigen preparation. Because of the life-long persistence of oil in the tissues and the occasional production of sterile abscesses, attention has been focused on the replacement of incomplete Freund's with a new biodegradable formulation, Adjuvant 65, which contains highly refined peanut oil and chemically pure mannide monooleate and aluminium monostearate as emulsifier and stabilizer respectively. Claims that antibody titres are comparable to those obtained with Freund's and no long-term adverse effects in man have yet been encountered must be treated with caution.

(ii) *Macrophage activation.* Under the influence of the repository adjuvants, macrophages form granulomata which provide sites for interaction with antibody-forming cells. The maintenance by the depot of consistent antigen concentrations, particularly on the macrophage surface, ensures that as antigen-sensitive cells divide within the granuloma, their progeny are highly likely to be further stimulated by antigen. Virtually all adjuvants stimulate macrophages, the majority probably through direct action, but complete Freund's adjuvant appears to act on the macrophage through the T-cell (cf. p. 94; it will be recalled that complete Freund's is made from the incomplete adjuvant by addition of killed mycobacterium, or more recently the water soluble muramyl dipeptide, MDP, isolated from its active components). The activated macrophages are thought to act by improving immunogenicity through an increase in the amount of antigen on their surface and the efficiency of its presentation to lymphocytes, by the provision of accessory signals to direct lymphocytes towards an immune response rather than tolerance, and by the secretion of soluble stimulatory factors (e.g. lymphocyte activating factor, LAF) which influence the proliferation of lymphocytes.

(iii) *Specific effects on lymphocytes.* The immunopotentiating and other effects of the mycobacterial component in complete Freund are so striking that their use in man is not normally countenanced; enhancement of T-cell function is seen in helper activity, delayed type hypersensitivity and the production of autoimmune disease. In man, BCG is a potent stimulator of T,B and reticuloendothelial cell activity. Levamisole boosts delayed hypersensitivity while polyanions such as poly A:U, and the fungal polysaccharide lentinan, promote T-helper cells. By contrast, bacterial lipopolysaccharide and polyanions such as dextran sulphate are B-cell mitogens with a preferential effect on Bμ cells.

Although the role of modulatory leucocyte mediators such as transfer factor and interferon in these interactions is unclear, it is of interest that polylysine stabilized poly-I:C, which produces good interferon levels in primates, is said to be an effective adjuvant for immunization to influenza virus.

(iv) *Anti-tumour action.* This will be discussed in chapter 9 but one may summarize by saying that the major effect is mediated through a cytostatic action of activated macrophages on tumours with the stimulation of specific T-cell immunity to the tumour antigens as a further possibility.

Recent interest has centred on the use of small lipid membrane vesicles (liposomes) as agents for the presentation of antigen to the immune system. It may be that the liposome acts as a storage vacuole within the macrophage or perhaps fuses with the macrophage membrane to provide a suitably immunogenic complex. One envisages the possibility of selecting the type of lymphocyte activated by incorporating accessory signalling agents into the liposome membrane, e.g. MDP derivatives, polyanions or levamisole to stimulate T-cells, components of ascaris or *Bordetella pertussis* to exaggerate IgE production, T-cell soluble factors for the triggering of Bγ cells, C3b for homing to lymph node follicles and so on.

Some general problems

Vigorous public health immunization programmes have virtually eliminated diseases like diphtheria and poliomyelitis from many communities (figures 7.14 & 7.16), while a global effort by the World Health Organisation combining widespread vaccination and selective epidemiological control methods, has eradicated smallpox. With certain vaccines there is a very small, but still real, risk of developing complications such as the encephalitis which can occur following rabies or measles immunization. With live viral vaccines there is a possibility that the nucleic acid might be incorporated into the host's genome or that the strain

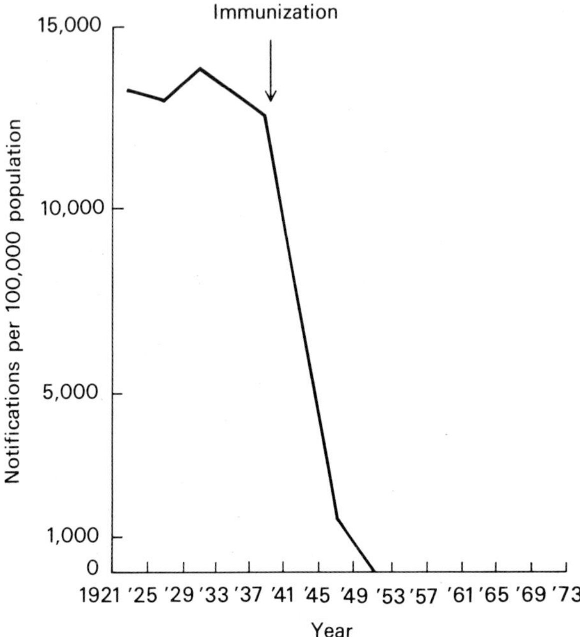

FIGURE 7.16. Notifications of diphtheria in England and Wales per 100,000 population showing dramatic fall after immunization. (Reproduced from '*Immunisation*' by G. Dick, Update Books with kind permission of author and publishers.)

may revert to a virulent form, although to some extent this latter eventuality can be countered by injection of appropriate antiserum. Another disadvantage of attenuated strains is the difficulty and expense of maintaining appropriate cold storage facilities. In diseases such as viral hepatitis and cancer, the dangers associated with live vaccines would make their use unthinkable. Generally speaking, the risk of complication must be balanced against the expected chance of contracting the disease. Where this is minimal some may prefer to avoid general vaccination and to rely upon a crash course backed up if necessary by passive immunization in the localities around isolated outbreaks of infectious disease.

It is important to recognize those children with immunodeficiency before injection of live organisms; a child with impaired T-cell reactivity can become overwhelmed by BCG and die. Perhaps this is only a sick story, but it is said that in one particular country there are no adults with T-cell deficiency. The reason? All children had been immunized with live BCG as part of a community health programme(!)

The extent to which children with partial deficiencies are at risk has yet to be assessed. It is also inadvisable to give live vaccines to patients being treated with steroids, immunosuppressive drugs or radiotherapy or who have malignant conditions such as lymphoma and leukaemia; pregnant mothers must also be included here because of the vulnerability of the foetus.

A worrying feature of immunization with viruses grown on monkey kidney culture is the presence of simian viruses which could be potentially oncogenic; SV-40, for example, is known to cause transformation of human cells in culture. More attention is being paid to the use of human diploid cell lines as viral hosts in the hope that this will limit the risk of oncogenic virus contamination.

One should mention the difficulty in producing adequate vaccines for respiratory viruses because of the multitude of antigenic variants which arise. Problems stemming from the competition of several antigens used concurrently in multiple vaccines, and the possible deviating influence of maternally derived antibody have been discussed in earlier chapters.

Primary immunodeficiency

In accord with the dictum that 'most things that can go wrong, do', a multiplicity of immunodeficiency states in man have been recognized. These are classified in table 7.3 together with some of the most clear-cut (and correspondingly rare) examples. We have earlier stressed the manner in which the interplay of complement, antibody and phagocytic cells constitutes the basis of a tripartite defence mechanism against pyogenic (pus-forming) infections with bacteria which require prior opsonization before phagocytosis. It is not surprising then, that deficiency in any one of these factors may predispose the individual to repeated infections of this type. Patients with T-cell deficiency of course present a markedly different pattern of infection, being susceptible to those viruses and moulds which are normally eradicated by cell-mediated immunity.

A relatively high incidence of malignancies and of autoantibodies with or without autoimmune disease, have been documented in patients with immunodeficiency but the reason for this association is not yet clear, although failure

TABLE 7.3. Classification of immunodeficiency states with examples

Deficiency	Example	Immune Response		Infection	Treatment
		Humoral	Cellular		
Complement	C3 deficiency	Normal	Normal	Pyogenic bacteria	Antibiotics
Myeloid cell	Chronic granulomatous disease	Normal	Normal	Catalase-positive bacteria	Antibiotics
B-cell	Infantile sex-linked a-γ-globulinaemia (Bruton)	↓↓	Normal	Pyogenic bacteria Pneumocystis carinii	γ-Globulin
T-cell	Thymic hypoplasia (DiGeorge)	↓	↓↓	Certain viruses Candida	Thymus graft
Stem cell	Severe combined deficiency (Swiss-type)	↓↓	↓↓	All the above	Bone marrow graft

of T-cell regulation or inability to control key viral infections are among the suggestions canvassed.

Deficiency of innate immunity

In chronic granulomatous disease the monocytes and polymorphs fail to produce hydrogen peroxide due to a defect in the NADPH oxidase normally activated by phagocytosis. Many bacteria oblige by generating H_2O_2 through their own metabolic processes but if they are catalase positive, the peroxide is destroyed and the bacteria will survive. Thus, polymorphs from these patients readily take up catalase positive staphylococci in the presence of antibody and complement but fail to kill them intracellularly. In Chediak-Higashi disease (what a lovely name!), the lysosomes are structurally and functionally abnormal and the patients suffer from pyogenic infections which can be fatal. Among other rare conditions, myeloperoxidase deficiency is associated with susceptibility to systemic candidiasis, while a defective polymorph response to chemotactic stimuli characterizes the lazy leucocyte syndrome.

Defects in complement, the other major components of the innate immune system, were dealt with in chapter 6.

B-cell deficiency

In Bruton's congenital a-γ-globulinaemia the production of immunoglobulin in affected males is grossly depressed and there are few lymphoid follicles or plasma cells in lymph node biopsies. The children are subject to repeated infection by pyogenic bacteria—*Staphylococcus aureus*, *Streptococcus pyogenes* and *pneumoniae*, *Neisseria meningitidis*, *Haemophilus influenzae*—and by a rare protozoon, *Pneumocystis carinii*, which produces a strange form of pneumonia. Cell-mediated immune responses are normal and viral infections such as measles and smallpox are readily brought under control. Therapy involves repeated administration of human γ-globulin to maintain adequate concentrations of circulating immunoglobulin.

IgA deficiency is encountered with relative frequency and these patients often have detectable antibodies to IgA. It is uncertain whether these antibodies prevented development of the IgA system or whether lack of tolerance resulting from an absent IgA system allowed the body to make antibodies to exogenous determinants immunologically related to IgA.

The most common form of immunodeficiency, late onset hypogammaglobulaemia (also known as common, variable immunodeficiency), probably includes many entities. The marrow contains normal numbers of immature B-cells, but a third of the patients lack circulating B-cells with surface Ig and of the remainder, half have subnormal numbers. Where present they are unable to differentiate to plasma cells in some cases or to secrete antibody in others. T-cells are also affected however; each lymphocyte has a low surface 5-nucleotidase, the T_M cells lack the characteristic non-specific esterase spot, around 30% have poor responses to PHA and a small proportion have marked suppressor activity for B-cells. Thus there are maturation defects in the lymphocyte populations which affect B-cell performance predominantly.

Immunoglobulin deficiency occurs naturally in human infants as the maternal IgG level wanes and may become a serious problem in very premature babies.

T-cell deficiency

The DiGeorge and Nezelof syndromes are characterized by a failure of the thymus to develop properly from the third and fourth pharyngeal pouches during embryogenesis

(DiGeorge children also lack parathyroids and have severe cardiovascular abnormalities). Consequently, stem cells cannot differentiate to become T-lymphocytes and the 'thymus dependent' areas in lymphoid tissue are sparsely populated; in contrast lymphoid follicles are seen but even these are poorly developed (figure 7.17). Cell-mediated immune responses are undetectable and although the infants can deal with common bacterial infections they may be overwhelmed by vaccinia or measles, or by BCG if given by mistake. Humoral antibodies can be elicited but the response is subnormal presumably reflecting the need for the co-operative involvement of T-cells. (The similarity of this condition to neonatal thymectomy and of B-cell deficiency to neonatal bursectomy in the chicken should not go unmentioned.) Treatment by grafting neonatal thymus leads to restoration of immunocompetence but unless graft and donor are well matched, the thymus is ultimately rejected by the ungrateful host cells it has helped to maturity; in any event, some matching between the major histocompatibility antigens on the non-lymphocytic thymus cells and peripheral cells is essential for the proper functioning of the T-lymphocytes (p. 281).

Complete absence of the thymus is pretty rare and more often one is dealing with a 'partial DiGeorge' in which the T-cells may rise from 6% at birth to around 30% of the total circulating lymphocytes by the end of the first year; antibody responses are adequate. Selective T-cell depression can arise from deficiency in the enzyme, purine nucleoside phosphorylase. Their poor T-cell responses make them especially susceptible to infection with varicella and vaccinia viruses but despite having less than 10% circulating T-cells, they have normal B-cell immunity suggesting that T-B collaboration can operate at much lower T-cell levels in the human than in the mouse.

Cell-mediated immunity is depressed in immunodeficient patients with ataxia telangiectasia or with thrombocytopenia and eczema (Wiskott-Aldrich syndrome) and it is of great

FIGURE 7.17. Lymph node cortex. (a) from patient with DiGeorge syndrome showing depleted thymus-dependent area (TDA) and small primary follicles (PF), (b) from normal subject: the populated T-cell area and the well-developed secondary follicle with its mantle of small lymphocytes (M) and pale staining germinal centre (GC) provide a marked contrast. (DiGeorge material kindly supplied by Dr. D. Webster; photograph by Mr. C.J. Sym.)

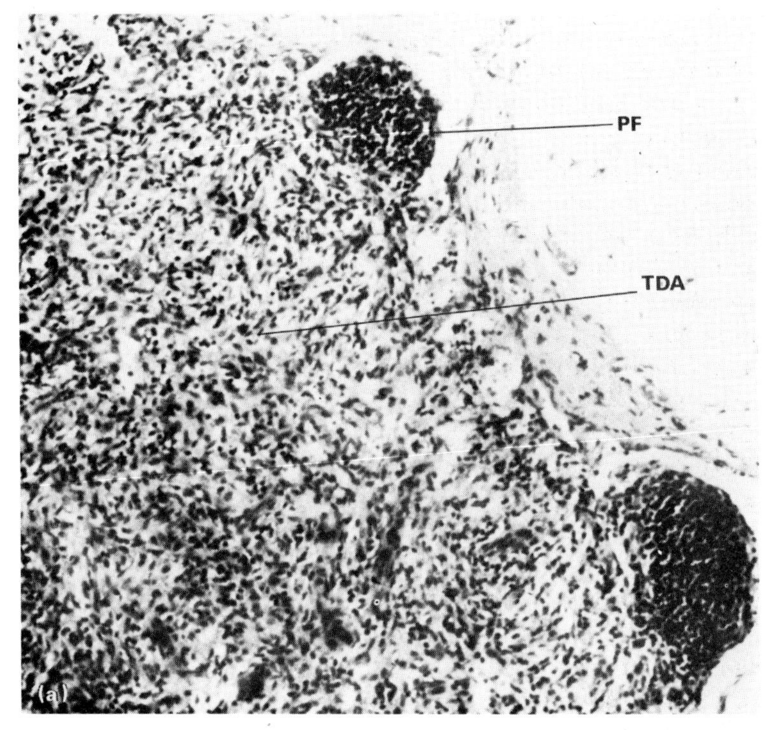
PF
TDA
(a)

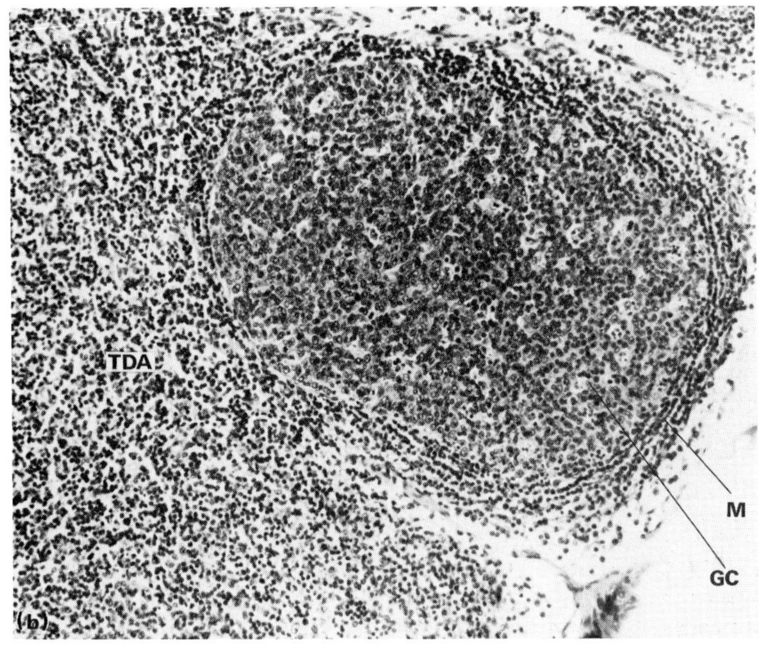
TDA
M
GC
(b)

interest that in both conditions about 10% of the patients so far studied have died of malignancies of the lymphoid system or of epithelial tumours. Wiskott-Aldrich is associated with a low IgM and poor antibody responses to many polysaccharides; evidence that a vital defect in macrophage presentation of antigen underlies the disorder has been presented. The concomitant lack of IgE with IgA may be partly responsible for the greater susceptibility to upper respiratory infections in ataxia telangiectasia as compared with individuals deficient in IgA alone. Treatment by injection of transfer factor has been attempted and some success reported.

Isolated cases of T-cell deficiency have been described where the serum contains a lymphocytotoxic antibody which presumably must be selective for T- rather than B-lymphocytes.

T-cells from some patients with mucocutaneous candidiasis are unable to produce MIF when stimulated *in vitro* and it is conceivable that other selective failures of lymphokine synthesis may be uncovered.

Stem-cell deficiency

Without proper differentiation of the common lymphoid stem cell, both T- and B-lymphocytes will fail to develop and there will be a severe combined immunodeficiency of cellular and humoral responses. Normal immune function can be established in the children by grafting with histocompatible bone marrow from a sibling. Cells from other donors too readily initiate a potentially lethal graft-vs-host reaction (cf. p. 260) even when reasonably well-matched, unless steps are first taken to rid the graft of any immunocompetent T-lymphocytes. Some patients lack the enzyme adenosine deaminase which affects both B- and T-cells but predominantly the latter. Half the patients do well on transfusions of normal red cells containing the enzyme whereas others with a longer-standing more severe deficiency which might have affected the thymus epithelium, also require treatment with thymic extracts (thymosin).

The rapidly fatal variant of severe combined immunodeficiency associated with lack of myeloid cell precursors is termed reticular dysgenesis. An attempt has been made to summarize the cellular basis of the various deficiency states in figure 7.18.

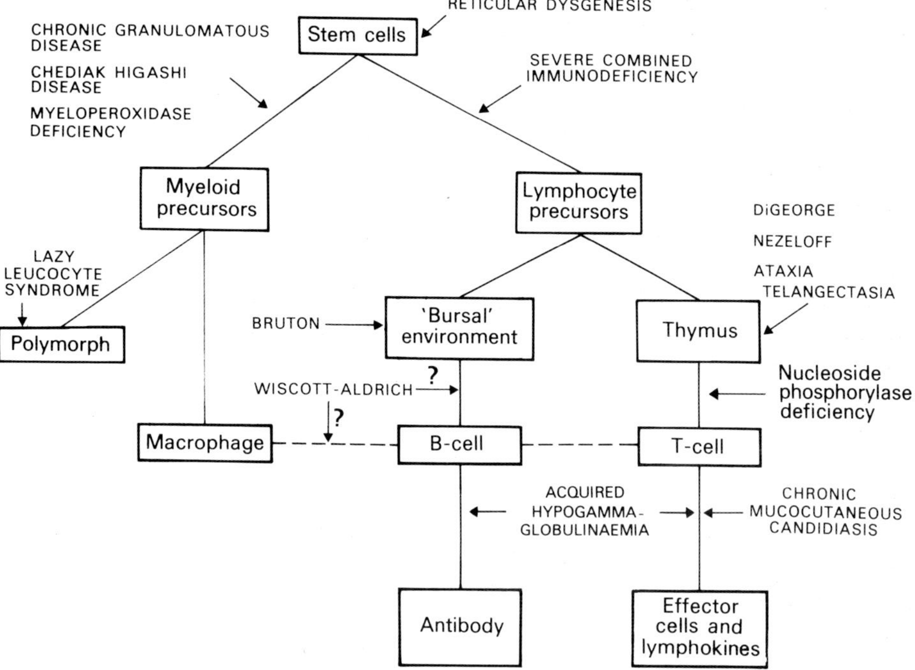

FIGURE 7.18. The cellular basis of immunodeficiency stated. The arrow indicates the cell type or differentiation process which is defective.

Recognition of immunodeficiencies

Defects in immunoglobulins can be assessed by quantitative estimations; levels of 200 mg/100 ml arbitrarily define the practical lower limit of normal. The humoral immune response can be examined by first screening the serum for natural antibodies (A and B isohaemagglutinins, hetero-antibody to sheep red cells, bactericidins against *E. coli*) and then attempting to induce active immunization with diphtheria, tetanus, pertussis and killed poliomyelitis—but no live vaccines.

Patients with T-cell deficiency will be hypo- or unreactive in skin tests to such antigens as tuberculin, candida, tricophytin, streptokinase/streptodornase and mumps. Active skin sensitization with dinitrochlorobenzene may be undertaken. The reactivity of peripheral blood mononuclear cells to phytohaemagglutinin is a good indicator of T-lymphocyte reactivity as is also the one-way mixed lymphocyte reaction (see chapter 9). Enumeration of T-cells is most readily achieved by counting the number of cells forming spontaneous rosettes with sheep erythrocytes (cf. p. 59).

In vitro tests for complement and for the bactericidal and other functions of polymorphs are available while the reduction of nitroblue tetrazolium (NBT) provides a measure of the oxidative enzymes associated with active phagocytosis.

Secondary immunodeficiency

Immune responsiveness can be depressed non-specifically by many factors. Cell-mediated immunity in particular may be impaired in a state of malnutrition even of the degree which may be encountered in urban areas of the more affluent regions of the world. Iron deficiency is particularly important in this respect.

Viral infections are not infrequently immunosuppressive and in the case of measles in man, Newcastle disease in chickens and rinderpest in cattle this has been attributed to a direct cytotoxic effect of virus on the lymphoid cells. In lepromatous leprosy and malarial infection there is evidence for a constraint on immune responsiveness imposed by distortion of the normal lymphoid traffic pathways and additionally, in the latter instance, macrophage function appears to be aberrant. Plasma factors from patients with secondary syphilis which block phytohaemagglutinin transformation of lymphocytes from normal subjects could be responsible for the general reduction in CMI seen in this disease.

Many agents such as X-rays, cytotoxic drugs and corticosteroids, although often used in a non-immunological context, can nonetheless have dire effects on the immune system (p. 271). B-Lymphoproliferative disorders like chronic lymphatic leukaemia, myeloma and Waldenström's macroglobulinaemia are associated with varying degrees of hypo-γ-globulinaemia and impaired antibody responses. Their common infections with pyogenic bacteria contrast with the situation in Hodgkin's disease where the patients display all the hallmarks of defective cell-mediated immunity—susceptibility to tubercle bacillus, brucella, cryptococcus and herpes zoster virus.

Summary

Micro-organisms are kept out of the body by the skin, the secretion of mucous, ciliary action, the lavaging action of bactericidal fluids (e.g. tears), gastric acid and microbial antagonism. If penetration occurs, bacteria are destroyed by soluble factors such as lysozyme and by phagocytosis with intracellular digestion. By activating the alternative complement pathway, phagocytic cells are attracted to the bacteria which adhere to the C3b receptors and are engulfed if they activate the surface of the polymorph. Complement activation also causes mast cell release of a further polymorph chemotactic factor and mediators of vascular permeability which increase the flow of more complement and antibody to the site. The influx of polymorphs and the increase in vascular permeability constitute the potent antimicrobial *acute inflammatory response* (figure 7.19). The antibody molecule is designed as a flexible adaptor to attach to foreign substances which fail to activate the alternative pathway or the surface of the phagocytic cell; the Ig domains fix complement by the classical pathway and stimulate the phagocyte through its Fc receptor.

Humoral immunity to bacteria depends largely upon this opsonizing mechanism of antibody to enhance phagocytosis,

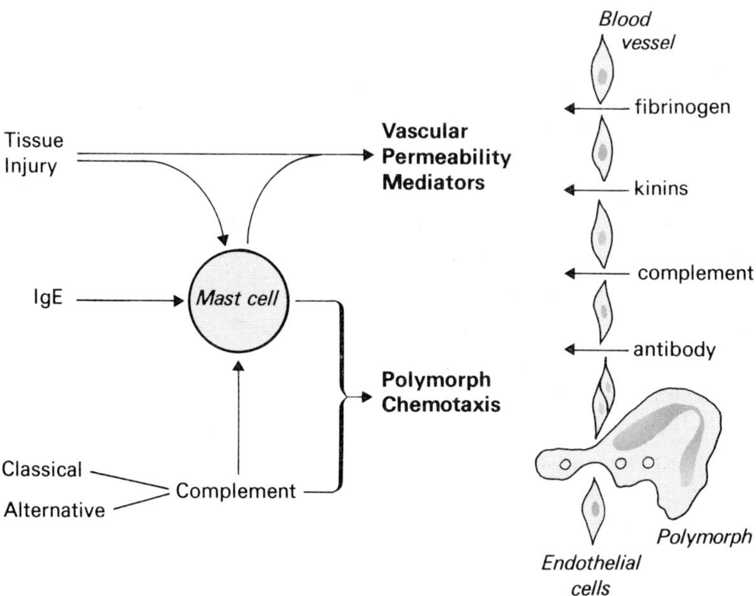

FIGURE 7.19. Production of a protective acute inflammatory reaction by microbes either (i) through tissue injury (e.g. bacterial toxin) or direct activation of the alternative complement pathway or (ii) by antibody-dependent triggering of the classical complement pathway or mast cell degranulation.

the lysis of cells through the terminal complement components plus lysozyme, and the neutralization of bacterial toxins. Intracellular facultative parasites such as the tubercle bacillus can grow happily within the macrophage which only becomes able to kill the organisms it harbours if activated by a lymphokine released by the reaction of sensitized T-cells with the antigen: this is one mechanism of cell-mediated immunity.

Antibodies can neutralize viruses by blocking their combination with cellular receptor sites and by encouraging their destruction by mechanisms similar to those described for bacteria. Antibodies are very effective in *preventing* reinfection with many viruses, serum antibody being important where the virus has to pass through the bloodstream before reaching its target organ and local antibody being essential where the target organ is the same as the portal for entry (e.g. influenza); however, interferon may be more effective in the *recovery* from these infections. Cells infected with non-cytopathic viruses which 'bud', have altered surface antigens and can be destroyed by cytotoxic T-cells. Free 'budded' viral particles can be destroyed by antibody but the other route of intercellular virus spread can only be stopped by macrophages (recruited and activated by lymphokines from viral stimulated specific T-cells) which inhibit intercellular bridges and make local cells resistant to infection by bathing them in interferon.

Circulating antibody can offer protection against the blood-borne forms of protozoa, but antigenic variation and suppression of the host's immune response favour survival of the parasites. Organisms such as leishmania and toxoplasma which prefer an intracellular life, elicit cell-mediated immunity. Helminths provoke a high IgE response which may mediate a cytotoxic attack by eosinophils. Schistosomes protect themselves by mimicking the host.

Generally speaking, the acquired response operates to amplify and enhance innate immune mechanisms; the interactions are summarized in figure 7.20.

Immunity can be acquired passively, from the mother or by injection of preformed antibody, or induced actively either by natural infection or vaccination using killed or live attenuated organisms and toxoids. Live replicating vaccines provide a larger and more potent stimulus in the tissues relevant to the natural infection. Attenuated viral strains are being produced by genetic recombination. The efficiency of non-living antigens may be enhanced by adjuvants which act as antigen depots and activate macrophages. The risk of complications attendant upon vaccination must be weighed against the chance of contracting the disease.

Primary immunodeficiency states affecting the comple-

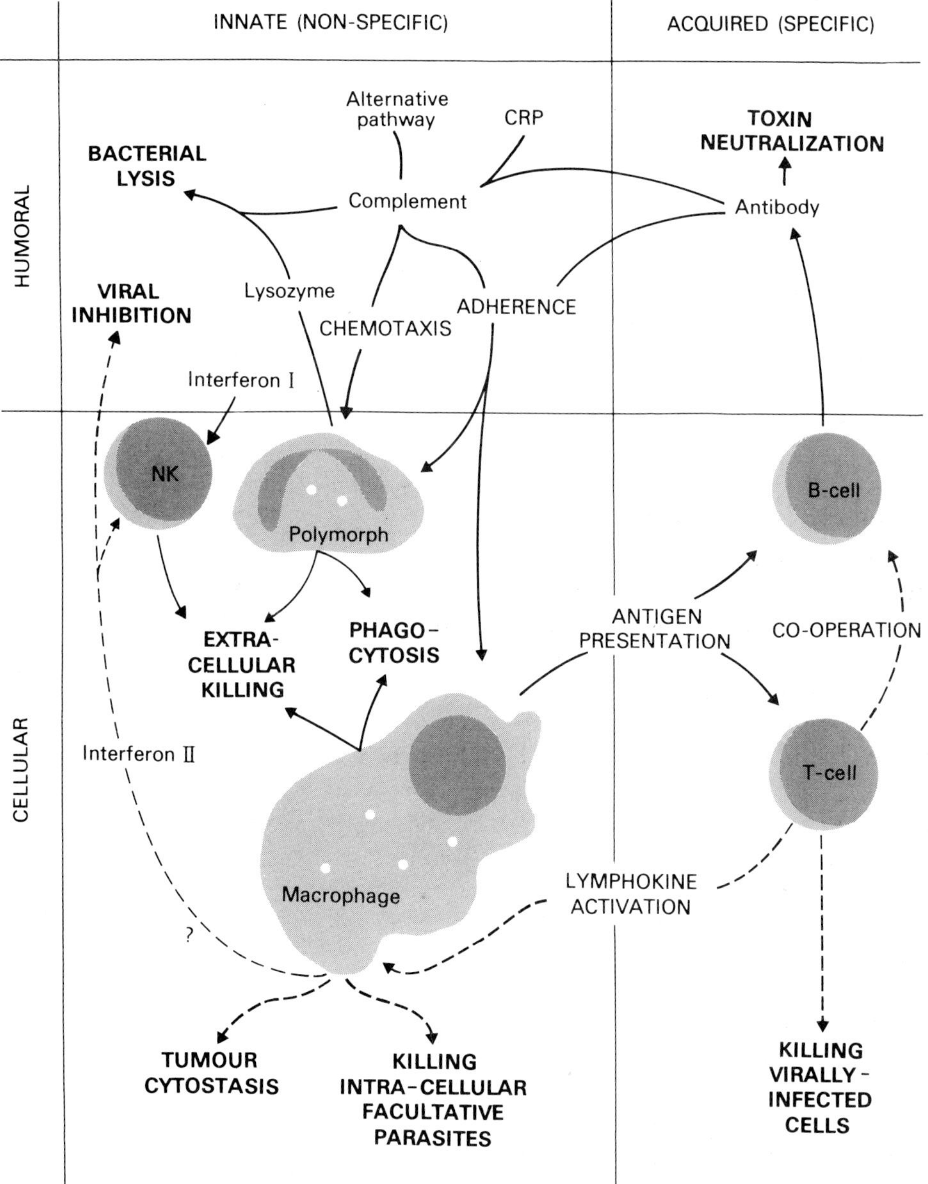

FIGURE 7.20. Simplified scheme to emphasize the interactions between natural and specific immunity mechanisms. Reactions influenced by T-cells are indicated by a broken line. (Developed from Playfair J.H.L. *Brit. Med. Bull.*, 1974, **30**, 24.)

ment system, phagocytic cells or antibody synthesis lead to infection by pyogenic bacteria. Children with T-cell deficiency cannot deal adequately with 'budding' viruses (e.g. pox type) and fungi. Severe combined immunodeficiency occurs where there is a failure in differentiation of lymphoid stem cells. In many instances replacement therapy is possible: Ig for B-cell, thymus graft for T-cell and bone marrow (stem cells) or adenosine deaminase for severe combined immunodeficiency. The deficiency may arise secondarily as a consequence of malnutrition, viral and other infection, cytotoxic drugs, or lymphoproliferative disorders.

Further reading

Bergsma D., Good R.A., Finstad J. & Paul N.W. (eds) (1975) *Immunodeficiency in man and animals* (Birth Defects Series), Vol. 11, No. 1. National Foundation, March of Dimes, New York.

Cohen S. & Sadun E. (eds) (1976) *Immunology of parasitic infections.* Blackwell Scientific Publications, Oxford.

Davis B.D., Dulbecco R., Eisen H.N., Ginsberg H.S. & Wood W.B. (1973) *Microbiology* (Including Immunology) Harper International (2nd) Edition.

Dick. G. (1978) *Immunisation.* Update Books, London.

Fongereau M. & Dansset J. (Eds) (1980) *Progress in Immunology IV.* Academic Press, London.

van Furth R. (ed.) (1975) *Mononuclear phagocytes in immunity, infection and pathology.* Blackwell Scientific Publications, Oxford.

Gell P.G.H., Coombs R.R.A. & Lachmann P.J. (1975) *Clinical Aspects of Immunology* 3rd ed. See chapters on immunity to infection and immunoprophylaxis. Blackwell Scientific Publications, Oxford.

Gray A. R. (1969) Antigenic variation in trypanosomes. *Bull.World Health Organization*, **41**, 805.

Mims C.A. (1976) *The pathogenesis of infectious disease.* Academic Press, London.

Notkins A.L. (ed) (1975) *Viral immunology and immunopathology.* Academic Press, New York.

Porter, Ruth & Knight, Julie (1974) *Parasites in the Immunized Host.* Ciba Foundation Symposium, Elsevier, Amsterdam.

Shvartsman Ya.S & Zykov M.P. (1976) Secretory anti-influenza immunity. *Adv.Immunol.*, **22**, 291.

Taussig M.J. (1979) *Processes in Pathology.* Blackwell Scientific Publications, Oxford.

Wheelock E.F. & Toy S.T. (1973) Participation of lymphocytes in viral infections. *Adv.in Immunology*, **16**, 124.

Wilson G.S. (1967) *The Hazards of Immunization.* Athlone Press, London.

(1973) Cell mediated immunity and resistance to infection. *W.H.O. Technical Report Series*, Geneva.

8 Hypersensitivity

When an individual has been immunologically primed, further contact with antigen leads to secondary boosting of the immune response. However, the reaction may be excessive and lead to gross tissue damage (*hypersensitivity*) if the antigen is present in relatively large amounts or if the humoral and cellular immune state is at a heightened level. It should be emphasized that the mechanisms underlying these excessive reactions are those normally employed by the body in combating infection as discussed in Chapter 7. We speak of *hypersensitivity reactions* and a state of *hypersensitivity.* Coombs and Gell defined four types of hypersensitivity, to which can be added a fifth, viz. 'stimulatory', which they mention. Types I, II, III and V depend on the interaction of antigen with humoral antibody and tend to be called 'immediate' type reactions although some are more immediate than others! Type IV involves receptors bound to the lymphocyte surface and because of the longer time course this has in the past been referred to as 'delayed-type sensitivity'. The essential basis of these reactions are summarized below and then each considered separately in more detail.

TYPE I—ANAPHYLACTIC SENSITIVITY

The antigen reacts with antibody bound to mast cells or circulating basophils through a specialized region of the Fc piece. This leads to degranulation of the mast cells and release of vasoactive amines (figure 8.1). These antibodies are termed homocytotropic (also referred to as reagins).

TYPE II—ANTIBODY-DEPENDENT CYTOTOXIC HYPERSENSITIVITY

Antibodies binding to an antigen on the cell surface cause (i) phagocytosis of the cell through opsonic (Fc) or immune (C3) adherence, (ii) non-phagocytic extracellular cytotoxicity

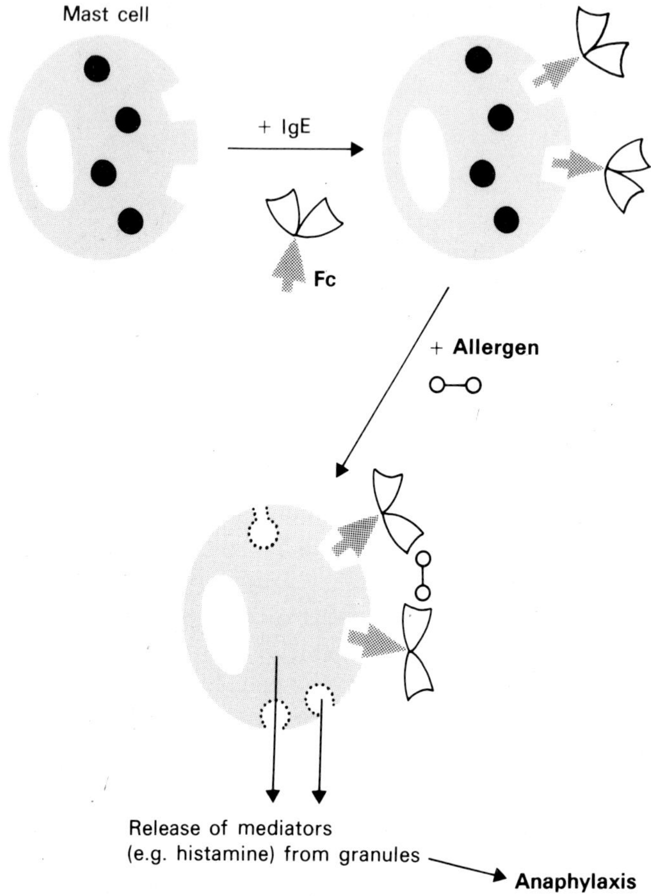

FIGURE 8.1. Type I—Anaphylactic hypersensitivity. Mast-cell degranulation following interaction of antigen with bound homocytotropic (reaginic) antibodies.

by killer cells with receptors for IgFc and (iii) lysis through the operation of the full complement system up to C8, 9 (figure 8.2).

TYPE III—COMPLEX-MEDIATED HYPERSENSITIVITY

The formation of complexes between antigen and humoral antibody can lead to activation of the complement system and to the aggregation of platelets with the consequences listed in figure 8.3.

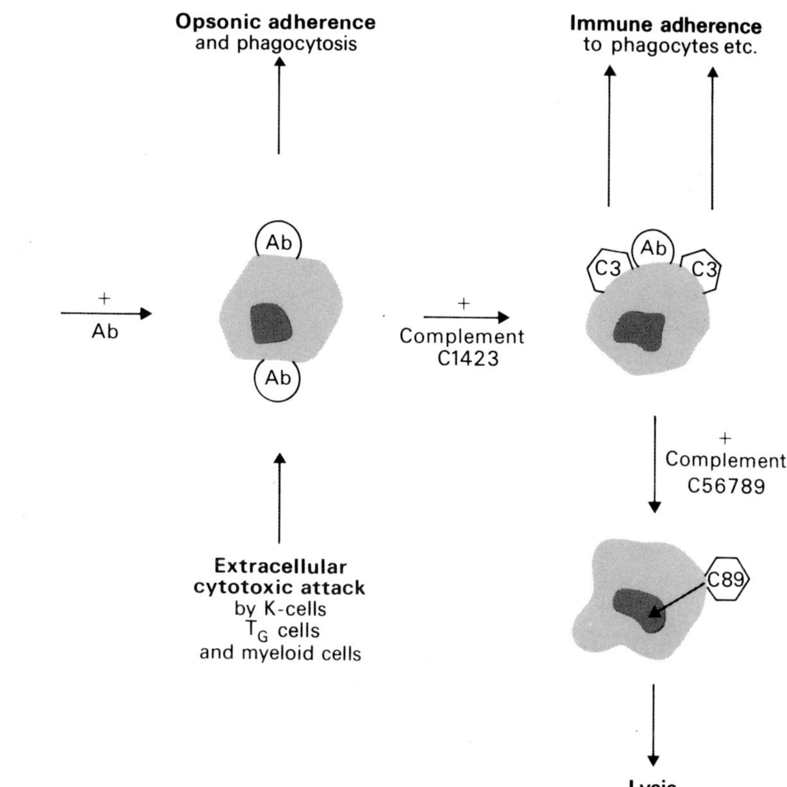

FIGURE 8.2. Type II—Antibody-dependent cytotoxic hypersensitivity. Antibodies directed against cell surface antigens cause cell death not only by C-dependent lysis but also by adherence reactions leading to phagocytosis or through non-phagocytic extracellular killing by certain lymphoreticular cells (antibody-dependent cell-mediated cytotoxicity).

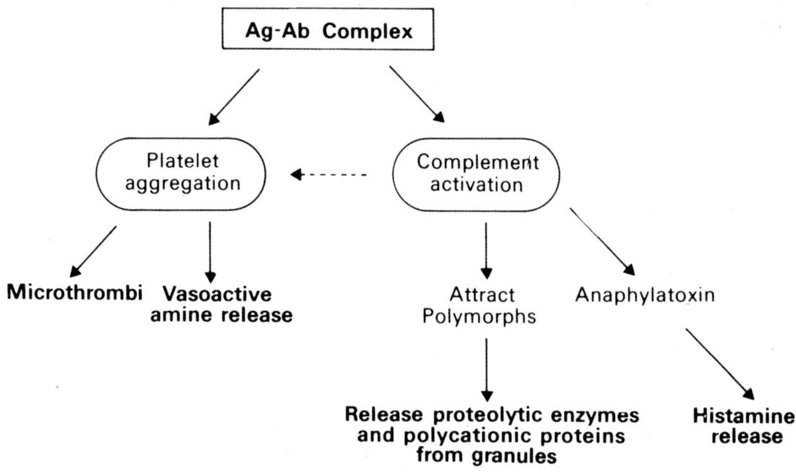

FIGURE 8.3. Type III—Complex-mediated hypersensitivity.

TYPE IV—CELL-MEDIATED (DELAYED-TYPE) HYPERSENSITIVITY

Thymic derived T-lymphocytes bearing specific receptors on their surface are stimulated by contact with macrophage-bound antigen to release lymphokines (cf. p. 77) which mediate delayed-type hypersensitivity (e.g. Mantoux test for tuberculin sensitivity); in the reaction against virally-infected cells or transplants, the stimulated lymphocytes transform into blast-like cells capable of killing target cells bearing the sensitizing antigens. Failure to eliminate the antigen will cause an accumulation of macrophages and the formation of a granuloma (figure 8.4).

TYPE V—STIMULATORY HYPERSENSITIVITY

Non-complement fixing antibodies directed against certain cell surface components may actually stimulate rather than destroy the cell (figure 8.5). Theoretically stimulation could also occur through the development of antibodies to naturally occurring mitotic inhibitors in the circulation.

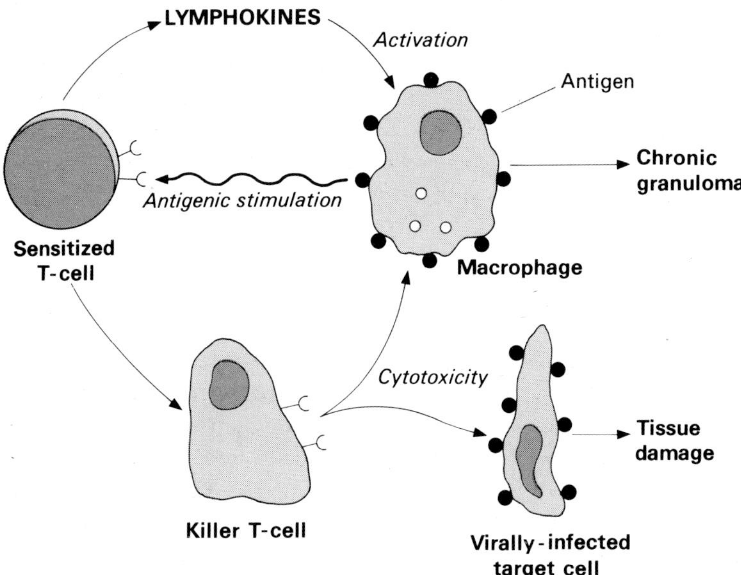

FIGURE 8.4. Type IV—Cell-mediated (delayed-type) hypersensitivity.

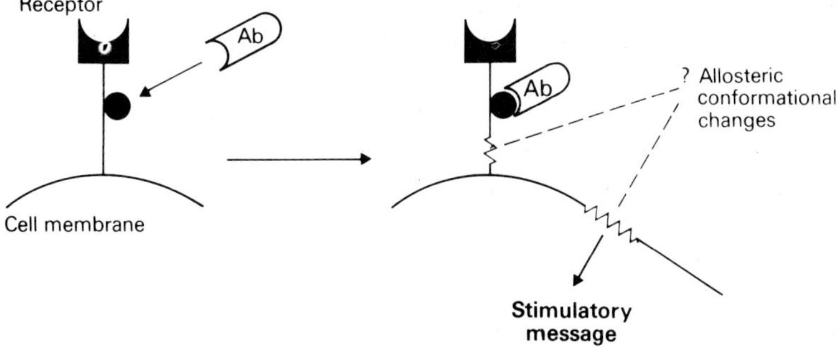

FIGURE 8.5. Type V—Stimulatory hypersensitivity.

Type I—Anaphylactic sensitivity

SYSTEMIC ANAPHYLAXIS

A single injection of 1 mg of an antigen such as egg albumin into a guinea-pig has no obvious effect. However, if the injection is repeated two to three weeks later, the sensitized animal reacts very dramatically with the symptoms of generalized anaphylaxis; almost immediately the guinea-pig begins to wheeze and within a few minutes dies from asphyxia. Examination shows intense constriction of the bronchioles and bronchi and generally there is (a) contraction of smooth muscle and (b) dilatation of capillaries.

Similar reactions can occur in human subjects and have been observed following insect bites or injections of penicillin in appropriately sensitive individuals. In many instances only a timely intravenous injection of adrenaline to counter the smooth muscle contraction and capillary dilatation can prevent death.

MECHANISM OF ANAPHYLAXIS

Sir Henry Dale recognized that histamine mimics the systemic changes of anaphylaxis and furthermore that the uterus from a sensitized guinea-pig releases histamine and contracts on exposure to antigen (Schultz–Dale technique). Serum from such an animal can passively sensitize the uterus from a normal guinea-pig so that it, too, will contract on addition of the specific antigen. Contraction is associated with an explosive degranulation of the mast cells (figure 8.6a & b) which is responsible for the release of histamine

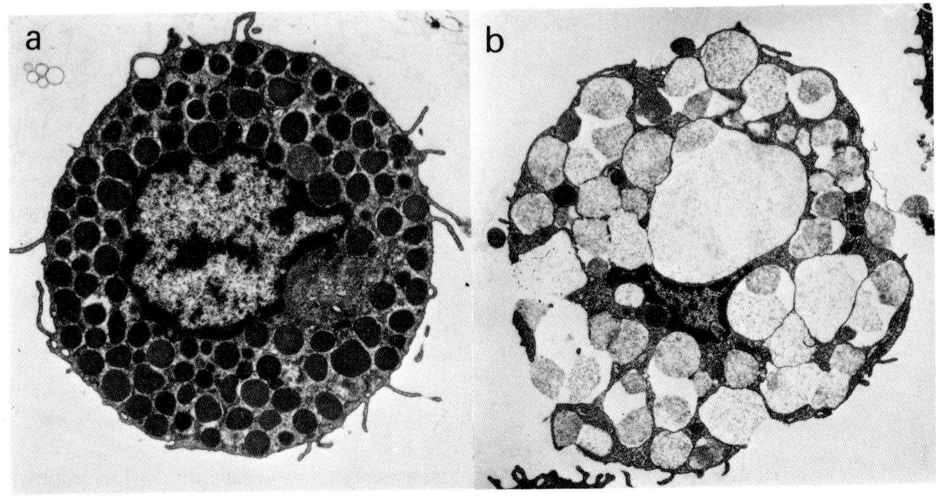

FIGURE 8.6. The mast cell. (a) An unreleased cell containing many membrane-bound, histamine-containing granules (× 5,400). (b) A mast cell degranulated by treatment with anti-Ig for 30 sec. at 37°. Note that the granules have released their histamine and are morphologically altered, being larger and less electron dense. Although most of the altered granules remain within the circumference of the cell, they are open to the extracellular space (× 5,400). (By courtesy of Drs. D. Lawson, C. Fewtrell, B. Gomperts & M. Raff: from *J. Exp. Med.* 1975, **142**, 391.)

and, in certain species, of another mediator of anaphylaxis, 5-hydroxytryptamine (serotonin). Other mediators which are released include slow reacting substance (SRS-A) capable of inducing a prolonged contraction of certain smooth muscles, platelet activating factor (PAF), heparin and chemotactic factors for both neutrophils and eosinophils. The eosinophils are thus attracted to the site of mast cell degranulation where they proceed to neutralize the effects of the released mediators; histamine is defused by histaminase, SRS-A by aryl sulphatase B and PAF by phospholipase D. In this way eosinophils modulate the reactions consequent upon mast cell activation (figure 8.7).

It seems clear that the mast cells become coated by a particular type of antibody whose Fc region can bind specifically to sites on the mast cell surface. The most effective homocytotropic antibodies belong to the IgE class but it is clear that IgG antibodies can also act as reagins although the extent of their contribution to the allergic state in the human is not yet resolved. IgG reagins differ from IgE in their relative insensitivity to mild heat and 2-mercaptoethanol reduction and especially in their lower

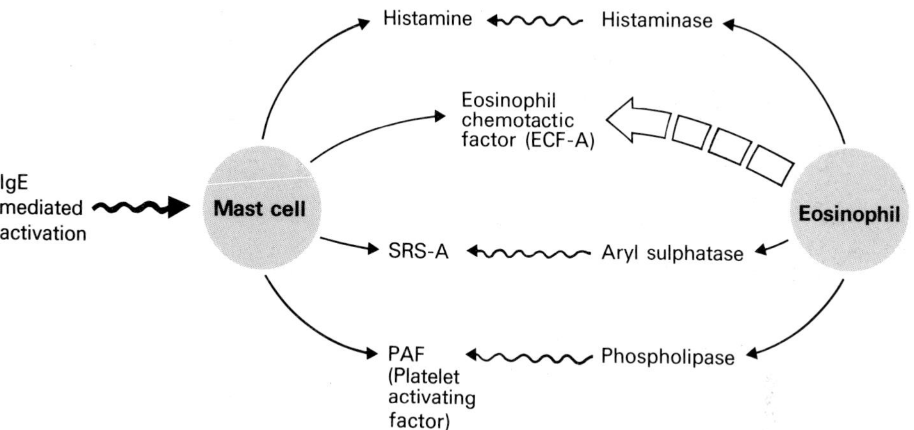

FIGURE 8.7. The mast cell response and its modulation by eosinophils. ECF-A is a very potent tetrapeptide of structure Val (or Ala). Gly. Ser. Glu. which binds to the eosinophil surface through hydrophobic (Val/Ala), H-bonding (Ser.) and ionic (Glu.) interactions. There is a negative feedback of histamine with the mast cell through combination with the surface histamine receptor (H_2). (After Austen F. & colleagues.)

binding affinity for mast cells; whereas IgE antibodies can be detected at the site of an intradermal injection into a normal individual for several weeks, IgG disperses within a day or so. The technique of *passive cutaneous anaphylaxis* (PCA) introduced by Ovary utilizes this dermal reaction as a highly sensitive indicator for reaginic antibodies. For example, high dilutions of guinea-pig serum containing γ_1-globulin antibodies may be injected into the skin of a normal animal and following the intravenous injection of antigen with a dye such as Evans' Blue, the anaphylactic reaction in the skin will lead to release of vasoactive amines and hence a local 'blueing'.

Degranulation of the mast cell occurs when the bound homocytotropic antibodies are cross-linked either by specific antigen (figure 8.1) or by the corresponding divalent anti-immunoglobulin (e.g. anti-IgE or anti-light chain); univalent (Fab) anti-IgE will not cause degranulation. This cross-linking reaction induces a membrane signal which leads to an influx of calcium ions and changes in cyclic nucleotide levels. A fall in cAMP or a rise in cGMP favours degranulation whereas high concentrations of cAMP stabilize the mast cell granules. The effects of different hormones and drugs on the control of mediator release by cyclic nucleotides are summarized in figure 8.8.

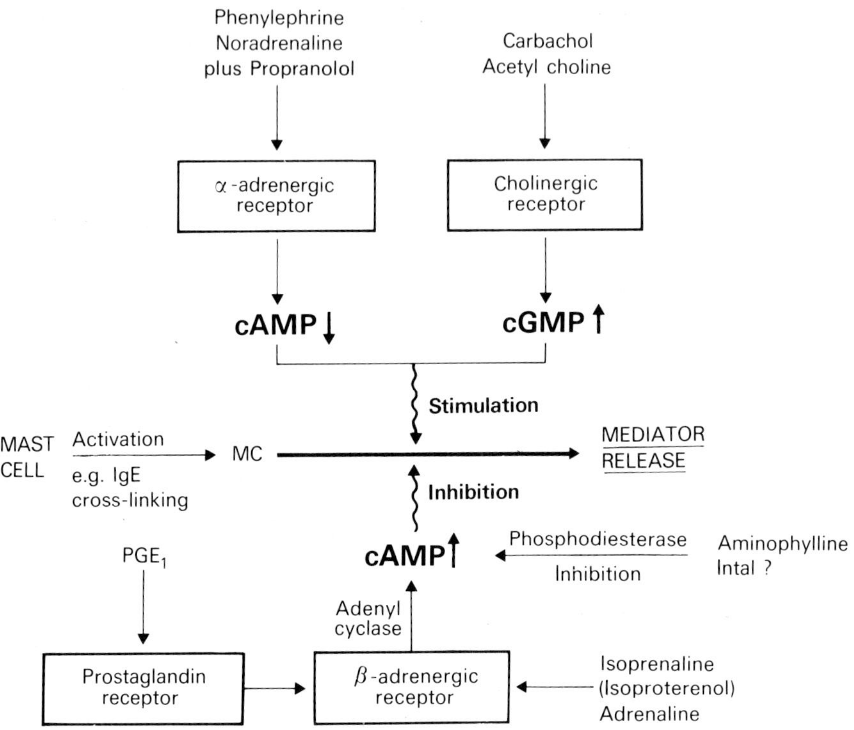

FIGURE 8.8. Factors affecting cyclic nucleotide control of mediator release from mast cells. Release is encouraged by a fall in cAMP or a rise in cGMP concentrations, and inhibited by an increase in cAMP level. (It should be noted that evidence for these hormone receptors has been more unequivocally established for the basophil than the mast cell.) (After Austen, F.)

ATOPIC ALLERGY

Nearly 10 per cent of the population suffer to a greater or lesser degree with allergies involving localized anaphylactic reactions to extrinsic allergens such as grass pollens, animal danders, mites in house dust and so on. Contact of the allergen with cell-bound IgE in the bronchial tree, the nasal mucosa and the conjunctival tissues releases mediators of anaphylaxis and produces the symptoms of asthma or hay fever as the case may be. For those unfortunates sensitized to foods such as the strawberry, the price of indulgence may be a generalized urticaria caused by reaction in the skin to materials absorbed from the gut into the blood stream. Acute anaphylaxis although rare may occur in highly sensitive subjects after an insect bite or injections of penicillin or procaine.

Sensitivity is normally assessed by the response to intradermal challenge with antigen. The release of histamine and other mediators rapidly produces a wheal and erythema (figure 8.13a), maximal within 30 minutes and then subsiding. The responsible IgE antibodies can be demonstrated by the ability of patient's serum to passively sensitize the skin of normal humans (Praüsnitz–Kustner or 'P–K' test) or preferably of monkeys. This passive sensitization of human skin can be blocked most effectively by prior injection of a myeloma of IgE rather than of any other class. The interpretation is that the specialized sites on the skin mast cells become fully saturated by binding to the Fc regions of the IgE myeloma globulin which blocks the subsequent attachment of specific IgE antibodies. In some instances, intranasal challenge with allergen provokes a response even though skin tests and the radioallergosorbent test (RAST, p. 146) for specific serum IgE are negative, a phenomenon attributable to local synthesis of IgE antibodies.

The lymphocytes from patients with atopic allergy undergo blast-cell transformation and release a migration inhibition factor on contact with allergen. These are thought to be indicators of cell-mediated immunity, and delayed-type hypersensitivity reactions (see below) have been elicited in some patients in whom the immediate response had been suppressed with anti-histamines.

The symptoms of atopic allergy are largely but not always completely controllable by anti-histamines. Other effective drugs such as Isoprenaline and disodium cromoglycate (Intal) probably act by stabilizing the adenyl cyclase–cyclic-AMP system to prevent vasoactive amine release. Attempts to desensitize patients immunologically by repeated treatment with allergen have at least the merit of a long history and in a significant but as yet unpredictable proportion of patients can lead to worthwhile improvement. It has generally been assumed that the purpose of these inoculations was to boost the synthesis of 'blocking' IgG antibody whose function was to divert the allergen from contact with tissue-bound IgE. This would be of unquestioned value were the increase in protective antibody (? particularly IgA) to occur locally at the sites vulnerable to allergen exposure. However, if T-lymphocyte co-operation is important for IgE synthesis, the beneficial effects of antigen injection may also be mediated through induction of tolerant or even suppressor T-cells. An especially hopeful finding is the observation that IgE-producing cells or their precursors can be switched off with comparative ease by haptens coupled to thymus-independent carriers such as poly-D-Glu. Lys. or isologous IgG, or by substitution of the allergen by polyethylene glycol. Better results must ultimately be attainable when we understand the rationale of 'hyposensitization' through the use of purified allergens, assessment of T-cell reactivity and quantitative measurement of specific IgG, IgA and IgE antibodies in individuals undergoing treatment. The affinity of these antibodies and their availability at local sites of allergen challenge such as the nasal mucosa are factors which cannot be ignored.

There is a strong familial predisposition to the development of these disorders but although this is linked to inheritance of a given HL-A haplotype within any one family, no association with specific HL-A types has so far come to light. Curiously, it is said that patients with allergy are less likely than their non-atopic counterparts to develop tumours.

Type II—Antibody-dependent cytotoxic hypersensitivity

Where an antigen is present on the surface of a cell, combination with antibody will encourage the demise of that cell by promoting contact with phagocytes either by reduction in surface charge, by opsonic adherence directly through the Fc or by immune adherence through bound C3. Cell death may also occur through activation of the full complement system up to C8 and C9 producing direct membrane damage. Although in the case of haemolytic antibodies, the generation of a single active complement site is enough to cause erythrocyte lysis, other cells appear to have repair mechanisms and it is likely that several complement sites need to be recruited in order to overwhelm the cell's defences.

The operation of a quite distinct cytotoxic mechanism is suggested by Perlmann's finding that target cells coated with low concentrations of IgG antibody can be killed 'non-specifically' through an extracellular non-phagocytic mechanism involving nonsensitized lymphoreticular cells which bind to the target by their specific receptors for IgG Fc (figure 8.9). This so-called antibody-dependent cell-mediated cytotoxicity (ADCC) may be exhibited by both phagocytic and nonphagocytic myeloid cells (polymorphs and monocytes) and by a weakly glass-adherent cell with

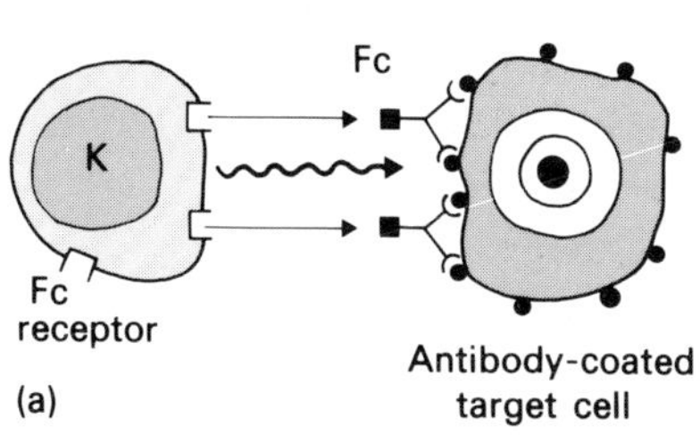

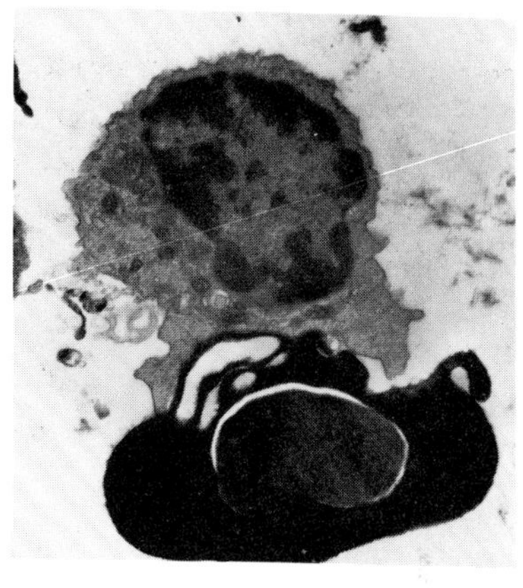

FIGURE 8.9. Killing of antibody-coated target by antibody-dependent cell-mediated cytotoxicity (ADCC). The surface receptors for Ig Fc region bind the effector cell to the target which is then killed by an extracellular mechanism. Several different cell types may display ADCC activity. (a) Diagram of effector and target cells. (b) Electron micrograph of attack on antibody-coated chick red cell by a mouse K-cell showing close apposition of effector and target and vacuolation in the cytoplasm of the latter (courtesy of P. Penfold).

Fc receptors dubbed the 'K-cell'. Although morphologically similar to a fairly small lymphocyte, the precise lineage of the K-cell is still uncertain. A proportion of human effector cells bear T-markers and therefore belong to the T_G subpopulation. The remainder are 'null' cells in the sense that they lack the presently employed surface markers of mature B- or T-lymphocytes and it will be of interest to see whether they represent stages in the differentiation of lymphoid (or myeloid) lines or belong to an entirely distinct cell type.

Contact between the effector and target cells is essential and activity is inhibited by cytochalasin B which interferes with cell movement, and aggregated IgG which binds firmly to the Fc receptors and blocks their ability to interact with antibody on the surface of the target. ADCC is not affected by inhibitors of protein synthesis and the presence of complement components has not so far been found to be mandatory although Nature would have shown a certain tidiness had the complement system been utilized to provide the cytotoxic effector molecule.

So far, ADCC has been studied exclusively as a phenomenon *in vitro*; to give examples, human K-cells have been shown to be strikingly unpleasant to chicken red cells coated with rabbit antibody, Chang liver cells coated with human antibody and human lymphocytes bearing anti-HLA. Whether ADCC is merely a curiosity of the laboratory test-tube or plays a positive role *in vivo* remains an open question. Functionally, this extracellular cytotoxic mechanism would be expected to be of significance where the target is too large for ingestion by phagocytosis, e.g. large parasites (p. 195) and solid tumours. It could also act as a back-up system for T-cell killing when antibody production might otherwise lead to protection of the target from attack by T-cells through blocking of the surface antigens; the evolution of ADCC mechanisms would ensure that the antibody-coated target was still vulnerable.

ISOIMMUNE REACTIONS

Transfusion reactions

Of the many different polymorphic constituents of the human red cell membrane, ABO blood groups form the dominant system. The antigenic groups A and B are derived from H substance (figure 8.10) by the action of glycosyl transferases encoded by A or B genes respectively. Individuals with both genes (group AB) have the two antigens on their red cells while those lacking these genes (group O) synthesize H substance only. Antibodies to A or to B occur

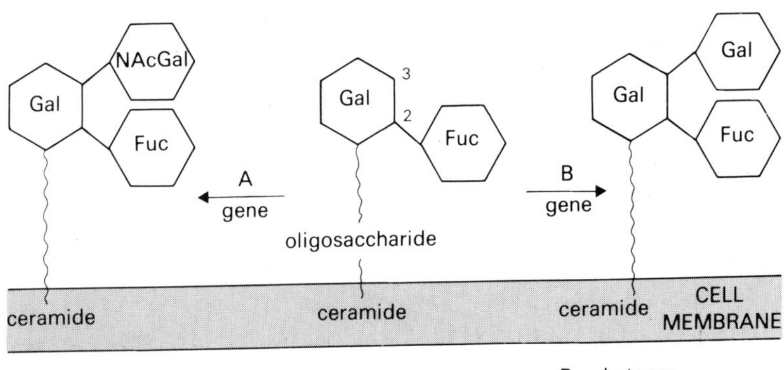

FIGURE 8.10. The ABO system. The allelic genes A and B code for transferases which add either N-acetylgalactosamine or galactose respectively to H substance. The oligosaccharide is anchored to the cell membrane by coupling to a sphingomyelin called ceramide. 85% of the population secrete blood group substances in the saliva where the oligosaccharides are present as soluble polypeptide conjugates formed under the action of a secretor (se) gene.

when the antigen is absent from the red cell surface; thus a person of blood group A will possess anti-B and so on. These *isohaemagglutinins* are usually IgM and are thought to arise through immunization against antigens of the gut flora which are similar to the blood group substances so that the antibodies formed cross-react with the appropriate red cell type. If an individual is blood group A, he will be tolerant to antigens closely similar to A and will only form cross-reacting antibodies capable of agglutinating B red cells; similarly an O individual will make anti-A and anti-B. On transfusion, mismatched red cells will be coated by the isohaemagglutinins and cause severe reactions.

Rhesus incompatibility

The Rhesus (Rh) blood groups form the other major antigenic system, the RhD antigen being of the most consequence for isoimmune reactions. A mother with an RhD negative blood group can readily be sensitized by red cells from a baby carrying RhD antigens. This occurs most often at the birth of the first child when a placental bleed can release a large number of the baby's erythrocytes into the mother. The antibodies formed are predominantly of the IgG class and are able to cross the placenta in any subsequent pregnancy. Reaction with the D-antigen on the fetal red cells leads to their destruction through opsonic adherence giving haemolytic disease of the newborn (figure 8.11).

These anti-D antibodies fail to agglutinate RhD + red cells *in vitro* ('incomplete antibodies') because the low density of antigenic sites does not allow sufficient antibody bridges to be formed between the negatively charged erythrocytes to overcome the electrostatic repulsive forces. Erythrocytes coated with anti-D can be made to agglutinate by addition of albumin or of an anti-immunoglobulin serum (Coombs' reagent).

If a mother has natural isohaemagglutinins which can react with any fetal erythrocytes reaching her circulation, sensitization to the D antigens is less likely due to 'deviation' of the red cells away from the antigen sensitive cells. For example, a group O Rh − ve mother with a group A Rh + ve baby would destroy any fetal erythrocytes with her anti-A before they could immunize to produce anti-D. In an extension of this principle, Rh − ve mothers are now treated prophylactically with small amounts of avid IgG anti-D

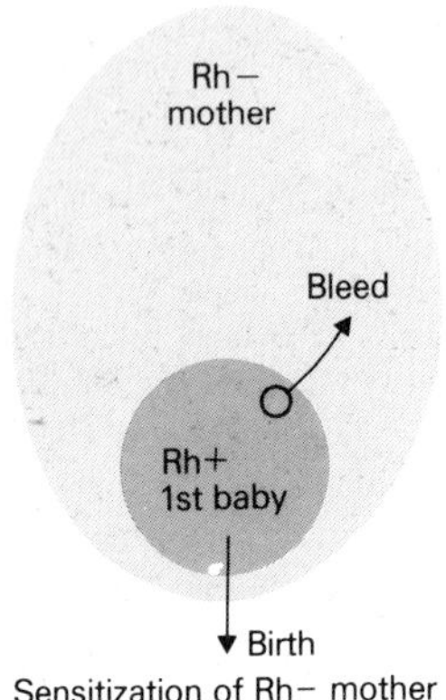

Sensitization of Rh− mother by bleed at birth of 1st Rh+ baby leading to synthesis of anti–D.

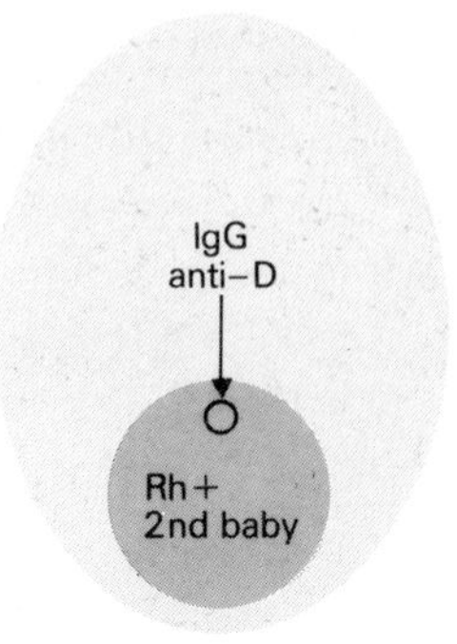

D+ erythrocytes in 2nd child affected by IgG anti–D crossing the placenta.

FIGURE 8.11. Haemolytic disease of the newborn due to rhesus incompatibility.

at the time of birth of the first child, and this greatly reduces the risk of sensitization.

Organ transplants

A long-standing homograft which has withstood the first onslaught of the cell-mediated reaction can evoke humoral antibodies in the host directed against surface transplantation antigens on the graft. These may be directly cytotoxic, or cause adherence of phagocytic cells or 'non-specific' attack by K cells (cf. figure 8.2). They may also lead to platelet adherence when they combine with antigens on the surface of the vascular endothelium.

AUTOIMMUNE REACTIONS

Autoantibodies to the patient's own red cells are produced in autoimmune haemolytic anaemia. Red cells coated with these antibodies have a shortened half-life largely through their adherence to phagocytic cells. Similar mechanisms account for the anaemia in patients with cold haemagglutin disease who have monoclonal anti-I after infection with *Mycoplasma pneumoniae*, and in some cases of paroxysmal cold haemoglobinuria associated with the actively lytic Donath-Landsteiner antibodies of specificity anti-blood group P.

The sera of patients with Hashimoto's thyroiditis contain antibodies which in the presence of complement are directly

(a)

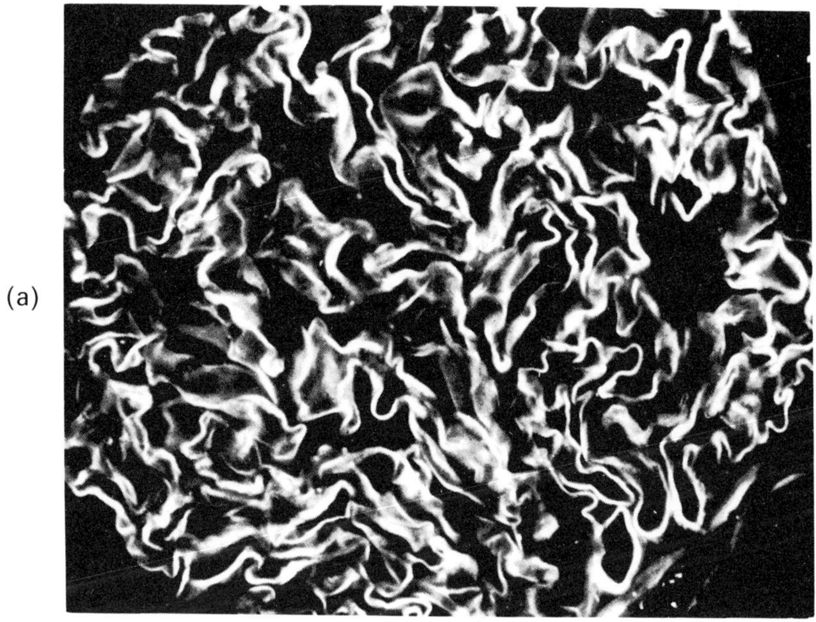

(b)

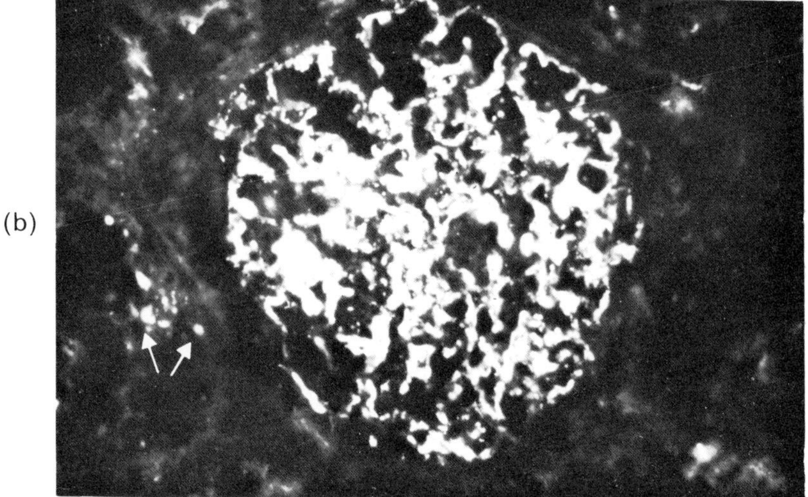

FIGURE 8.12. Glomerulonephritis: (a) due to linear deposition of antibody to glomerular basement membrane here visualized by staining the human kidney biopsy with a fluorescent anti-IgG (courtesy of Dr. F.J. Dixon) and (b) due to deposition of antigen–antibody complexes which can be seen as discrete masses lining the glomerular basement membrane following immunofluorescent staining with anti-IgG; patches of blue autofluorescence are present in the extraglomerular tissue arrowed) (courtesy of Dr. D. Doniach). Similar patterns to these are obtained with a fluorescent anti-C3.

cytotoxic for isolated human thyroid cells in culture. In Goodpasture's syndrome (included here for convenience), antibodies to kidney glomerular basement membrane are present. Biopsies show these antibodies together with complement components bound to the basement membranes where the action of the full complement system leads to serious damage (figure 8.12a).

DRUG REACTIONS

Very complicated. Drugs may become coupled to body components and thereby undergo conversion from a hapten to a full antigen which will sensitize certain individuals (we don't know which). If IgE antibodies are produced, anaphylactic reactions can result. In some circumstances, particularly with topically applied ointments, cell-mediated hypersensitivity may be induced. In other cases where coupling to serum proteins occurs, the possibility of type III complex-mediated reactions may arise. In the present context we are concerned with those instances where the drug appears to form an antigenic complex with the surface of a formed element of the blood and evokes the production of antibodies which are cytotoxic for the cell-drug complex. When the drug is withdrawn, the sensitivity is no longer evident. Examples of this mechanism have been seen in the *haemolytic anaemia* sometimes associated with continued administration of chlorpromazine or phenacetin, in the *agranulocytosis* associated with the taking of amidopyrine or of quinidine, and the classic situation of *thrombocytopenic purpura* which may be produced by Sedormid. In the latter case, freshly drawn serum from the patient will lyse platelets in the presence but not in the absence of Sedormid; inactivation of complement by preheating the serum at 56°C for 30 minutes abrogates this effect.

Type III—Complex-mediated hypersensitivity

The union of soluble antigens and antibodies within the body may give rise to an acute inflammatory reaction (cf. figure 8.3). If complement is fixed, anaphylatoxins will be released as split products of C3 and C5 and these will cause histamine release with vascular permeability changes.

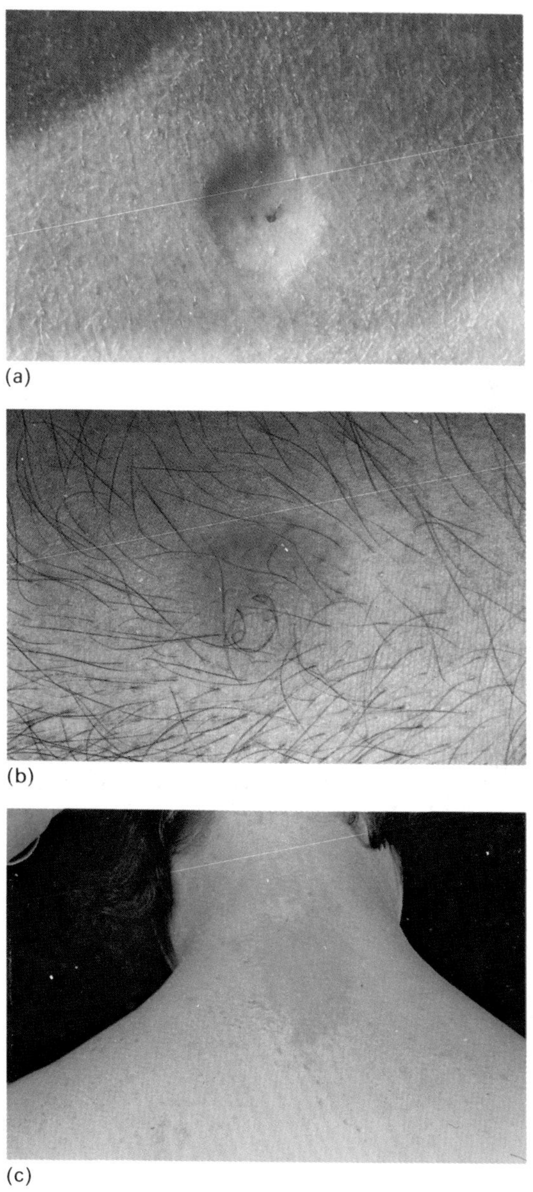

FIGURE 8.13. Hypersensitivity reactions. (a) Type I anaphylactic intradermal reaction to pollen allergen showing well-developed wheal and a degree of erthema (flare). (b) Type IV cell-mediated hypersensitivity reaction to tuberculin, characterized by induration and erythema. (c) Type IV contact hypersensitivity reaction to nickel caused by the clasp of a necklace. (a & b kindly provided by Dr. J. Brostoff, photographed by Mr. B.N. Rice; c reproduced from Brit. Soc. Immunol. teaching slides with permission of the Society and Dermatology Department, London Hospital.)

The chemotactic factors also produced will lead to an influx of polymorphonuclear leucocytes which begin the phagocytosis of the immune complexes; this in turn results in the extracellular release from the polymorph granules of proteolytic enzymes (including neutral proteinases and collagenase), kinin-forming enzymes and polycationic proteins which increase vascular permeability through both mastocytolytic and histamine-independent mechanisms. These will damage local tissues and intensify the inflammatory responses. Further damage may be mediated by reactive lysis (chapter 6, p. 164) in which activated C567 becomes attached to the surface of nearby cells and binds C8,9. Under appropriate conditions, platelets may be aggregated with two consequences: they provide yet a further source of vasoactive amines and may also form microthrombi which can lead to local ischaemia. (The discerning reader will appreciate the need for the complex system of inhibitors present in the body.)

The outcome of the formation of immune complexes *in vivo* depends not only on the absolute amounts of antigen and antibody, which determine the intensity of the reaction, but also on their *relative* proportions which govern the nature of the complexes (cf. precipitin curve, p. 6) and hence their distribution within the body. Between *antibody excess* and *mild antigen excess*, the complexes are rapidly precipitated and tend to be localized to the site of introduction of antigen, whereas in *moderate* to *gross antigen excess*, soluble complexes are formed which circulate and may cause systemic reactions and be widely deposited in the kidneys, joints and skin.

LOCALLY FORMED COMPLEXES

Maurice Arthus found that injection of soluble antigen intradermally into hyperimmunized rabbits with high levels of precipitating antibody produced an erythematous and oedematous reaction reaching a peak at 3–8 hours and then usually resolving. The lesion was characterized by an intense infiltration with polymorphonuclear leucocytes (figure 8.14a). The injected antigen precipitates with antibody often within the venule and the complex binds complement; using the appropriate fluorescent reagents, antigen, immunoglobulin and complement components can all be demonstrated in this lesion. Anaphylatoxin is soon generated and causes histamine

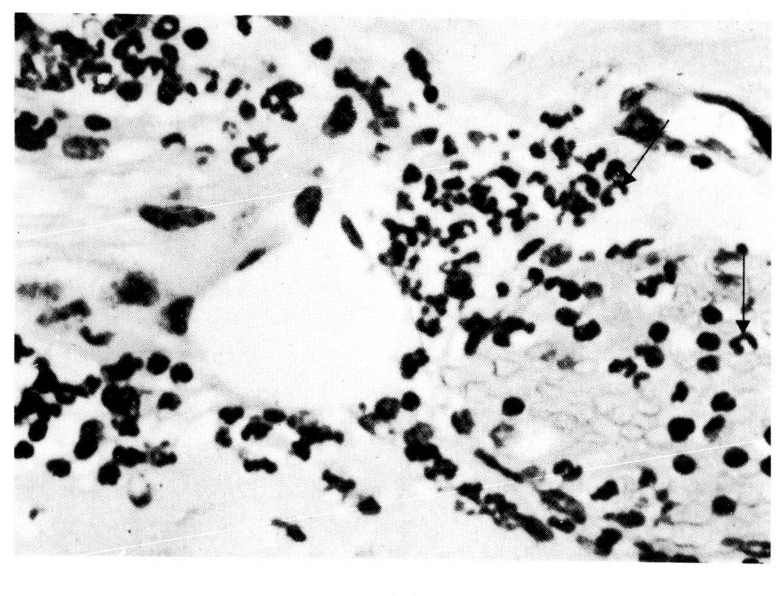

(a)

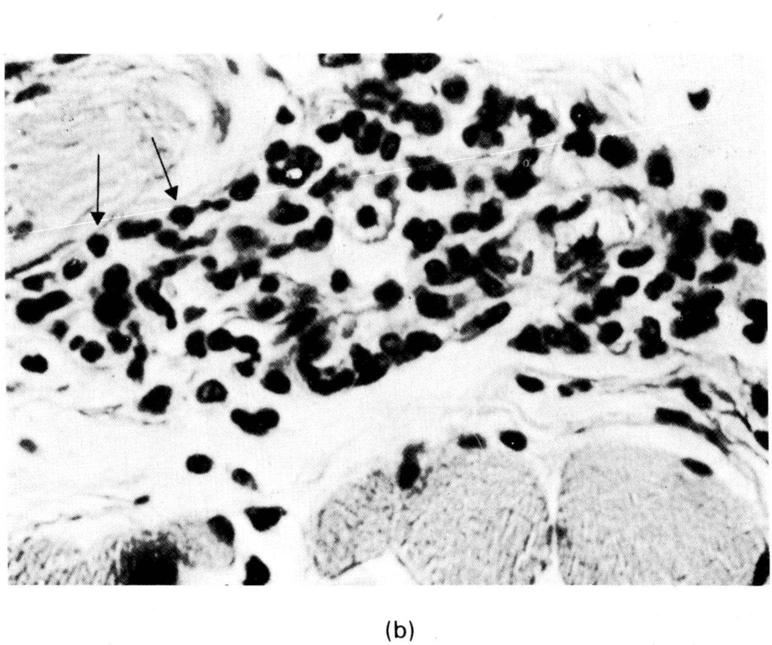

(b)

FIGURE 8.14. Histology of intradermal hypersensitivity reactions: (a) Acute inflammatory response in Arthus reaction (Type III) in rabbit skin with predominance of polymorphs (arrows), and (b) Type IV cell-mediated (delayed type) hypersensitivity reaction to intradermal antigen revealing the mononuclear cell infiltration (arrows).

liberation. Local intravascular complexes will cause platelet aggregation and vasoactive amine release. The formation of chemotactic factors leads to the influx of polymorphs and, as a result, erythema and oedema increase. The Arthus reaction can be blocked by depletion of complement or of the neutrophil polymorphs (by nitrogen mustard or specific anti-polymorph sera).

Intrapulmonary Arthus-type reactions to exogenous inhaled antigen appear to be responsible for a number of hypersensitivity disorders in man. The severe respiratory difficulties associated with Farmer's lung occur within 6–8 hours of exposure to the dust from mouldy hay. The patients are found to be sensitized to thermophilic actinomycetes which grow in the mouldy hay, and extracts of these organisms give precipitin reactions with the subject's serum and Arthus reactions on intradermal injection. Inhalation of bacterial spores present in dust from the hay introduces antigen into the lungs and a complex-mediated hypersensitivity reaction occurs. A similar situation arises in pigeon-fancier's disease where the antigen is probably serum protein present in the dust from dried faeces, and in many other quaintly named cases of allergic alveolitis resulting from continual inhalation of organic particles, e.g. cheese washer's disease (*Penicillium casei* spores), furrier's lung (fox fur proteins) and maple bark stripper's disease (*Cryptostroma* spores). Evidence that an immediate anaphylactic type I response may sometimes be of importance for the initiation of an Arthus reaction comes from the study of patients with allergic bronchopulmonary aspergillosis who have high levels of IgE and precipitating IgG antibodies to *Aspergillus* species.

Type III reactions are often provoked by the local release of antigen from infectious organisms within the body, for example, living filarial worms such as *Wuchereria bancrofti* are relatively harmless, but the dead parasite found in lymphatic vessels initiates an inflammatory reaction thought to be responsible for obstruction of lymph flow and the ensuing, rather monstrous, elephantiasis. Chemotherapy may cause an abrupt release of microbial antigens in individuals with high antibody levels producing quite dramatic immune complex-mediated reactions such as erythema nodosum leprosum in the skin of dapsone-treated lepromatous leprosy patients and the Jarisch–Herxheimer reaction in syphilitics on penicillin.

An interesting variant of the Arthus reaction is seen in rheumatoid arthritis where complexes are formed locally in the joint due to the production of self-associating IgG anti-IgG by synovial plasma cells (cf. p. 319).

It has also been recognized that complexes could be generated at a local site by a quite different mechanism involving non-specific adherence of an antigen to tissue structures followed by the binding of soluble antibody—in other words, the antigen becomes fixed in the tissue *before* not *after* combining with antibody. Although it is not clear to what extent this mechanism operates in patients with immune complex disease, let me describe the experimental observation on which it is based. After injection with bacterial endotoxin, mice release DNA into their circulation which binds specifically to the collagen in the basement membrane of the glomerular capillaries: infusion of anti-DNA now gives rise to antigen-antibody complexes in the kidney.

CIRCULATING COMPLEXES (SERUM SICKNESS)

Injection of relatively large doses of foreign serum (e.g. horse anti-diphtheria) used to be employed for various therapeutic purposes. It was not uncommon for a condition known as 'serum sickness' to arise some eight days after the injection. A rise in temperature, swollen lymph nodes, a generalized urticarial rash and painful swollen joints associated with a low serum complement and transient albuminuria could be encountered. These result from the deposition of soluble antigen–antibody complexes formed in antigen excess.

Some individuals begin to synthesize antibodies against the foreign protein—usually horse globulin. Since the antigen is still present in gross excess at that time (figure 8.15), circulating soluble complexes of composition Ag_2Ab, Ag_3Ab_2, Ag_4Ab_3, etc. will be formed (cf. precipitin curve, figure 1.3, p. 6). To be pathogenic, the complexes have to be of the right size—too big and they are snapped up smartly by the macrophages of the reticuloendothelial system, and too small ($< 19S$) they fail to induce an inflammatory reaction. Even when they are the right size, it seems that they will only localize in vessel walls if there is a change in vascular permeability. This may come about through release of 5-hydrotryptamine from platelets reacting with larger complexes or through an IgE-mediated degranulation of basophils and mast cells to produce histamine and platelet activating factor. As a result of the vascular changes which are generated, the appropriately sized complexes deposit in

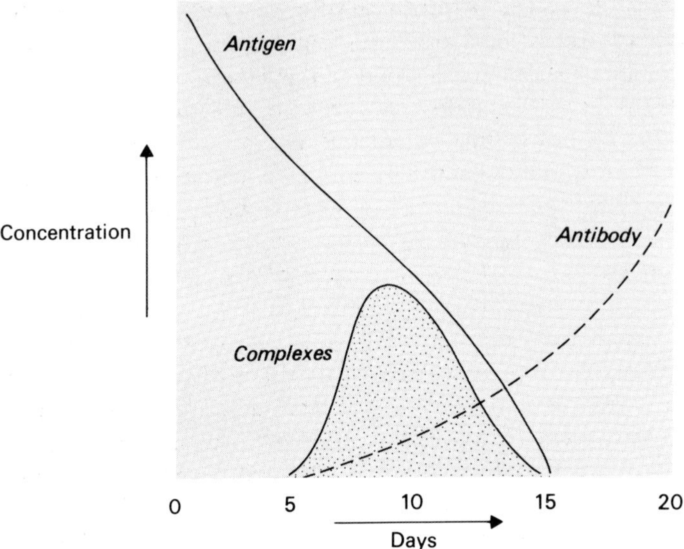

FIGURE 8.15. Formation of soluble complexes after injection of large amount of antigen (e.g. horse serum) as antibody is first synthesized. The complexes cause 'serum sickness'.

different blood vessels particularly those in the skin, joints and kidneys. They build up as 'lumpy' granules staining for antigen, immunoglobulin and complement (C3) by immunofluorescence (figure 8.12b) and may be seen as large amorphous masses associated with the glomerular basement membrane in the electron microscope. As antibody synthesis increases, antigen is cleared and the patient normally recovers.

The deposition of complexes is a dynamic affair and long lasting disease is only seen when the antigen is persistent as in chronic infections and autoimmune diseases. Experimentally, Dixon produced chronic glomerular lesions by repeated administration of foreign proteins to rabbits. Not all animals showed the lesion and perhaps only those genetically capable of producing low affinity antibody (Soothill & Steward) or antibodies to a restricted number of determinants (Christian) formed soluble complexes in the right size range. The smallest complexes reach the epithelial side but progressively larger complexes are retained in or on the endothelial side of the glomerular basement membrane.

It should be said that persistence of circulating complexes does not invariably lead to type III hypersensitivity (e.g. in many cancer patients). Perhaps these individuals lack the factors required for complex deposition, but some hold the alternative view that deposited complexes are not preformed in the circulation but are laid down sequentially by the binding to the tissues first of antigen, then of antibody as described in the section on 'locally formed complexes' above. Be that as it may, many cases of glomerulonephritis are associated with circulating complexes and biopsies give a fluorescent staining pattern similar to that of figure 8.12b which depicts DNA/anti-DNA/complement deposits in the kidney of a patient with systemic lupus erythematosus (cf. p. 316). Well known is the disease which can follow infection with certain strains of so-called 'nephritogenic' streptococci and the nephrotic syndrome of Nigerian children associated with quartan malaria where complexes with antigens of the infecting organism have been implicated. Immune complex nephritis can arise in the course of chronic viral infections; for example, mice infected with lymphocytic choriomeningitis virus develop a glomerulonephritis associated with circulating complexes of virus and antibody. This may well represent a model for many cases of glomerulonephritis in man.

The choroid plexus is also a favoured site for immune complex deposition and this could account for the frequency of central nervous disorders in systemic lupus. Neurologically affected patients tend to have depressed C4 in the cerebrospinal fluid and at post-mortem, SLE patients with neurological disturbances and high titre anti-DNA were shown to have scattered deposits of immunoglobulin and DNA in the choroid plexus. Subacute sclerosing panencephalitis is associated with a high c.s.f. to serum ratio of measles antibody and deposits containing Ig and measles Ag may be found in neural tissue.

The necrotizing arteritis produced in rabbits by experimental serum sickness closely resembles the histology of polyarteritis nodosa and it has recently been reported that in some of these patients, immune complexes containing the HBs antigen of hepatitis B virus are present in the lesions. Another example is the haemorrhagic shock syndrome found with some frequency in South-East Asia during a second infection with a dengue virus. There are 4 types of virus, and antibodies to one type produced during a first infection may not neutralize a second strain but rather facilitate its entry into and replication within human monocytes by attachment of the complex to Fc receptors. The enhanced production of virus leads to immune complex formation and a massive intravascular activation of the classical complement pathway. In some instances drugs such as penicillin become antigenic after conjugation with body proteins and form complexes which mediate hypersensitivity reactions.

DETECTION OF IMMUNE COMPLEX FORMATION

Tissue-bound complexes are usually visualized by the immunofluorescent staining of biopsies with conjugated anti-immunoglobulins and anti-C3 (cf. figure 8.12b).

Many techniques for the detection of circulating complexes have been described and because of variations in the size, complement-fixing ability and Ig class of different complexes, it is useful to apply more than one method. In our laboratory we tend to prefer:

(i) precipitation of complexed IgG from serum at concentrations of polyethylene glycol which do not bring down significant amounts of IgG monomer, followed by estimation of IgG in the precipitate by single radial diffusion or laser nephelometry, and

(ii) binding of serum complexes to plastic tubes coated with Clq and estimation of the amount and class of Ig in the complex with radio- or enzyme-labelled class-specific anti-Ig (cf. method used for determination of antibody-binding capacity, p. 144).

Other major techniques include (a) estimation of the binding of ^{125}I-Clq to complexes by coprecipitation with polyethylene glycol, (b) inhibition by complexes of rheumatoid factor-induced aggregation of IgG-coated particles and (c) detection with radiolabelled anti-Ig of serum complexes capable of binding to the C3b (and to a lesser extent the Fc) receptors on the Raji cell line. Sera from patients with immune complex disease often form a cryoprecipitate when allowed to stand at 4°. Measurement of serum C3 and its conversion product C3c are sometimes useful.

TREATMENT

The avoidance of exogenous inhaled antigens inducing type III reactions is obvious. Elimination of micro-organisms associated with immune complex disease by chemotherapy may provoke a further reaction due to copious release of antigen. Suppression of the accessory factors thought to be necessary for deposition of complexes would seem logical; for example, the development of serum sickness is prevented by histamine and 5HT antagonists. Disodium cromoglycate, heparin and salicylates are often used, the latter being an effective platelet stabilizer as well as a potent anti-inflammatory agent. Corticosteroids are particularly powerful inhibitors of inflammation and are immunosuppressive. In many cases, particularly those involving autoimmunity, conventional immunosuppressive agents may be justified. Where type III hypersensitivity is thought to arise from an inadequate immune response, the more aggressive approach of immunopotentiation to boost avidity is being advocated, but that is a path that will be trod gently.

Type IV—Cell-mediated (delayed-type) hypersensitivity

This form of hypersensitivity is encountered in many allergic reactions to bacteria, viruses and fungi, in the contact dermatitis resulting from sensitization to certain simple chemicals and in the rejection of transplanted tissues. Perhaps the best known example is the Mantoux reaction obtained by injection of tuberculin into the skin of an individual in whom previous infection with the mycobacterium had induced a state of cell-mediated immunity (CMI). The reaction is characterized by erythema and induration (figure 8.13b) which appears only after several hours (hence the term 'delayed') and reaches a maximum at 24–48 hours, thereafter subsiding. Histologically the earliest phase of the reaction is seen as a perivascular cuffing with mononuclear cells followed by a more extensive exudation of mono- and polymorphonuclear cells. The latter soon migrate out of the lesion leaving behind a predominantly mononuclear cell infiltrate consisting of lymphocytes and cells of the monocyte–macrophage series (figure 8.14b). This contrasts with the essentially 'polymorph' character of the Arthus reaction (figure 8.14a).

Comparable reactions to soluble proteins are obtained when sensitization is induced by incorporation of the antigen into complete Freund's adjuvant (p. 202). In some but not all cases, if animals are primed with antigen alone or in incomplete Freund's adjuvant (which lacks the mycobacteria), the delayed hypersensitivity state is of shorter duration and the dermal response more transient. This is known as 'Jones-Mote' sensitivity but has recently been termed cutaneous basophil hypersensitivity on account of the high proportion of basophils infiltrating the skin lesion.

CELLULAR BASIS

Unlike the other forms of hypersensitivity which we have discussed, delayed-type reactivity cannot be transferred from a sensitive to a non-sensitized individual with serum antibody; lymphoid cells, in particular the T-lymphocytes, are required. Thus a guinea-pig with negative skin reactions to tuberculin gives a positive response after injection of peritoneal exudate cells (containing lymphocytes and macrophages), lymph node cells, or peripheral blood cells from a donor previously sensitized to the tubercle bacillus provided donor and recipient share major histocompatibility antigens in the I region. Transfer of delayed hypersensitivity has also been achieved in the human using viable blood white cells and interestingly, by a low molecular weight material extracted from them (Lawrence's transfer factor). The nature of this substance is, however, a mystery. It appears to be capable of stimulating precommitted T-cells mediating delayed hypersensitivity, but its role as an informational molecule conferring antigen-specific reactivity is still a highly contentious issue.

It cannot be stressed too often that the hypersensitivity lesion results from an exaggerated interaction between antigen and the *normal* cell-mediated immune mechanisms (cf. p. 78). Following earlier priming, memory T-cells recognize the antigen together with I-region molecules on a macrophage and are stimulated into blast cell transformation and proliferation. A proportion of the stimulated T-cells release a number of soluble factors which function as mediators of the ensuing hypersensitivity response while a separate population develops cytotoxic powers.

The cytotoxic drug, cyclophosphamide, enhances cell-mediated hypersensitivity and converts the Jones-Mote reaction to a full tuberculin-type response. This has been attributed to a selective depletion of suppressor B-cells but one should bear in mind also that suppressor T-cells are known to be vulnerable to this drug. CMI is also potentiated by a drug called levamisole whose mechanism of action is unknown, but which might be functioning like transfer factor (possibly not an illuminating comparison at this stage).

Migration inhibition tests

The production of macrophage migration inhibition factor (MIF) by peritoneal exudate cells from sensitized guinea-pigs on incubation with antigen is widely accepted as an *in vitro* correlate of cell-mediated hypersensitivity. The cells are packed into capillary tubes which are placed in small tissue culture chambers. On incubation the macrophages migrate out to form a fan of cells on the bottom of the chamber. If specific antigen is present in the medium, MIF is produced and the migration is inhibited. The degree of inhibition is assessed from the area of the macrophage fan obtained in the presence of antigen expressed as a percentage of that in the control chambers lacking antigen (figure 8.16) and this correlates with the intensity of the delayed hypersensitivity state.

The macrophages act as non-specific indicators of the reaction between antigen and specifically sensitized lymphocytes. Thus a purified small lymphocyte population isolated from the peritoneal exudate of a sensitized pig is able to induce migration inhibition in the presence of antigen when mixed with as many as 50 times its number of macrophages

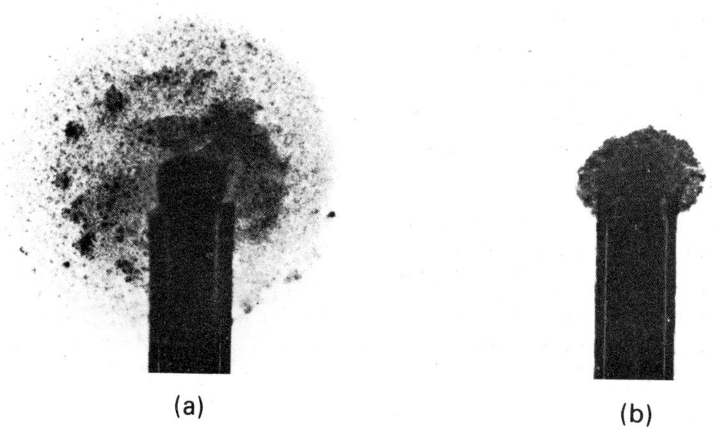

FIGURE 8.16. Migration inhibition as an *in vitro* test for cell-mediated hypersensitivity. Migration of peritoneal exudate cells from a sensitized guinea-pig: (a) control in absence of antigen and (b) in the presence of antigen. (Courtesy of Dr. J. Brostoff.)

taken from unsensitized animals; purified macrophages from the sensitized animal however are unable to produce MIF when mixed with lymphocytes from normal donors and incubated with antigen.

Greater difficulties have been encountered in attempting migration inhibition tests in the human. One variant is to incubate blood lymphocytes with antigen for several days and then to assay for MIF in the supernatant by addition to guinea-pig macrophages. Another is to mix the lymphocytes directly with the guinea-pig macrophages and to assess the effect of antigen on the migratory properties of the macrophages either in a MIF test or in the electric field of a cytopherometer. Inhibitory tests involving migration of buffy coat cells are potentially most useful but the conditions required to define when this represents a direct expression of T-cell reactivity have yet to be rigidly established.

Transformation

The proliferation of sensitized cells on contact with specific antigen and their change in morphology to larger blast-like cells with paler staining nuclei and basophilic cytoplasm (figure 3.6c, p. 61) has frequently been used as an *in vitro* test for cell-mediated hypersensitivity and several studies have shown reasonable correlation with *in vivo* results. The degree of stimulation is assessed either by the percentage of blast-like cells surviving in the culture or by the incorporation of labelled thymidine into newly synthesized DNA. The test is complicated by the possibility of recruitment into division of non-sensitized lymphocytes through release of a mitogenic factor from stimulated cells and also by the fact that B-lymphocytes may also be transformed.

Comparable changes can be induced in lymphocytes by certain plant mitogens of which the best known are phytohaemagglutinin (PHA) and concanavalin A (conA). These are termed polyclonal activators because they react with the cell surface non-specifically (i.e. not as an antigen) and produce the same series of cellular events as does antigen locking on to its specific surface receptor. Unlike the situation with antigen stimulation where only a small fraction of the cells are sensitive, PHA transforms a major proportion of the T-cells. Additionally some B-cells are affected although their response appears to be T-cell dependent. The picture is emerging that helper T-cells are preferentially stimulated by PHA and suppressors by conA. Pokeweed activates both T- and B-lymphocytes while lipopolysaccharide (in the mouse at least) is a B-cell mitogen.

Cytotoxicity

The degree of cytolysis produced by cytotoxic cells is assessed by measuring the release of radioactive chromium from pre-labelled target cells into the supernatant fluid at varying ratios of effector to target cells. The T-cell dependence of the phenomenon can be established by depletion with anti-θ plus complement in the mouse, or by rosetting with sheep red cells in the human. Direct killing by T-cells using their endogenous receptors for target cell recognition is not inhibited by anti-light chain sera unlike K-cell cytotoxicity.

Some tests appraise cytotoxicity in terms of a reduction in target cell division (e.g. inhibition of radioactive thymidine uptake into DNA) and this will measure both *cytolysis* and *cytostasis*, two quite different processes.

TISSUE DAMAGE

Infection

The development of a state of cell-mediated hypersensitivity to bacterial products is probably responsible for the lesions associated with bacterial allergy such as the cavitation, caseation and general toxaemia seen in human tuberculosis and the granulomatous skin lesions found in patients with the tuberculoid form of leprosy. When the battle between the replicating bacteria and the body defences fails to be resolved in favour of the host, persisting antigen provokes a chronic local delayed hypersensitivity reaction. Continual release of lymphokines from sensitized T-lymphocytes leads to the accumulation of large numbers of macrophages, many of which give rise to arrays of epithelioid cells, while others fuse to form giant cells. Macrophages bearing bacterial antigen on their surface become targets for killer T-cells and are destroyed. Further tissue damage will occur as a result of indiscriminate cytotoxicity by lymphokine activated macrophages (and NK cells?) and perhaps lymphotoxin itself. Morphologically, this combination of cell types with proliferating lymphocytes and fibroblasts associated with areas of fibrosis and necrosis is termed a *chronic granuloma* and represents an attempt by the body to wall-off a site of persistent infection.

The skin rashes in smallpox and measles and the lesions of herpes simplex may be largely attributed to delayed type allergic reactions with extensive damage to virally infected cells by cytotoxic T-lymphocytes. Cell-mediated hypersensitivity has also been demonstrated in the fungal diseases, candidiasis, dermatomycosis, coccidioidomycosis and histoplasmosis, and in the parasitic diseases, leishmaniasis and schistosomiasis where the pathology has been attributed to a reaction against soluble enzymes derived from the eggs which lodge in the liver capillaries.

Contact dermatitis

The dermal route of inoculation tends to favour the development of a T-cell response through processing by Langerhans' cells which migrate to the lymph nodes and present antigen to T-lymphocytes (p. 64). Thus, delayed-type reactions in the skin are often produced by foreign materials capable of binding to body constituents, possibly surface molecules of the Langerhans cell, to form new antigens. Thus contact hypersensitivity can occur in people who become sensitized while working with chemicals such as picryl chloride and chromates, or who repeatedly come into contact with the substance urushiol from the poison ivy plant. *p*-Phenylene diamine in certain hair dyes, neomycin in topically applied ointments and nickel salts formed from articles such as nickel suspenders can provoke similar reactions.

Other examples

Delayed hypersensitivity contributes significantly to the prolonged reactions which result from insect bites. The possible implication of homograft rejection by cytotoxic T-cells as a mechanism for the control of cancer cells is discussed in chapter 9. The contribution made by cell-mediated hypersensitivity reactions to different autoimmune diseases is even now rather uncertain (cf. p. 321).

Type V—Stimulatory hypersensitivity

Many cells receive instruction by agents such as hormones through surface receptors which specifically bind the external agent presumably through complementarity of structure. This combination may lead to allosteric changes in configuration of the receptor or of adjacent molecules which become activated and transmit a signal to the cell interior. For example, when thyroid stimulating hormone (TSH) of pituitary origin binds to the thyroid cell receptors there appears to be an activation of adenyl cyclase in the membrane which generates cyclic-AMP from ATP and this substance acts to stimulate activity in the thyroid cell. The thyroid stimulating antibody present in the sera of thyrotoxic patients (cf. p. 312) is an autoantibody directed against an antigen on the thyroid surface which stimulates the cell and produces the same changes as TSH, similarly utilizing the cyclic-AMP pathway. It is likely that the antibody combines with a site on the TSH receptor or an adjacent molecule to produce the allosteric change required for adenyl cyclase activation. The situation is analogous to lymphocyte stimulation; B-lymphocytes with immunoglobulin surface receptors can be stimulated by changes induced through the receptor molecules either by binding of specific antigen or by an antibody to the immunoglobulin (even anti-Fc) as shown in figure 8.17. Other experimental examples of stimulation by antibodies to cell surface antigens may be cited: the transformation of lymphocytes by heterologous anti-lymphocyte serum (ALS); the induction of pinocytosis by anti-macrophage serum; and the mitogenic effect of antibodies to sea-urchin eggs. It is worthy of note that although antibodies to enzymes directed against deter-

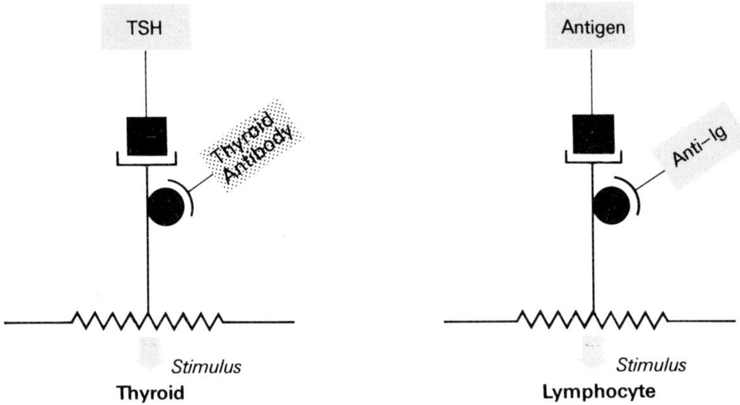

FIGURE 8.17. Stimulation of thyroid cell and of lymphocyte by physiological agent or by antibody both of which cause comparable membrane changes leading to cell activation by reacting with surface receptors.

minants near to the active site can exert a blocking effect, combination with more distant determinants can sometimes bring about allosteric conformational changes which are associated with a considerable increase in enzymic activity as has been described for certain variants of penicillinase and β-galactosidase.

Summary

The normal effector mechanisms for cell-mediated and humoral immunity are dependent upon the activation of T- and B-cells respectively (figure 8.18). Excessive stimulation of these effector mechanisms by antigen in a sensitized host can lead to tissue damage and we speak of hypersensitivity reactions of which 5 main types can be distinguished.

Type I—anaphylactic hypersensitivity depends upon the reaction of antigen with specific IgE antibody bound through its Fc to the mast cell, leading to release from the granules of the mediators histamine, slow reacting substance-A and platelet activating factor, plus an eosinophil chemotactic factor. Eosinophils neutralize the mast cell mediators. Hay fever and extrinsic asthma represent the most common atopic allergic disorders. The offending antigen is identified by intradermal prick tests giving immediate wheal and erythema reactions or by provocation testing. Symptomatic treatment involves the use of mediator antagonists or agents which maintain intracellular cAMP and thereby stabilize the mast cell granules. Courses of antigen injection may desensitize by formation of blocking IgG or IgA antibodies or by turning off IgE production.

Type II—antibody-dependent cytotoxic hypersensitivity involves the death of cells bearing antibody attached to a surface antigen. The cells may be taken up by phagocytic cells to which they adhere through their coating of IgG or C3b or lysed by the operation of the full complement system. Cells bearing IgG may also be killed by myeloid cells (polymorphs and macrophages) or by non-adherent lymphoid K cells through an extracellular mechanism (antibody-dependent cell-mediated cytotoxicity). Examples are: transfusion reactions, haemolytic disease of the newborn through Rhesus incompatibility, antibody mediated graft destruction, autoimmune reactions directed against the

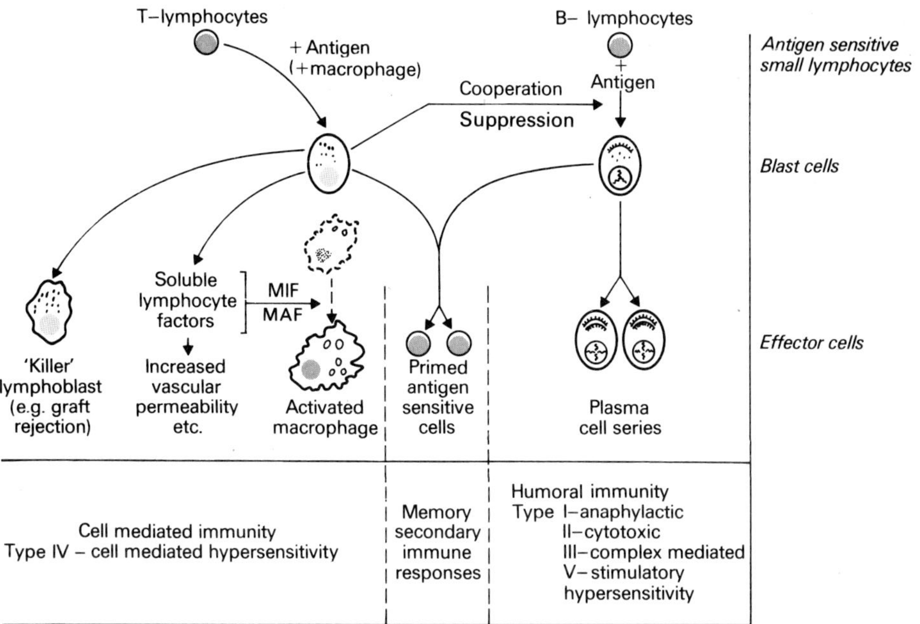

FIGURE 8.18. Relationship of B- and T-cell activity to different forms of hypersensitivity and immunity. Different T-cell functions are mediated by distinct sub-populations.

formed elements of the blood and kidney glomerular basement membranes, and hypersensitivity resulting from the coating of erythrocytes or platelets by a drug.

Type III—complex-mediated hypersensitivity results from the effects of antigen–antibody complexes through (a) activation of complement and attraction of polymorphonuclear leucocytes which release tissue damaging enzymes on contact with the complex and (b) aggregation of platelets to cause microthrombi and vasoactive amine release. Where circulating antibody levels are high, the antigen is precipitated near the site of entry into the body. The reaction in the skin is characterized by polymorph infiltration, oedema and erythema maximal at 3–8 hours (Arthus reaction). Examples are Farmer's lung, pigeon fancier's disease and pulmonary aspergillosis where inhaled antigens provoke high antibody levels, reactions to an abrupt increase in antigen caused by microbial cell death during chemotherapy for leprosy or syphilis, and an element of the synovial lesion in rheumatoid arthritis. In relative *antigen excess*, soluble complexes are formed which circulate and are deposited under circumstances of increased vascular permeability at certain preferred sites, the kidney glomerulus, the joints, the skin and the choroid plexus. Complexes can be detected in tissue biopsies by immunoflorescence and in serum by precipitation with polyethylene glycol, reaction with C1q, changes in C3 and C3c, and binding to the C3 receptor on the Raji cell line. Examples are: serum sickness following injection of large quantities of foreign protein, glomerulonephritis associated with systemic lupus or infections with streptococci, malaria and other parasites, neurological disturbances in systemic lupus and subacute sclerosing panencephalitis, polyarteritis nodosa linked to hepatitis B virus, and haemorrhagic shock in dengue viral infection.

Type IV—cell-mediated or delayed-type hypersensitivity is based upon the interaction of antigen with primed T-cells. A number of soluble mediators (lymphokines) are released which account for the events which occur in a typical delayed hypersensitivity response such as the Mantoux reaction to tuberculin, namely, the delayed appearance of an indurated and erythematous reaction which reaches a maximum at 24–48 hours and is characterized histologically by infiltration first with polymorphs and subsequently with mononuclear phagocytes and lymphocytes. The lymphokines include: macrophage migration inhibition (MIF), macrophage activation (MAF), mononuclear chemotactic, skin reactive, lymphocyte mitogenic, and cytostatic (lymphotoxin) factors. Interferon is also generated. Another sub-population of T-cells are activated by major histocompatibility antigens to become directly cytotoxic to target cells bearing the appropriate antigen; they also react to viral determinants on the surface of infected cells which are recognized in association with these MHC antigens. *In vitro* tests for cell-mediated hypersensitivity include macrophage migration inhibition, assessment of blast cell transformation and direct cytotoxicity. Examples are: tissue damage occuring in bacterial (tuberculosis, leprosy), viral (smallpox, measles, herpes), fungal (candidiasis, histoplasmosis) and parasitic (leishmaniasis, schistosomiasis) infections, contact dermatitis from exposure to chromates and poison ivy, and insect bites. Continuing provocation of delayed hypersensitivity by persisting antigen leads to formation of chronic granulomata.

Type V—stimulatory hypersensitivity where the antibody reacts with a key surface component such as a hormone

TABLE 8.1. Comparison of different types of hypersensitivity

	I Anaphylactic	II Cytotoxic	III Complex-mediated	IV Cell-mediated	V Stimulatory
Antibody mediating reaction	Homocytotropic Ab Mast-cell binding	Humoral Ab ±CF*	Humoral Ab ±CF	Receptor on T-lymphocyte	Humoral Ab Non-CF
Antigen	Usually exogenous (e.g. grass pollen)	Cell surface	Extracellular	Associated with MHC antigens on macrophage or target cell	Cell surface
Response to intradermal antigen:					
Max. reaction	30 min.	—	3–8 hr.	24–48 hr.	—
Appearance	Wheal and flare	—	Erythema and oedema	Erythema and induration	—
Histology	Degranulated mast cells; oedema; eosinophils	—	Acute inflammatory reaction; predominant polymorphs	Perivascular inflammation: polymorphs migrate out leaving predominantly mononuclear cells	—
Transfer sensitivity to normal subject	←———	Serum antibody	———→	Lymphoid cells Transfer factor	Serum antibody
Examples:	Atopic allergy, e.g. hay fever	Haemolytic disease of newborn (Rh)	Complex glomerulonephritis Farmer's lung	Mantoux reaction to TB Killing virally infected cells Contact sensitivity	Thyrotoxicosis

* CF = Complement fixation.

receptor and 'switches on' the cell. An example is the thyroid hyper-reactivity in Graves' disease due to a thyroid stimulating autoantibody.

Features of the 5 types of hypersensitivity are compared in Table 8.1.

Further reading

Brostoff J. (1973) Atopic allergy. *Brit.J.Hosp.Med.*, **9**, p. 29.

Cochrane C.G. & Koffler D. (1973) Immune complex disease in experimental animals and man. *Adv.in Immunology*, **16**, 186.

Fudenberg, H.H., Stites D.P., Caldwell J.L. & Wells J.V. (1978) *Basic and Clinical Immunology*, 2nd ed. Lange Medical Publications, Los Altos, California.

Gell P.G.H., Coombs R.R.A. & Lachmann R. (eds) (1975) *Clinical Aspects of Immunology*, 3rd ed., Section IV. Blackwell Scientific Publications, Oxford.

Ling N.R. (1975) *Lymphocyte Stimulation*, 2nd ed. North Holland, Amsterdam.

Maini R.N. & Holborow E.J. (eds) (1977) Detection and measurement of circulating soluble antigen–antibody complexes and anti-DNA antibodies. *Ann.Rheum.Dis.*, **36**, Suppl. No. 1.

Mollison P.L. (1970) Red cell destruction. *Brit.J.Haematol.*, **18**, 249.

O'Regan S., Smith M. & Drumond K.N. (1976) Antigens in human immune complex nephritis. *Clin.Nephrol.*, **6**, 417.

Pepys J. (1969) *Hypersensitivity Diseases of the Lungs due to Fungi and Organic Dusts.* Karger, Basle.

Roitt I.M., Shen L. & Greenberg A.H. (1976) Antibody-dependent cell-mediated cytotoxicity. In *The role of immunological factors in infectious, allergic and autoimmune processes.* Beers R.F. & Bassett E.G. (eds). Raven Press, New York.

Rose N.R. & Friedman H. (1976) *Manual of clinical immunology.* Amer. Soc. Microbiology, Washington, D.C.

Stanworth D.S. (1973) *Immediate Hypersensitivity.* North Holland, Amsterdam.

Turk J.L. (1975) *Delayed Hypersensitivity*, 2nd ed. North Holland, Amsterdam.

Turk J.L. (1978) *Immunology in Clinical Medicine*, 3rd ed. Heinemann, London.

9 Transplantation

The replacement of diseased organs by a transplant of healthy tissue has long been an objective in medicine but has been frustrated to no mean degree by the unco-operative attempts by the body to reject grafts from other individuals. Before discussing the nature and implications of this rejection phenomenon, it would be helpful to define the terms used for transplants between individuals and species:

Autograft—tissue grafted back onto the original donor.

Isograft—graft between syngeneic individuals (i.e. of identical genetic constitution) such as identical twins or mice of the same pure line strain.

Allograft (old term, homograft)—graft between allogeneic individuals (i.e. members of the same species but different genetic constitution), e.g. man to man and one mouse strain to another.

Xenograft (heterograft)—graft between xenogeneic individuals (i.e. of different species), e.g. pig to man.

It is with the allograft reaction that we have been most concerned although it should one day be possible to use grafts from other species. The most common allografting procedure is probably blood transfusion where the unfortunate consequences of mismatching are well known. Considerable attention has been paid to the rejection of solid grafts such as skin and the sequence of events is worth describing. In mice, for example, the skin allograft settles down and becomes vascularized within a few days. Between three and nine days the circulation gradually diminishes and there is increasing infiltration of the graft bed with lymphocytes and monocytes but very few plasma cells. Necrosis begins to be visible macroscopically and within a day or so the graft is sloughed completely (figure 9.1).

Evidence that rejection is immunological

First and second set reactions

It would be expected if the reaction has an immunological basis, that the second contact with antigen would represent

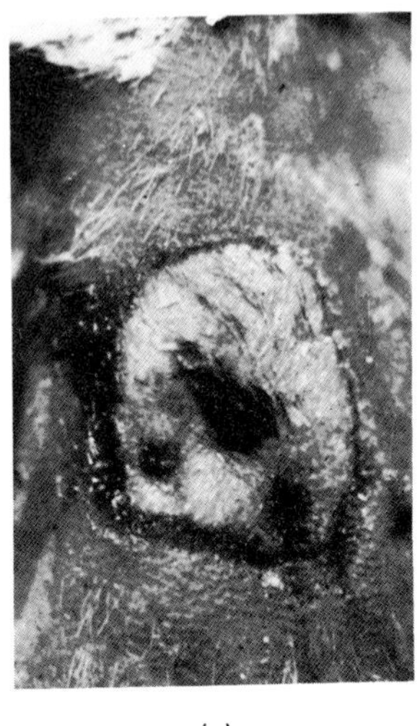

(a)

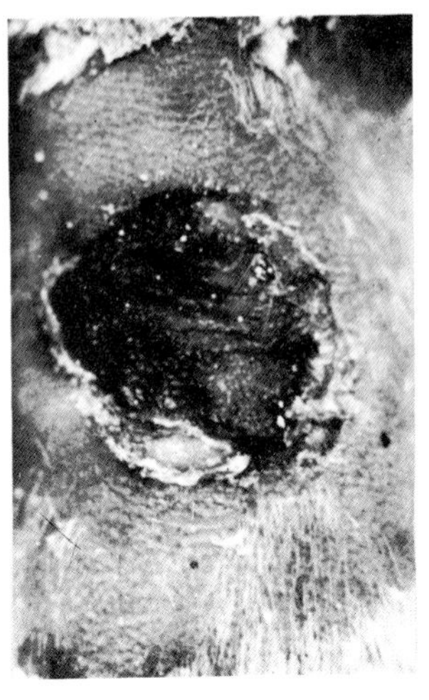

(b)

FIGURE 9.1. Rejection of CBA skin graft by strain A mouse. (a) 10 days after transplantation; discoloured areas caused by destruction of epithelium and drying of the exposed dermis. (b) 13 days after transplantation; the scabby surface indicates total destruction of the graft. (Courtesy Prof. L. Brent.)

a more explosive event than the first and indeed the rejection of a second graft from the same donor is much accelerated. The initial vascularization is poor and may not occur at all. There is a very rapid invasion by polymorphonuclear leucocytes and lymphoid cells including plasma cells. Thrombosis and acute cell destruction can be seen by three to four days.

Specificity

Second set rejection is not the fate of all subsequent allografts but only of those derived from the original donor or a related strain. Grafts from unrelated donors are rejected as first set reactions.

Role of the lymphocyte

Neonatally thymectomized animals have difficulty in rejecting skin grafts but their capacity is restored by injection of lymphocytes from a syngeneic normal donor, suggesting that T-cells are implicated. The recipient of lymphoid cells from a donor which has already rejected a graft will give

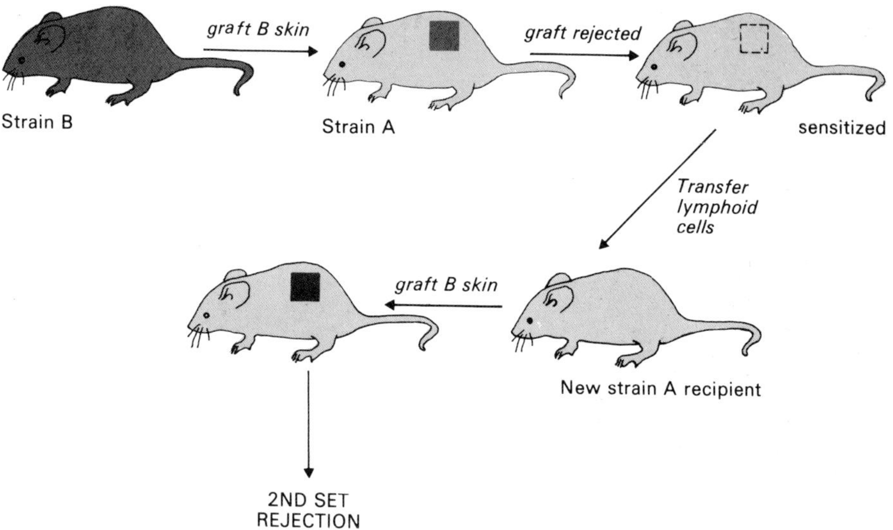

FIGURE 9.2. Transfer of ability to give accelerated graft rejection with lymphoid cells from a sensitized animal.

accelerated rejection of a further graft of the same type (figure 9.2) showing that the lymphoid cells are primed and retain memory of the first contact with graft antigens.

Production of antibodies

After rejection, humoral antibodies with specificity for the graft donor may be recognized. In the mouse where the erythrocytes carry transplantation antigens, haemagglutination tests become positive; in the human, lymphocytotoxins are found. A Jerne plaque test using donor strain thymocytes in place of sheep erythrocytes will often demonstrate the presence of antibody-forming cells in the lymphoid tissues of grafted animals.

Transplantation antigens

GENETICS

The specificity of the antigens involved in graft rejection is under genetic control. Genetically identical individuals such as mice of a pure strain or uniovular twins have identical transplantation antigens and grafts can be freely exchanged between them. The Mendelian segregation of the genes controlling these antigens has been revealed by interbreeding experiments between mice of different pure strains. Since these mice breed true within a given strain and always accept grafts from each other, they must be homozygous for the 'transplantation' genes. Consider two such strains A and B with allelic genes differing at one locus. In each case paternal and maternal genes will be identical and they will have a genetic constitution of, say, AA and BB respectively. Crossing strains A and B gives a first familial generation (F1) of constitution AB. These accept grafts from either parent; they must therefore be tolerant to the antigens expressed by both A and B genes and in fact these genes are codominant, i.e. individual cells carry both types of transplantation antigen (figure 9.3) as may be shown by immunofluorescent studies. By intercrossing the F1 generation, it will be seen from figure 9.3 that three out of four of the F2 generation accept parental strain grafts. Extending the analysis, if instead of one locus with a pair of allelic genes, there were *n* loci, the fraction of the F2 generation accepting parental strain grafts would be $(3/4)^n$. In this way an estimate of the number of loci controlling transplantation antigens can be made.

In the mouse at least 20 such loci have been established, but of these, one complex locus termed H-2 predominates in the sense that it controls the 'strong' transplantation antigens which provoke intense allograft reactions that are the most difficult to suppress. This H-2 locus constitutes the *major histocompatibility complex* (MHC), and it is a

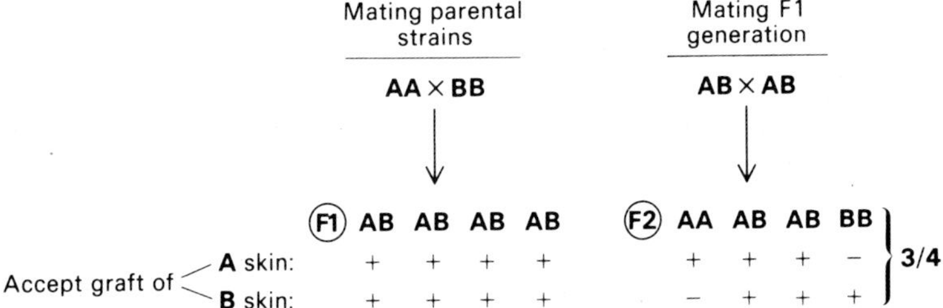

FIGURE 9.3. Inheritance of genes controlling transplantation antigens. A represents a gene expressing the 'A' antigen and B the corresponding allelic gene at the same genetic locus. The pure strains are homozygous for AA and BB respectively. Since the genes are codominant, an animal with an AB genome will express both antigens, become tolerant to them and therefore accept grafts from either A or B donors. The illustration shows that for each gene controlling a transplantation antigen specificity, three-quarters of the F2 generation will accept a graft of parental skin. For *n* genes the fraction is $(\frac{3}{4})^n$.

feature of all the vertebrate species so far studied that each possesses a single MHC which dominates allo-transplantation reactivity.

THE MAJOR HISTOCOMPATIBILITY COMPLEX IN MICE

Classical transplantation antigens

Although the H-2 locus appeared to be a single entity, it is now seen to be far more complicated and may be broken down into regions which are separable by genetic recombination (i.e. by chromosomal crossing over between the subregions). Alloantisera obtained by grafting or immunization between different mouse strains identify two major regions K and D (figure 9.4) each defined by a major genetic locus (with numerous alleles) which encodes a single 'strong' transplantation antigen. Each chromosome therefore controls the synthesis of an H-2K and an H-2D antigenic specificity. Because they are the most potent antigens of the H-2 complex in provoking an antibody response, they were the first to be recognized by sera from allografted animals and the term classical transplantation antigens is appropriate, and as it turns out, useful. A third locus codes for H-2L, a minor series of polymorphic antigens structurally similar to H-2D/K. All lymphoid cells are rich in H-2D/K antigens; liver, lung and kidney have moderate amounts whereas brain and skeletal muscle have relatively little. The antigens are evidently on the cell surface since lymphocytes are readily lysed by antibody in the presence of complement. Capping experiments and SDS-polyacrylamide gel analysis of immunoprecipitates of radiolabelled, detergent-solubilized H-2 show the K and D specificities to be associated with separate molecules. They are located on peptides of molecular weight 43,000 which are associated non-covalently with β_2-microglobulin (cf. HLA-A, figure 9.8). Both β_2-microglobulin and the H-2D/K peptides show a high degree of homology with the immunoglobulin constant region domains and appear to adopt a similar tertiary configuration suggesting a common evolutionary origin. There is evidence that in the absence of β_2-microglobulin, the classical transplantation antigens fail to be expressed on the cell surface. These antigens are transmembrane glycoproteins and the serological specificity lies in the amino acid sequence rather than the carbohydrate moiety.

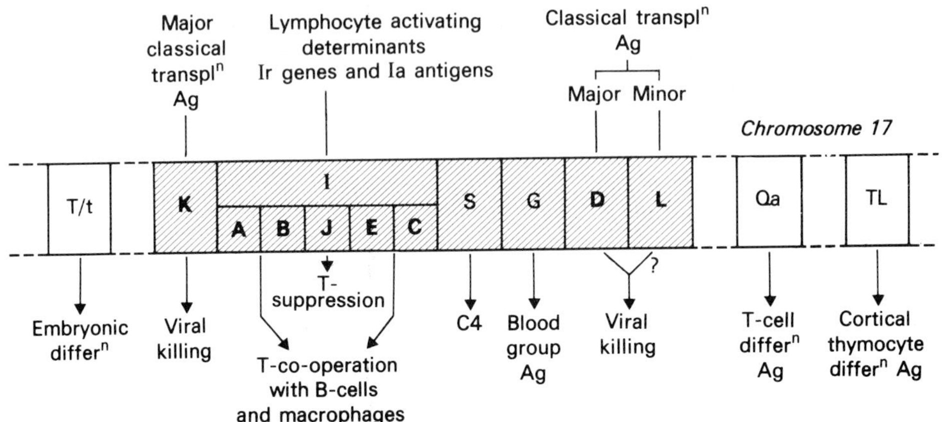

FIGURE 9.4. The H-2 major histocompatibility gene complex (▨) and its subregions in the mouse (bold letters encode antigens concerned in transplantation reactions; differ^n = differentiation, Ag = antigen). The complex spans 0·5 centimorgans equivalent to a recombination frequency between the D and K ends of 0·5%. The genes making up a given H-2 complex are termed a haplotype, usually represented by a superscript, e.g. DBA has the H-2^d haplotype. Because the genes are close together, the haplotype appears to segregate as a single Mendelian trait, the complexity only being revealed by recombination through crossing over. Each H-2K and D molecule possesses several antigenic specificities corresponding with a number of different antigenic determinants and these are classed as (i) private specificities unique for a given haplotype, (ii) public specificities shared between different haplotypes but unique for K or D regions and (iii) public specificities shared between K and D regions. The H-2K product provokes a more powerful transplantation reaction than H-2D. Other genes within the H-2 complex control: (a) levels of C2, C3 and factor B, (b) resistance to Gross leukaemia virus (Rgv-1) and mammary tumour virus (RMTV), (c) innate resistance to bone marrow grafts in non-syngeneic irradiated recipients (*Hh* factors) e.g. parent into F1 (presumably reflecting non-codominant expression of Hh genes), and (d) the level of testosterone and testosterone-binding protein (Hom-1). Near to the H-2 complex are genes coding for the Tl antigens specific for thymocytes and certain thymus leukaemic cells, another region controlling the Qa antigens which segregate between various T-cell subsets (p. 101) and the T-t region (T = normal, t = tailless) which affects complex differentiation events in the embryo. The T/t antigens are present on sperm and in early ontogeny and are probably replaced by H-2K and D which they resemble biochemically. Recombination with H-2 is suppressed.

Lymphocyte activating determinants

Mixed lymphocyte reaction (*MLR*). When lymphocytes from genetically dissimilar mice are cultured together, blast cell transformation and mitosis occurs (MLR), each population of lymphocytes reacting against 'foreign' determinants on the surface of the other population. For the 'one-way MLR', the stimulator cells are made unresponsive by treatment with mitomycin C or X-rays and then added to the responder lymphocytes from the other donor. The responding cells belong predominantly to a subpopulation of Ly1 positive T-lymphocytes and they are stimulated by lymphocyte activating determinants (Lad) present mostly on B-cells and macrophages, the genes which code for them lying within the I region (figure 9.4). Antisera to I region antigens (anti-Ia) block the Lad of the stimulator cells and thereby inhibit the MLR, suggesting that the Lad are present on Ia molecules. It will be recalled that the Ia antigens are concerned in T help and T suppression. Cells bearing I-J evoke suppressors and T-lymphocytes positive for I-A and I-E/C mediate delayed sensitivity and B-cell help. I-A and I-E/C are transmembrane glycoproteins each consisting of an α- and a β-polypeptide, both of which are polymorphic (cf. figure 9.8).

The I-A genetic subregion encodes the two chains of the I-A molecule and the β chain of I-E/C, i.e. the I-E/C molecules are controlled by genes in two subregions of the H-2 complex. This may account for the phenomenon of gene complementation in the T-dependent responsiveness to certain antigens (p. 96) seen when mating two poor-responder strains produces a high responder Fl, since random association of maternal and paternally derived Ia peptides may yield a 'high response' I-E/C molecule.

Cell-mediated lympholysis (*CML*). The relevance of Lad to the provocation of transplantation rejection has been brought into some focus by the discovery of the phenomenon of *cell mediated lympholysis* (CML) which was developed as a possible test for histocompatibility. The principle is illustrated in figure 9.5. In short, if lymphocytes from donor X react against Y in one-way mixed lymphocyte culture because of Ia differences, the transformed lymphoblasts are cytotoxic for Y cells provided there are H-2K or D incompatibilities between them. With unrelated but H-2K and D matched strains, an MLR occurs but the resulting cells are not cytotoxic for the other member of the pair. The cytotoxic T-cell subpopulation which recognizes H-2K/D differences is not the same as that which responds to Ia. Nonetheless, they can only differentiate into cytotoxic effectors with the co-operation generated by a response to Ia; in other words, T helpers recognizing Ia produce the conditions required for triggering potentially cytotoxic cells by H-2K/D determinants (figure 9.5), a situation not unlike the two signal mechanism envisaged for B-cell

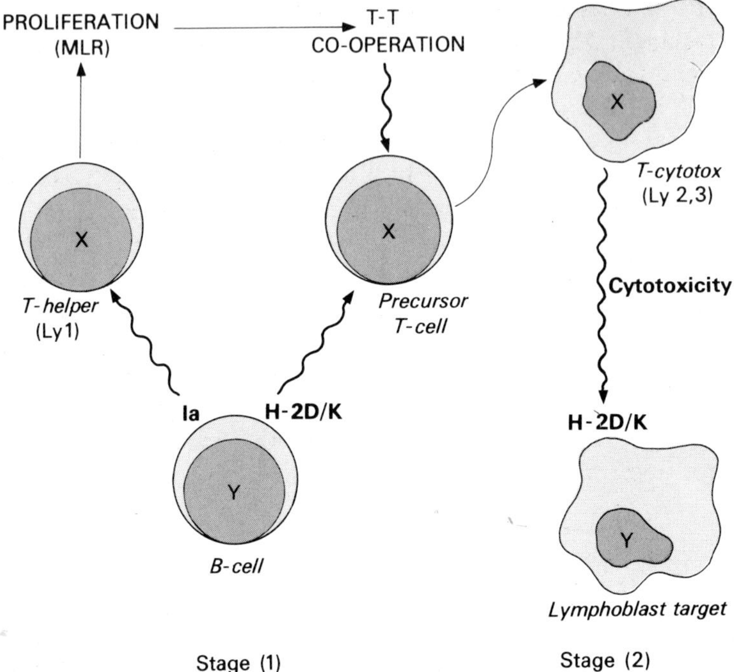

FIGURE 9.5. Cell-mediated lympholysis. *Stage* (1)—X's T_{helper} cells recognize Ia differences on Y (the target cell) but Y cannot react reciprocally since it has been blocked by mitomycin. The $T_{cytotox}$ cells bind H-2K/D determinants on Y and under the influence of the activated T_{helper} population, they differentiate into cytotoxic effectors. *Stage* (2)—Meanwhile a separate sample of Y's lymphocytes are transformed into blasts with PHA, labelled with radioactive chromium and added to cultures at the end of stage (1) to test for the presence of cytotoxic cells. Cytotoxicity is evaluated by the release of chromium from the blasts (which are more vulnerable as targets than small lymphocytes).

stimulation through T-lymphocyte co-operation in the carrier hapten system (p. 70).

Graft vs. host (g.v.h.) reaction. When competent lymphoid cells are transferred from a donor to a recipient which is incapable of rejecting them, the grafted cells survive and have time to recognize the host antigens and react immunologically against them. Instead of the normal transplantation reaction of host against graft, we have the reverse, the so-called graft vs. host reaction. In the young rodent there can be inhibition of growth (runting), spleen enlargement and haemolytic anaemia (due to production of red cell antibodies). In the human, fever, anaemia, weight loss, rash, diarrhoea and splenomegaly are observed. The 'stronger' the transplantation antigen difference, the more severe the reaction. Where donor and recipient differ at HLA or H-2 loci, the reaction can be fatal.

Two possible situations leading to g.v.h. reactions are illustrated in figure 9.6. In the human this may arise in immunologically anergic subjects receiving bone marrow grafts, e.g. for combined immunodeficiency (p. 210), for red cell aplasia after radiation accidents or as a possible form of cancer therapy. Competent lymphoid cells in blood or present in grafted organs given to immunosuppressed patients may give g.v.h. reactions; so could maternal cells which adventitiously cross the placenta, although in this case there is as yet no evidence of diseases caused by such a mechanism in the human.

THE MAJOR HISTOCOMPATIBILITY COMPLEX IN MAN

In man, as in the mouse, there is also one dominant group of antigens which provokes strong reactions—the HLA system. In addition, the ABO group provides strong transplantation antigens.

Of the four principal HLA loci identified, HLA-A and HLA-B probably represent the counterpart of the murine serologically-defined antigens H-2K and H-2D in that they

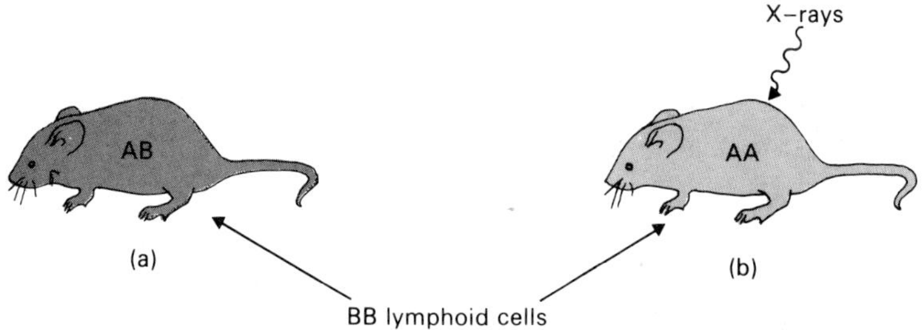

FIGURE 9.6. Graft vs. host reaction. When competent lymphoid cells are inoculated into a host incapable of reacting against them, the grafted cells are free to react against the antigens on the host's cells which they recognize as foreign. The ensuing reaction may be fatal. Two of many possible situations are illustrated: (a) the hybrid AB receives cells from one parent (BB) which are tolerated but react against the A antigen on host cells (b) an X-irradiated AA recipient restored immunologically with BB cells cannot react against the graft and a g.v.h. reaction will result.

most readily evoke the formation of complement-fixing cytotoxic antibodies which can be used for tissue typing. Operationally mono-specific sera are selected from patients transfused with whole blood and multigravidas who often become immunized with fetal antigens with specificities defined by paternally derived genes absent from the mother's genome. An individual is typed by setting up their lymphocytes against a panel of such sera in the presence of complement, cell death normally being judged by the inability to exclude

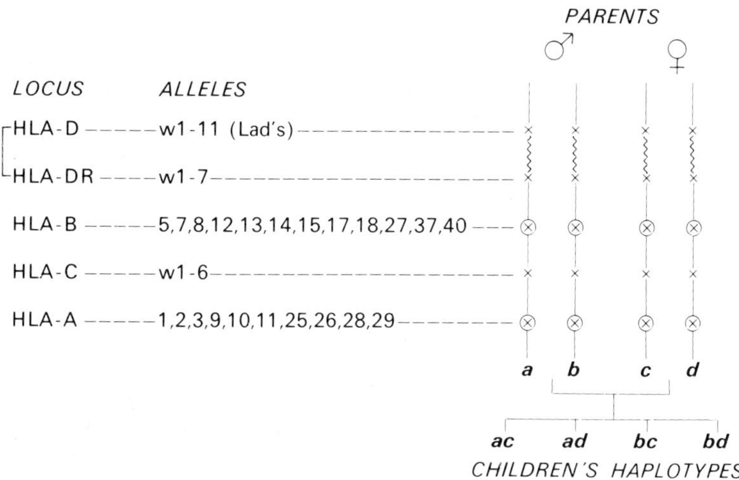

FIGURE 9.7. The major histocompatibility complex in man (HLA) and its inheritance. The 4 loci lie on chromosome 6, the D locus being closest to the centromere. ⊗ = Major loci originally defined by serological tissue typing which parallel the murine H-2K and H-2D classical transplantation loci; there are several more specificities at each locus but only the most solidly established are given. A further locus with just two alleles, HLA-Bw4 and Bw6 (formerly 4a/4b) is intimately linked to HLA-B. Specificities at the D locus (Lad's) are defined by their mixed lymphocyte reactions against homozygous typing cells, but closely related (HLA-DR), if not sometimes identical antigens, are also being characterized using cytotoxic antibodies. The small 'w' before a number stands for 'workshop' and indicates that the specificity concerned has not yet been characterized sufficiently for upgrading to full HLA-status.

Since there are several possible alleles at each locus, the probability of a random pair of subjects from the general population having identical HLA specificities is low. However, there is a 1:4 chance that two *siblings* will be identical in this respect because each group of specificities on a single chromosome forms a haplotype which will be inherited *en bloc* giving 4 possible combinations of paternal and maternal chromosomes. Parent and offspring can only be identical (1:2 chance) if the mother and father have one haplotype in common.

trypan blue. Antigens arbitrarily assigned the specificities 1, 2, 3, 9, 10, 11, 28 and 29 by this means are negatively associated with each other in population studies, no individual has more than two of these antigens and not more than one is transmitted to an offspring from each parent; they therefore form an allelic series referred to as the HLA-A locus (figure 9.7). HLA-B5, 7, 8, 12, 13, 14, 18 and 27 constitute a second locus. Thus, an individual heterozygous at each locus must express four *major* serologically-defined HLA specificities, two from maternally derived and two from the paternally derived chromosomes (figure 9.7). Serologically-defined antigens encoded by a third locus, HLA-C induce a somewhat weaker response.

The major lymphocyte activating determinants are controlled by alleles at a fourth locus, HLA-D. Typing is carried out by looking for non-reactivity in the MLR against a homozygous stimulating cell. Such typing cells may be

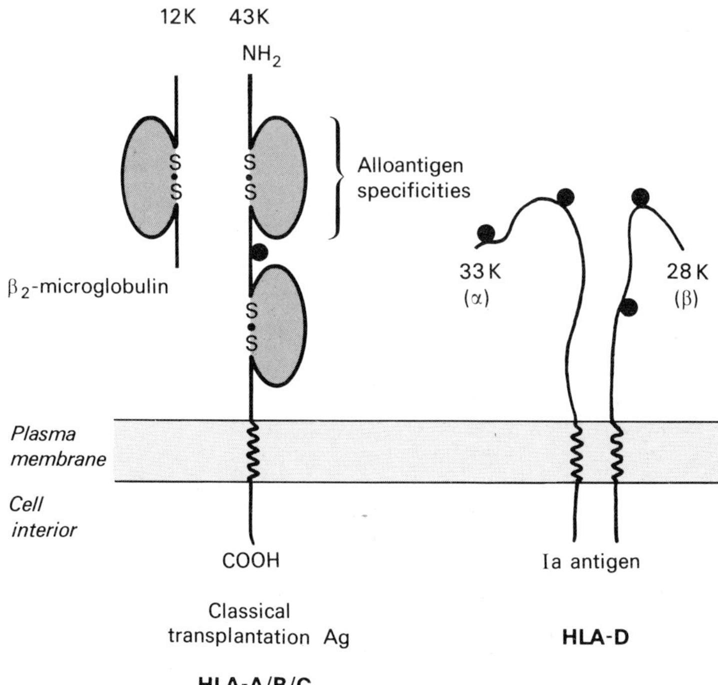

FIGURE 9.8. Structure of major HLA molecules. They are transmembrane glycoproteins (● = carbohydrate) with hydrophobic segments (〰) inserted into the plasma membrane (cf. figure 6.16). Regions with homology for Ig domains are shaded (▒). The molecular weight of each peptide in thousands is shown. (After Barnstable C.J., Jones E.A. & Crumpton M.J. *Brit med Bull.*, 1978, **34**, 241. Based on structures suggested by Strominger, Snarg & colleagues.)

obtained from the children of first cousin marriages (where there is a 1 : 16 chance of homozygosity) or from patients with a disease known to be strongly associated with certain D alleles, e.g. multiple sclerosis and HLA-Dw2. Another approach is to use spermatozoa as stimulators since they only carry one haplotype; spermatozoa expressing the other paternal haplotype can be eliminated by appropriate cytotoxic antisera directed against A or B locus antigens. Closely related, if not identical antigens are also being characterized by cytotoxic antibodies. These HLA-D related serologically defined specificities (HLA-DR) are most abundant on B-lymphocytes and are often termed B-cell alloantigens; however, they are also present on macrophages and are probably the equivalent of murine Ia antigens. The structures of the different HLA molecules are represented in figure 9.8.

Rejection mechanisms

LYMPHOCYTE-MEDIATED REJECTION

A great deal of the work on allograft rejection has involved transplants of skin or solid tumours because their fate is relatively easy to follow. In these cases there is little support for the view that humoral antibodies are instrumental in destruction of the graft although as we shall see later this is not necessarily so with transplants of other organs such as the kidney. Whereas passive transfer of *serum* from an animal which has rejected a skin allograft cannot usually accelerate the rejection of a similar graft on the recipient animal, injection of *lymphoid cells* (particularly recirculating small lymphocytes) is effective in shortening graft survival (cf. figure 9.2). Tissue culture studies have shown that such lymphoid cells taken from animals sensitized by a graft which they have rejected are able to kill target cells possessing the same transplantation antigens as the original graft. The sensitized lymphocytes recognize the target cells through specific surface receptors and this combination with antigen leads to surface membrane changes responsible for the cytotoxic potential of the lymphocytes.

A primary role of lymphoid cells in first set rejection would be consistent with the histology of the early reaction showing infiltration by mononuclear cells with very few polymorphs or plasma cells (figure 9.9). The dramatic effect of neonatal thymectomy in prolonging skin transplants, as mentioned

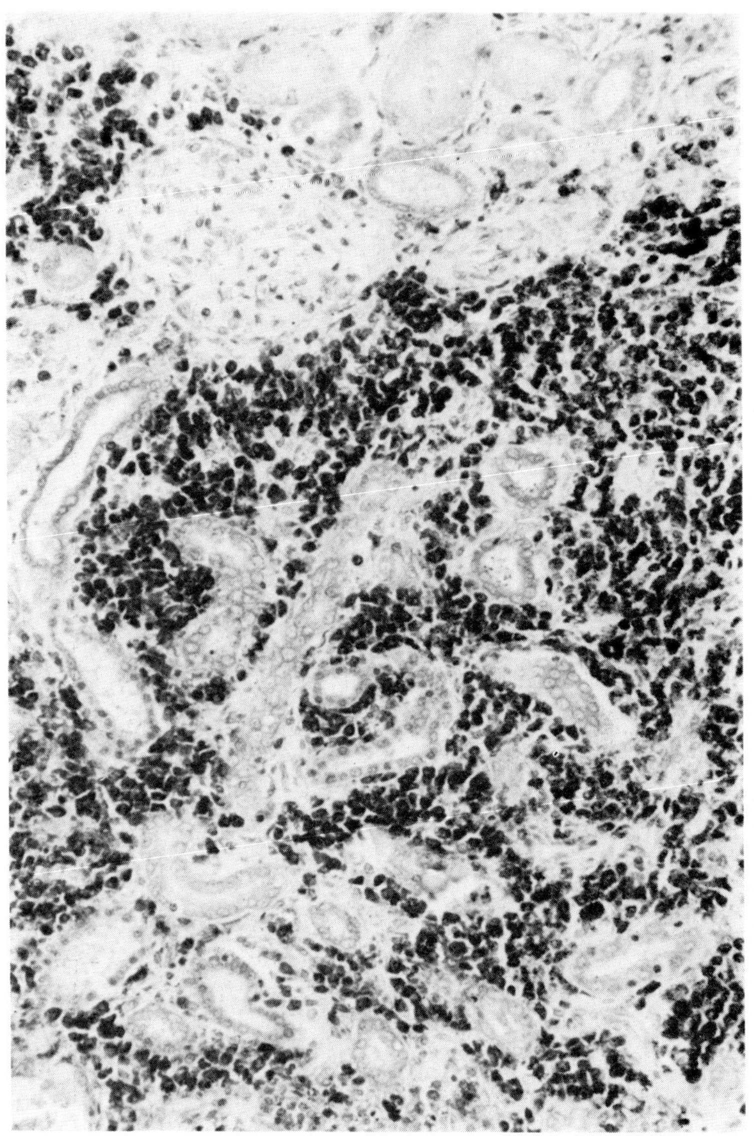

FIGURE 9.9. Acute early rejection of human renal allograft 10 days after transplantation showing dense cellular infiltration of interstitium by mononuclear cells (pyronin stain). (Courtesy Prof. K. Porter.)

earlier, and the long survival of grafts on children with thymic deficiencies implicate the T-lymphocytes in these reactions. In the chicken, homograft rejection and g.v.h. reactivity are influenced by neonatal thymectomy but not bursectomy. More direct evidence has come from *in vitro* studies showing that the sensitized mouse lymphocytes responsible for killing certain target allograft in tissue culture bear the Thy1 marker on their surface (see p. 59) and are therefore T-lymphocytes.

Lymphoid cells sensitized to a graft can release macrophage migration inhibition factor (MIF; see p. 78) when confronted with the appropriate histocompatibility antigens and it is possible that this test will give an early indication of sensitization in a grafted individual.

THE ROLE OF HUMORAL ANTIBODY

It has long been recognized that isolated allogeneic cells such as lymphocytes can be destroyed by cytotoxic (type II) reactions involving humoral antibody. However, although earlier experience with skin and solid tumour-grafts suggested that they were not readily susceptible to the action of cytotoxic antibodies, it is now clear that this does not hold for all types of organ transplants. Consideration of the different ways in which kidney allografts can be rejected illustrates the point:

(a) *Hyperacute rejection* within minutes of transplantation, characterized by sludging of red cells and microthrombi in the glomeruli, occurs in individuals with pre-existing humoral antibodies—either due to blood group incompatibility or presensitization through blood transfusion.

(b) *Acute early rejection* occurring up to 10 days or so after transplantation is characterized by dense cellular infiltration (figure 9.9) and rupture of peritubular capillaries and appears to be a cell-mediated hypersensitivity reaction involving T-lymphocytes.

(c) *Acute late rejection*, which occurs from 11 days onwards in patients suppressed with prednisone and azathioprine, is probably caused by the binding of immunoglobulin (presumably antibody) and complement to the arterioles and glomerular capillaries where they can be visualized by immunofluorescent techniques. These immunoglobulin deposits on the vessel walls induce platelet aggregation in the glomerular capillaries leading to acute renal shutdown (figure 9.10). The possibility of damage to antibody-coated cells through antibody-dependent cell-mediated cytotoxicity must also be considered.

(d) *Insidious and late* rejection associated with subendothelial deposits of immunoglobulin and C3 on the glomerular basement membranes which may sometimes be an expression of an underlying immune complex disorder (originally neces-

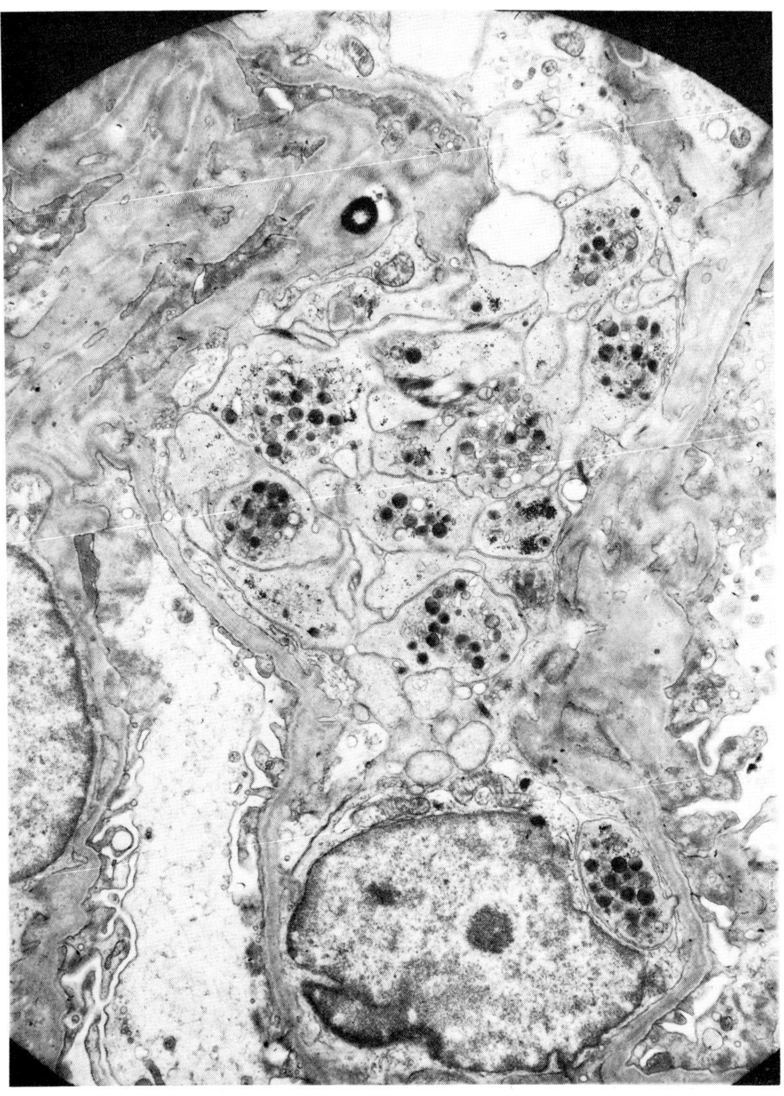

FIGURE 9.10. Acute late rejection of human renal allograft showing platelet aggregation in a glomerular capillary induced by deposition of antibody on the vessel wall (electron micrograph). (Courtesy Prof. K. Porter.)

sitating the transplant) or possibly complex formation with soluble antigens derived from the grafted kidney.

The complexity of the action and interaction of cellular and humoral factors in graft rejection is therefore considerable and an attempt to summarize the postulated mechanisms involved is presented in figure 9.11.

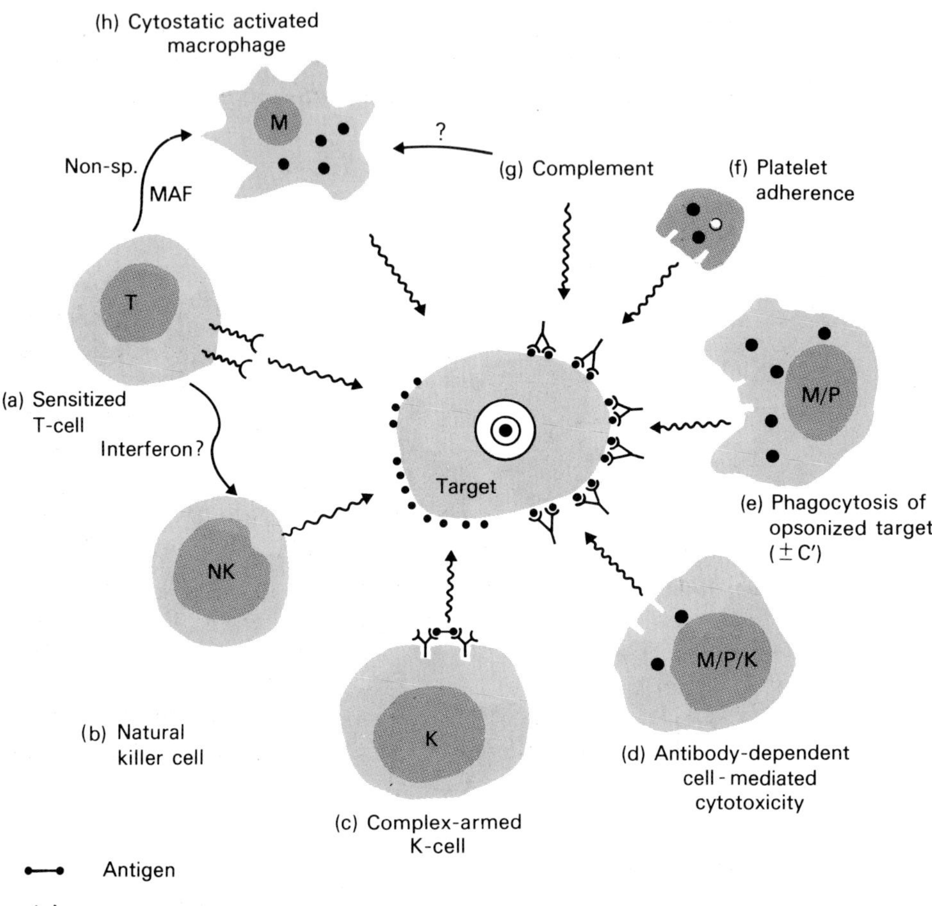

FIGURE 9.11. Mechanisms of target cell destruction. M = Macrophage; P = Polymorph; K = K cell. (a) Direct killing by sensitized T cells binding through specific surface receptors. In addition a non-specific soluble toxin is released. (b) Killing by NK cells (p. 285) enhanced by interferon. (c) Specific killing by immune-complex-armed K-cell recognizes target through free antibody valencies in the complex. (d) Attack by antibody-dependent cell-mediated cytotoxicity (in a–d the killing is extra-cellular). (e) Phagocytosis of target coated with antibody (heightened by bound C3). (f) Sticking of platelets to antibody bound to surface of graft vascular endothelium leading to formation of micro-thrombi. (g) Complement mediated cytotoxicity. (h) Macrophages activated non-specifically by agents such as BCG, endotoxin, poly-I:C, T-cell non-specific macrophage activating factor and (?) C3b are cytostatic and sometimes cytotoxic for dividing tumour cells perhaps through extracellular action of peroxide and O_2^- derived radicals generated at the cell surface (p. 176). In some situations *in vitro*, sensitized B cells secrete antibody which coats the target rendering it susceptible to attack by ADCC.

There are also circumstances when antibodies may actually *protect* a graft from destruction and this important phenomenon of *enhancement* will be considered further below.

Prevention of graft rejection

TISSUE MATCHING

Based upon experience of matching blood for transfusion and of transplantation between mice of similar specificities it could reasonably be expected that the chances of rejection in the human would be minimized by matching donor and recipient at the HLA loci. Indeed in the case of human kidney transplantation, the data based upon typing for HLA-A and -B specificities indicate that the closer the match, the better the survival of the graft. This is especially true with matched siblings (figure 9.12) but it would be wrong to conclude that full matching at A and B loci is all that is necessary since grafts between unrelated individuals who fulfil this condition are markedly less successful than those between siblings. Now we have seen that matched siblings have the same haplotypes (figure 9.7)

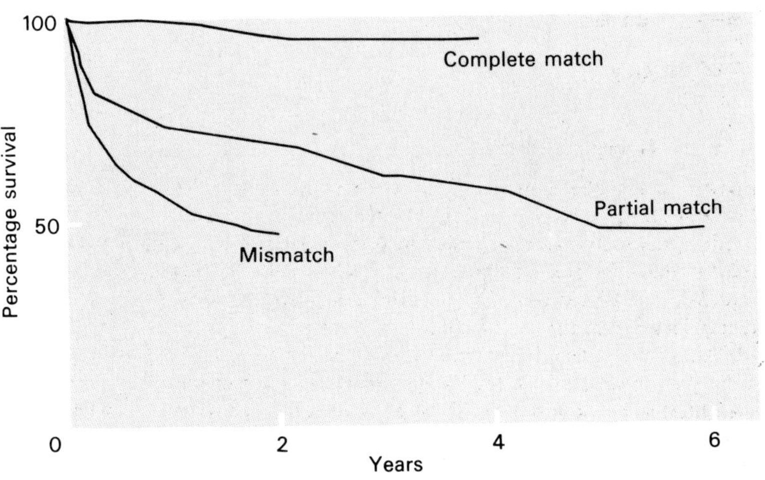

FIGURE 9.12. Survival of kidney transplants in relation to degree of matching at HLA-A and -B loci. Complete match (siblings) = all antigens identical; partial match (siblings and parent to child) = only antigens on one chromosome (haplotype) identical; mismatch (unrelated) = all antigens different. (Data taken from J. Dausset & J. Hors, *Transpl. Proc.* 1973, **V**, 223).

and are therefore identical at all *four* loci, and if we further recall that the generation of T helpers for cytotoxicity (and antibody?) is largely dependent upon D locus differences (p. 259), it seems likely that matching the D antigens will prove to be a major factor in improving graft survival.

Because of the many thousands of different HLA phenotypes possible (figure 9.7), it is usual to work with a large pool of potential recipients on a continental basis so that when graft material becomes available the best possible match can be made. The position will be improved when the pool of available organs can be increased through the development of long-term tissue storage banks but techniques are not good enough for this at present except in the case of bone marrow cells which can be kept viable even after freezing and thawing. With a paired organ such as the kidney, living donors may be used; siblings provide the best chance of a good match (cf. figure 9.7). However, the use of living donors poses difficult ethical problems and the objective must be to perfect the use of cadaver material (? or animal organs—or mechanical substitutes!).

GENERAL IMMUNOSUPPRESSION

Graft rejection can be held at bay by the use of agents which non-specifically interfere with the induction or expression of the immune response. Because these agents are non-specific, patients on immunosuppressive therapy tend to be susceptible to infections; they are also more prone to develop lymphoreticular cancers.

Lymphoid cell ablation

Thymectomy, splenectomy and lymphadenectomy in adult recipients do not appear to help, although extra-corporeal irradiation of blood, injections of anti-lymphocyte globulin (ALG) and thoracic duct cannulation have proved beneficial. Total lymphoid irradiation would appear somewhat Draconian but has been shown to prolong skin grafts in mice when given in divided doses over an extended period. The most striking feature of this work is that allogeneic bone marrow cells given at the end of this treatment schedule are fully accepted without the development of g.v.h. reactions (Strober & Slavin).

Immunosuppressive drugs

The development of an immunological response requires the active proliferation of a relatively small number of antigen-sensitive lymphocytes to give a population of sensitized cells large enough to be effective. Many of the immunosuppressive drugs now employed were first used in cancer chemotherapy because of their toxicity to dividing cells. Aside from the complications of blanket immunosuppression mentioned above, these antimitotic drugs are especially toxic for cells of the bone marrow and small intestine and must therefore be used with great care.

Perhaps the most commonly used drug in this field is *azathioprine* which has a preferential effect on T-cell mediated reactions. It is broken down in the body first to 6-mercaptopurine and then converted to the active agent, the ribotide. Because of the similarity in shape (figure 9.13), this competes with inosinic acid for enzymes concerned in the synthesis of guanylic and adenylic acids; it also inhibits the synthesis of 5-phosphoribosylamine, a precursor of inosinic acid, by a feedback mechanism. The net result is inhibition of nucleic acid synthesis. Another drug, methotrexate, through its action as a folic acid antagonist also inhibits synthesis of nucleic acid. The N-mustard derivative cyclophosphamide probably attacks DNA by alkylation and cross-linking so preventing correct duplication during cell division. These agents appear to exert their damaging effects on cells during mitosis and for this reason are most powerful when administered after presentation of antigen at a time when the antigen-sensitive cells are dividing. Cyclosporin A, a rather insoluble fungal metabolite, is of particular interest since not only will it act on these antigen-sensitive dividing cells and spare the resting cells which carry the vital memory for immunity to microbial infections, but it seems to be

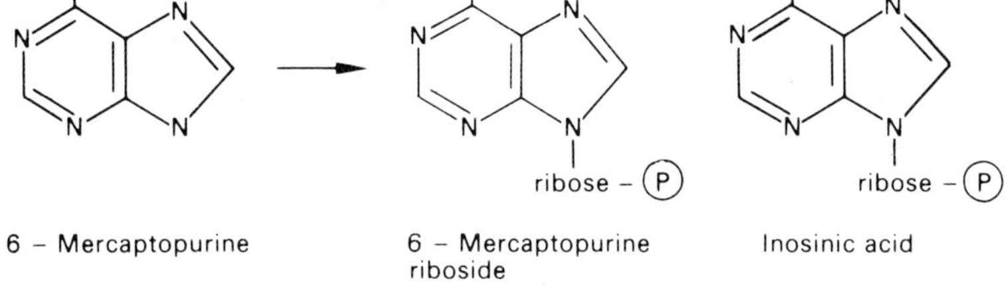

6 – Mercaptopurine | 6 – Mercaptopurine riboside | Inosinic acid

FIGURE 9.13. Metabolic conversion of azathioprine through 6-mercaptopurine to the ribotide: similarity to inosinic acid with which it competes.

differentially toxic to dividing lymphocytes as compared with other active cells in the gut and bone marrow. Whether or not Cyclosporin itself proves to be of permanent clinical value, it does seem to offer a new pathway towards the development of agents with selective action against dividing lymphocytes.

Steroids such as prednisone intervene at many points in the immune response, affecting lymphocyte recirculation and the generation of cytotoxic effector cells for example; in addition, their outstanding anti-inflammatory potency rests on features such as inhibition of neutrophil adherence to vascular endothelium in an inflammatory area and suppression of monocyte/macrophage functions such as microbicidal activity and response to lymphokines. The combination of azathioprine and prednisone is commonly employed in the long-term management of kidney grafts.

ANTIGEN-SPECIFIC DEPRESSION OF ALLOGRAFT REACTIVITY

Immunological tolerance

If the disadvantages of blanket immunosuppression are to be avoided, we must aim at knocking out only the reactivity of the host to the antigens of the graft leaving the remainder of the immunological apparatus intact. One approach is through the induction of tolerance in the patient. Through selective action on antigen-sensitive dividing cells, Cyclosporin A may induce clonal abortion. Total lymph node irradiation plus bone marrow (*vide supra*) is thought to induce specific T-suppression, and grafts of skin and heart from the same donor enjoy prolonged survival. Active suppression is probably also responsible for the long-lasting tolerance to a skin allograft seen in mice given donor liver extract 16 days before the graft and alternating procarbazine hydrochloride and antilymphocyte globulin for a few days afterwards (Brent). As purified histocompatibility antigens become available it should ultimately not be beyond the wit of *Homo sapiens* to juggle the relative timing and dosages of antigen and various immunosuppressants to produce a specific hyporesponsive state. On rather a different tack, it has been reported that tolerance between rodent strains can be established by autoimmunization with the idiotype of the host receptor for donor transplantation antigens.

Enhancement

There is another possible solution which may be easier to achieve and that is deliberate immunization with these antigens to evoke antibodies which protect rather than destroy the graft. It has long been recognized that such *enhancing* sera are responsible for the prolonged survival of tumour allografts after prior immunization with irradiated tumour cells. The precise mechanism has still to be revealed but explanations usually fall under two headings, masking by antibody and blocking by antigen (figure 9.14).

Masking by antibody. The killing of target cells by sensitized lymphocytes from an H-2 incompatible mouse is inhibited by addition of antibodies directed against the H-2K and D antigens of the target. Presumably the antibodies combine with the surface antigens of the target cells which are then no longer accessible to the receptors on the aggressor lymphocytes. The bound antibodies must avoid the activation of complement or indeed of non-specific aggressor K cells (p. 227). In the case of complement at least, this would occur if the determinants on the surface were too far apart to allow the Fc portions of adjacent antibodies to interact and bind complement (cf. p. 160) and might also be insufficient to allow effective interaction with K-cells; alternatively if the antigenic determinants were close together, no activation of C1 or of K-cells would be possible if there were a preponderance of antibodies belonging to inappropriate immunoglobulin classes such as IgA. Shedding of antigen from the cell surface due to complexing with antibody (p. 152) would also leave the cell resistant to attack.

A quite different situation arises in the presence of antibodies to the Ia lymphocyte activating determinants since these would block induction of T helper cells; not only would cytotoxic T-cells fail to differentiate, but they might conceivably become tolerized by interaction with serologically-defined determinants in the absence of the T helper signal. This raises another point: if the only Ia positive cells in an organ graft such as kidney are the passenger lymphocytes and macrophages, their removal before grafting or their destruction by preformed Ia antibodies in the recipient should prolong survival. Experience with rat kidney grafts pretreated with anti-lymphocyte serum supports this view, but it should be noted that X-irradiation of the organ will not prevent the passenger lymphocytes from provoking a strong transplantation reaction (cf. use of irradiated stimulators for cell-mediated lympholysis, figure 9.5). Culture of parathyroids and of islets of Langerhans for 7 to 10 days is said to reduce the immunogenicity of the tissue for grafting. Is this due to loss of residual lymphocytes?

Blocking by antigen. Graft or tumour antigen may be shed from the surface either spontaneously or as a result of stripping by antibody, in which case it will be released as a complex. The shed antigen may block the receptors on specific cytotoxic T-cells, the complex possibly being more effective in this than free antigen to the extent that it can establish multivalent linking to both antigen and Fc receptors. Alternatively, the antigen may pre-emptively neutralize antibody which would otherwise render the graft vulnerable to ADCC.

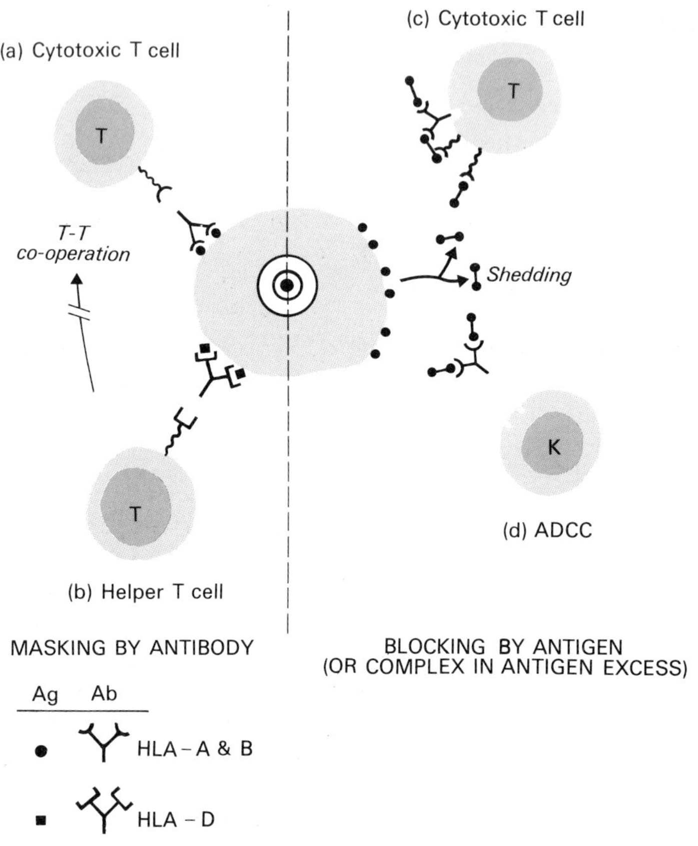

FIGURE 9.14. Enhancement: possible mechanisms. *Block by antibody*—(a) Masking the HLA-A or B antigens on the target surface inhibits attack by cytotoxic T-cells. (b) Masking of Ia on the target prevents the induction of T helpers and hence of cytotoxic T-cells. There is evidence that tolerance may be induced if classical transplantation antigens are presented in the absence of Ia-induced T-helpers (cf. the idea that 1 signal tolerizes and 2 signals trigger a B-cell, p. 75). *Block by antigen*—Sufficient antigen shed from the surface of the target, either free or as a complex in antigen excess, can (c) block the receptors on cytotoxic T-cells and possibly tolerize their precursors or (d) block the antibody involved in antibody-dependent cell-mediated cytotoxicity.

It has also been suggested that antibody could opsomize antigen-sensitive cells which had bound antigen to their surface, so causing their elimination.

Successful enhancement of kidney and bone-marrow grafts have been reported in isolated instances and one supposes this will inevitably be extended. There are indications that serum enhancing factors may inhibit tumour destruction by cell-mediated mechanisms in some cancer patients as will be discussed later.

Clinical experience in grafting

Privileged sites

Corneal grafts survive without the need for immunosuppression. Because they are avascular they do not sensitize the recipient although they become cloudy if the individual has been presensitized. Grafts of cartilage are successful in the same way but an additional factor is the protection afforded the chondrocytes by the matrix. With bone and artery it doesn't really matter if the grafts die because they can still provide a framework for host cells to colonize.

Kidney

Thousands of kidneys have been transplanted and with improvement in patient management there is a high survival rate (figure 9.12). Patients are partially immunosuppressed at the time of transplantation because uraemia causes a degree of immunological anergy. Recipients sharing 3 or 4 of the A and B locus antigens with the donor show improved results if they have previously been transfused with blood; will this prove to be a case of serendipitous enhancement through production of Ia antibodies? Unquestionably the importance of D-locus matching is widely recognized. If kidney function is poor during a rejection crisis renal dialysis can be used. When transplantation is performed because of immune complex induced glomerulonephritis, the usual immunosuppressive regimen of azathioprine and prednisone may help to prevent a similar lesion developing in the grafted kidney. Patients with glomerular basement membrane antibodies (e.g. Goodpasture's syndrome) are likely to destroy their renal transplants.

Heart

Something like 40–50% of transplant patients survive by one year. The results have not been as good as with kidney grafting but special factors should be taken into account. The recipient patients were in irreversible cardiac failure with wasting and advanced secondary changes of passive congestion, and the clinical urgency made it difficult to find well-matched donor organs. Aside from the rejection problem it is likely that the number of patients who would benefit from cardiac replacement is much greater than the number dying with adequately healthy hearts. More attention will have to be given to the possibility of xenogeneic grafts and mechanical substitutes.

Liver

Survival rates for orthotopic liver grafts are broadly in line with those receiving heart transplants. Three-quarters of the patients transplanted for hepatic cancer have had recurrence of their tumour within one year.

Experience with liver grafting between pigs revealed an unexpected finding. Many of the animals retained the grafted organs in a healthy state for many months without any form of immunosuppression. The transplanted liver represented a large antigen pool which induced a state of unresponsiveness to grafts of skin or kidney from the same donor. The mechanism is not clear but may involve true tolerance or enhancement. There is as yet no evidence that this highly desirable state can be established by a hepatic transplant in man.

Haematopoietic tissue

Certain immunodeficiency disorders and some forms of anaemia are obvious candidates for treatment with lymphoid stem cells. Successful results with bone marrow transfers require highly compatible donors if fatal graft vs. host reactions are to be avoided, and here siblings offer the best chance of finding a matched donor (figure 9.7). Matching for antigens quite distinct from those controlled by the major HLA loci may prove to be essential (cf. the murine Hh locus, figure 9.4 legend).

Other organs

It is to be expected that improvement in techniques of control of the rejection process will encourage transplantation in several other areas. Not, of course, in most cases of endocrine disorders where exogenous replacement therapy is available, but one looks forward to the successful transplantation of lungs, of skin for lethal burns, and even of bones and joints.

Biological significance of the major histocompatibility complex

POLYMORPHISM

With 4 loci on each of 2 chromosomes and several alleles at each locus, there are literally millions of different possible phenotypes, in other words the MHC is an extraordinarily polymorphic system. That this holds for widely divergent species like man, mouse and chicken implies that the maintenance of such polymorphism confers a survival advantage in evolutionary terms. One suggestion is that a polymorphic system provides a defence against microbial molecular mimicry in which a whole species might be put at risk by its inability to recognize as foreign an organism which displayed determinants similar in structure to those of the host. It is also possible that in some way the existence of a high degree of polymorphism helps to maintain the diversity of antigenic recognition within the lymphoid system of a given species.

One consequence of this multi-allelic complex is that it ensures *heterozygosity*, with its connotation of 'hybrid vigour' (yet another phenomenon whose mechanisms remain obscure but could involve almost anything from fertilization onwards).

IMMUNOLOGICAL RELATIONSHIP OF MOTHER AND FETUS

A further consequence of polymorphism in an outbred population is that mother and fetus will almost certainly have different MHC's. Some examples of selection for heterozygotes (where maternally and paternally derived haplotypes are different) over homozygotes (both fetal haplotypes identical with the mother's) in viviparous animals suggest that this is beneficial. Likewise, the placentae of F1 offspring are larger than normal when mothers are preimmunized to the paternal H-2 haplotype and smaller when mothers are tolerant to these antigens.

The threat posed to the fetus as a potential graft due to the possession of paternal transplantation antigens so intrigued Lewis Thomas that he was moved to suggest that rejection of the fetus might initiate parturition, although it would be difficult to account for the normal birth of female offspring to pure strain mating pairs where fetus and mother would have identical histocompatibility antigens without further postulating a placenta-specific surface antigen.

Nonetheless, in the human haemochorial placenta, maternal blood with immunocompetent lymphocytes does circulate in contact with the fetal trophoblast and we have to explain how the fetus avoids allograft rejection, despite the development of an immunological response in a proportion of mothers as evidenced by the appearance of anti-HLA antibodies and cytotoxic lymphocytes. In fact, prior sensitization with a skin graft fails to affect a pregnancy, showing that trophoblast cells are immunologically protected. Some of the many speculations which have been aired on this subject are summarized in figure 9.15. The low density or absence of classical transplantation antigens on the syncytiotrophoblast cells which are in front-line contact with the maternal circulation makes them an unattractive target for graft rejection. This alone might be sufficient to explain the invulnerability of the placenta to immunological attack, but in addition, trophoblast cells may be protected against cytotoxic lymphocytes by a surrounding barrier (admittedly incomplete) of sialic acid-rich mucopolysaccharide.

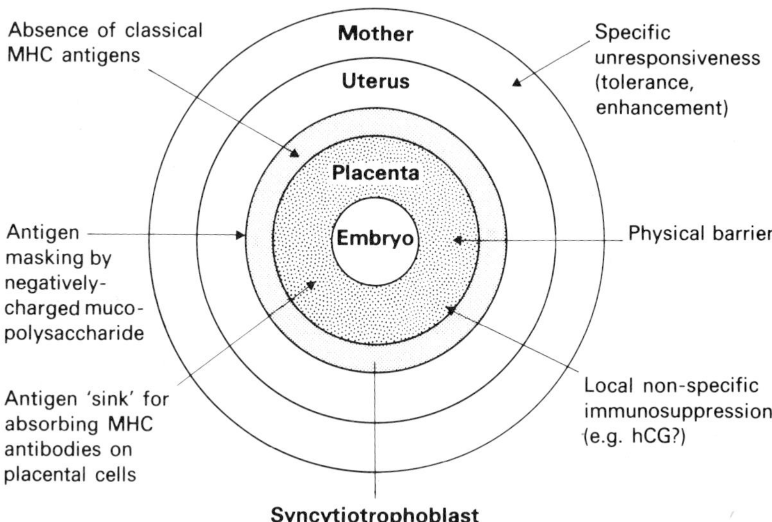

FIGURE 9.15. Mechanisms postulated to account for the survival of the fetus as an allograft in the mother. (After L. Brent).

It is becoming increasingly clear that the major transplantation antigens subserve an intercellular recognition function. We do not know whether they are involved in phenomena like the reassortment of dispersed kidney cells in culture which preferentially reaggregate with each other despite admixture with hepatocytes but they do undoubtedly play a central role in directing T-cell interactions.

Haplotype restriction

Of dramatic significance has been the revelation that the MHC is intimately involved in the T-cell recognition of macrophage-processed antigens (cf. p. 97), collaboration with B-cells (p. 98) and killing of virally-infected cells (cf. p. 191). In essence, T-cells recognize antigen in association with one of the products of the MHC complex. Memory T-cells are most effectively triggered by exposure to antigen in association with the MHC haplotype used for priming.

Let us look at an example of this phenomenon of so-called 'haplotype restriction' in more detail. If I may be permitted to refresh your mind, dear reader, cytotoxic T-cells provoked by a virus infection will only kill target cells infected with that virus *in vitro* if they share the same classical transplantation antigens as the original host. Thus cytotoxic T-cells arising in a mouse of H-2^d haplotype infected with lymphocytic choriomeningitis virus (LCM) will kill LCM infected cells of H-2^d but not H-2^k haplotype (figure 9.16a). By using target cells from strains derived by genetic recombination within the H-2 complex, the relevant MHC molecule recognized by the T-cell has been pinpointed as H-2D. With certain other viruses such as vaccinia, the target cell shows H-2K restriction. Various models have been proposed for these recognition processes: (i) two distinct receptors combine with self H-2D (or H-2K) and virally coded antigen respectively, (ii) a single receptor recognizes a determinant formed by association of H-2D/K and viral antigen, or (iii) the virus modifies the synthesis or configuration of the H-2D/K molecule to produce a new 'altered self' determinant. These are discussed further in the legend to figure 9.16b.

There is evidence that the T-cells are programmed to recognize the appropriate self MHC antigens during their differentiation in the thymus and they learn the haplotype of the cells they meet in the thymus gland.

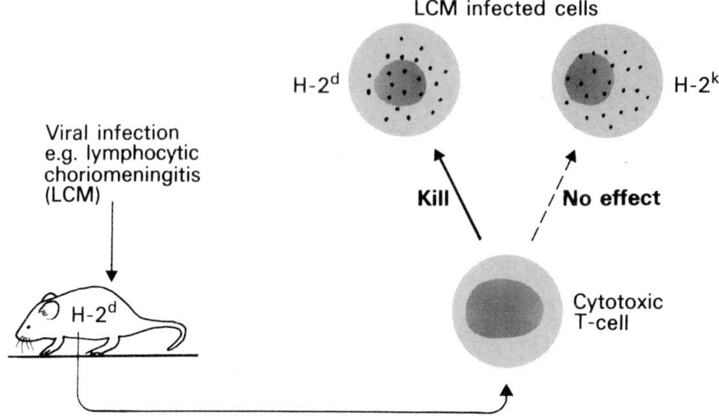

(a) MHC RESTRICTED CYTOTOXICITY OF T-CELLS FOR VIRALLY INFECTED TARGETS IN VITRO

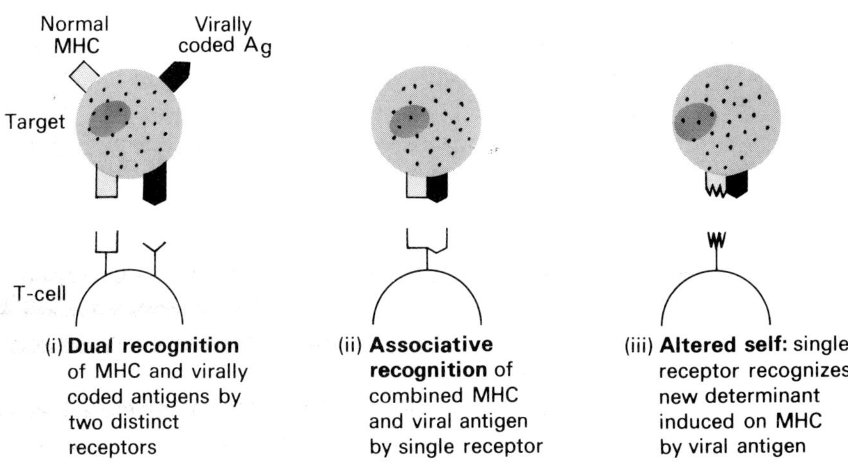

(b) POSSIBLE MECHANISMS

FIGURE 9.16. The Doherty and Zinkernagel phenomenon of haplotype restriction in recognition of virally infected targets by cytotoxic T-cells. The same mechanisms apply to the recognition of H-2 linked minor transplantation antigens such as the male (Y) antigen and to the response to Ia associated antigen on the macrophage surface.

A consequence of the altered self model is that there must be as many new determinants inducible on the MHC molecule as there are distinct cytotoxic T-cell specificities. Both dual and associative models involve recognition of self MHC + viral antigen; whether it is stereochemically likely that determinants on MHC and a separate surface antigen, even in a fluid membrane, can become sufficiently closely apposed to fit into a single receptor has not been established. I have proposed a 2 receptor model, each a single peptide using the V_H genes and a constant region gene characteristic for T-cells, there being no need for allelic exclusion as in B-cells. If many V_H segments have

This is shown by experiments in which thymectomized irradiated Fl offspring of two parental strains, A and B, injected with Fl bone marrow, are reconstituted with different thymuses and then tested in the LCM haplotype restriction system. Cytotoxic cells generated by LCM infection of mice given an Fl thymus could kill both A and B targets infected with virus; A strain thymus restricted killing to A targets and B thymus to B targets. However, similar results were not obtained when thymus grafted nude mice were used as bone marrow recipients and the situation awaits some clarification.

Facilitation of the appropriate immune response

When a cell is first infected with virus, there is an eclipse phase during which the machinery of the cell is being switched for viral replication and the only marker of the complete microbe is the viral antigen on the cell surface. At this stage, killing of the cell by a cytotoxic T-cell will prevent viral replication.

How does the killer T-cell know when it has reached its target? It has to recognize two features before striking: one is the presence of viral antigen and the other is its location on the surface of a body cell. The microbial antigen is recognized by the specific T-receptor and the cell through its marker, the classical transplantation antigens which are present on nearly every cell in the body. Thus, the killer cell in the mouse for example, operates on the basis that:

viral antigen + H-2D/K = virally infected cell

and that is why its receptor(s) has to see both antigens. The human utilizes the HLA-A and B (and probably C) loci in the same way.

The situation is quite different with intracellular bacteria and protozoa which do not go through an eclipse phase after phagocytosis by macrophages but are held as infectious entities; lysis by cytotoxic T-cells will merely release the organisms, not kill them. A separate strategy utilizing the delayed-type hypersensitivity T-cell population is required

---

specificity for the constant regions (framework) of the MHC, random combination with D and J segments (p. 132) would generate a diversity of receptors enabling at least some T-cells to recognize almost any MHC private specificity. Cells which recognize self MHC with receptor will be selected for and amplified probably by the thymus or perhaps by the MHC on the body cells which prime T-lymphocytes; thus the majority of differentiated T-cells will have one receptor able to recognize self and the other, randomly selected from the V_H repertoire, able to combine with virus, minor transplantation antigens, etc.

and in this case, the effector T-lymphocyte recognizes the infected macrophage by the presence of microbial antigen on the surface in association with an I-region molecule. This interaction triggers the release of lymphokines which enable the macrophage to kill the intracellular parasites (p. 186). Similarly, in T-B co-operation, the B-cell is recognized by an Ia molecule associated with the foreign antigen while I-J is used as a marker for T-cells mediating suppression. In summary, each T-lymphocyte subset has to communicate with a particular cell type in order to make the *appropriate* immune response and it does so by recognizing not only foreign antigen (or idiotype, cf. p. 102) but also the particular MHC molecule used as a marker of that cell (Table 9.1).

The Ia molecule used on the dendritic macrophages which present antigen to T-helpers is the same as that on the B-cell which is the final target of collaboration (p. 98); it might be expected that the Ia molecule for 'microbe-crunching' phagocytic macrophages will be encoded by a separate I-subregion.
In addition to the I region on chromosome 17, the quite separate M locus on chromosome 1 in the mouse, encodes strong Lad's as manifested by mixed lymphocyte reactivity and, following the theme of a link with recognition systems, it is exciting to note that a gene controlling susceptibility to leishmania infection maps in the close vicinity.

THE CANCER CELL AND THE ALLOGRAFT REACTION

The ability to reject transplants of tissue may be traced back a long way down the evolutionary tree—back even as far as the annelid worms. Long before the studies on the involvement of self-MHC in immunological responses, Lewis Thomas suggested that the allograft rejection mech-

TABLE 9.1. Guidance of T subpopulations to appropriate target cell by MHC molecules

Function	Cell interaction	MHC marker on target cell
T-help	T-B	I
T-proliferation	T-macrophage	I
T-delayed sensitivity	T-macrophage	I
T-suppression	T-T	I(J)
T-cytotoxic	T-Infected cell	D/K

anism represented a means by which the body's cells could be kept under *immunological surveillance* so that altered cells with a neoplastic potential could be identified and summarily eliminated. For this to operate, cancer cells must display a new surface antigen which can be recognized by the lymphoid cells and examples have been discovered.

Tumour surface antigens (figure 9.17)

(a) *Virally controlled.* Cells infected with oncogenic viruses usually display two new antigens on their surface, one (V) identical with an antigen on the isolated virion and the other (T), also a product of the viral genome, present only on infected cells; the latter represents a strong transplantation antigen and generates haplotype restricted cytotoxic T cells. All syngeneic tumours induced by a given virus carry the same surface antigen, irrespective of their cellular origin, so that

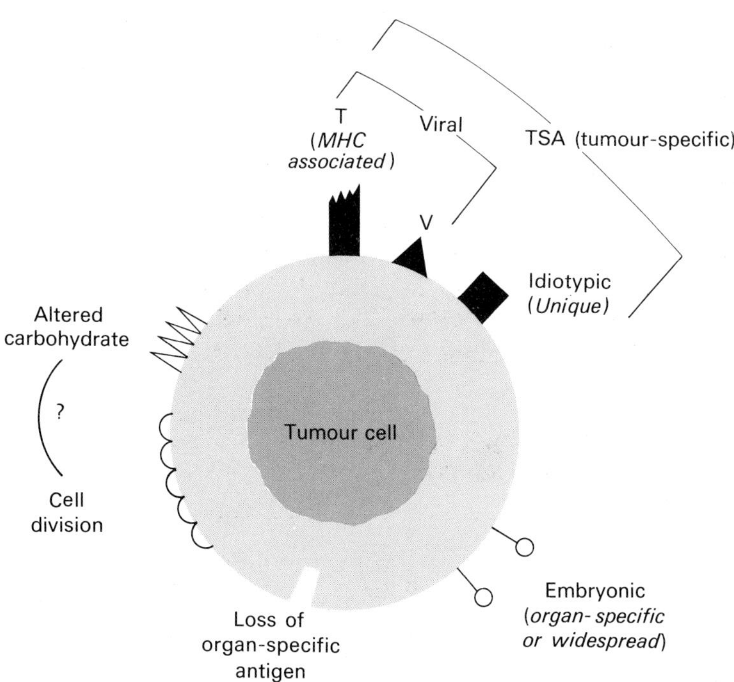

FIGURE 9.17. Tumour associated antigens. Even virally induced tumours may possess idiotypic specificities. If the tumour is cycling, surface components associated with mitosis may be detected and could be responsible for the lectin-binding carbohydrates thought at one time to be characteristic of transformed tumour cells.

immunization with any one of these tumours confers resistance to subsequent challenge with the others.

(b) *Embryonic.* Tumours derived from the same cell type often express a common differentiation antigen also present on embryonic cells (so-called oncofetal antigens). Examples would be α-fetoprotein in hepatic carcinoma and carcino-embryonic antigen (CEA) in cancer of the intestine.

(c) *Division.* The carbohydrate moiety of surface membrane glycoproteins may change during cell division. For example, Thomas found that the density of surface sugar determinants with blood group H specificity fell as murine mastocytoma cells moved into the G_1 phase of the division cycle while reciprocally, group B determinants increased; it was postulated that the continued expression of this latter component was related to a commitment to further division. We have found that surface components binding the lectin, wheat germ agglutinin, are abundant on myeloid cells (polys and macrophages) but poorly represented on resting T- and B-cells; however, within 24 hours of stimulation by lymphocyte polyclonal activators and before DNA synthesis begins, high concentrations of lectin binding sites appear on the surface.

(d) *Idiotypic.* Tumours induced by chemical agents, benzopyrene for example, also possess specific transplantation antigens, but each tumour produced by a given chemical carcinogen has its own individual idiotypic antigen; even when a carcinogen produces two different primary tumours in the same animal, they do not exhibit the same antigenic specificities and do not confer cross-resistance by immunization.

Immune response to tumours

These tumour antigens can provoke immune responses in experimental animals which lead to resistance against tumour growth but they vary tremendously in their efficiency. Powerful antigens associated with tumours induced by oncogenic viruses or ultraviolet-light generate strong resistance while chemically-induced tumours are weaker and somewhat variable; disappointingly, tumours which arise spontaneously in animals produce little or no response. This would seem to reason against the immune surveillance theory, although it might be argued that most tumours were silenced at their inception by immunological control and that only the very few which lacked a provocative surface component were 'successful'. However, athymic nude mice have a normal incidence of spontaneous tumours and this makes a single, exclusively T-cell surveillance system most unlikely. Furthermore, the only increase in cancer reported in immunosuppressed patients was related to the lympho-reticular system which could have been the direct target for the drugs employed; one exception was the considerable increase in skin cancer in immunosuppressed patients living in high sunshine regions north of Brisbane and we have already noted the 'antigen strength' of such tumours provoked in experimental animals.

Perhaps in speaking of immunity to tumours, one too readily thinks in terms of acquired responses whereas it is possible that innate mechanisms will prove to be of greater significance. Macrophages taken from BCG-infected animals, or activated by a diversity of factors, bacterial lipopolysaccharide, double-stranded RNA, T-cell lymphokine and so forth, will inhibit the division of tumour cells in tissue culture. There is an uncommon flurry of interest in the natural killer (NK) cell which is similar in many ways to the K cell of ADDC fame (p. 227). NK cells are spontaneously cytolytic for certain, but by no means all, tumour lines in culture as well as for cells infected with herpes and mumps viruses or *Listeria monocytogenes*. The target molecule might be a surface membrane glycoprotein with altered carbohydrate and the blocking of cytotoxicity by anti-Ly5 sera tentatively suggests that this differentiation antigen could be the NK receptor. Interferon markedly enhances the activity of NK cells and at the same time, increases the resistance of *normal* cells to lysis. Agents such as BCG and *C. parvum* which stimulate macrophages also increase NK activity. A recently described mouse strain with a mutant gene (*beige*) which leads to complete and selective impairment of NK activity should help to define the role of these cells in resistance to spontaneous tumours much the same as the nude mouse allowed more precise delineation of thymus function.

Immunotherapy

On one point all are agreed, if immunotherapy is to succeed, it is essential that the tumour load should first be reduced by surgery, irradiation or chemotherapy, since not only is it unreasonable to expect the immune system to cope with a large tumour mass, but considerable amounts of antigen released by shedding would prevent the generation of any significant response. This leaves the small secondary deposits as the proper target for immunotherapy.

For active immunization we need antigen. Based on the not unreasonable belief that certain forms of cancer (e.g. lymphoma) are caused by oncogenic viruses, attempts are being made to isolate the virus and prepare a suitable vaccine from it. In fact, large-scale protection of chickens against the development of Marek's disease lymphoma has been successfully achieved by vaccination with another herpes virus native to turkeys. In the human, patients with Burkitt's lymphoma develop antibodies which react with antigens on cells of their own and other Burkitt tumours which are controlled by a herpes group organism, the Epstein-Barr (EB) virus. The unique idiotype on monoclonal B-cell tumours with surface Ig also offers a potentially feasible target for immunotherapy.

Despite reports of cytotoxic antibodies in a proportion of patients with malignant melanoma and cytotoxic leukocytes from patients with neuroblastoma or bladder cancer, which indicate that some form of immunological response to tumour antigens is possible, it must be said that attempts to control human cancer by injection of tumours with adjuvants have had very mixed and in many ways somewhat disappointing results. Perhaps we have to devise new ways of boosting the inherently weak autoantigenicity of the oncofetal antigens when present, to generate an appropriate response? There have also been numerous, not very successful, attempts to boost 'non-specific' effector mechanisms mediated by macrophages and NK cells through the injection of BCG, *Corynebacterium parvum* and interferon. Intimate contact of the adjuvant with the tumour itself can produce dramatic results and one hopeful study records the beneficial effects of intrathoracic BCG in lung cancer.

Immunodiagnosis

Analysis of blood for the oncofetal antigens α-fetoprotein in hepatoma and carcinoembryonic antigen in tumours of the colon has provided valuable diagnostic information, but enthusiasm has been slightly curtailed by the knowledge that there is a high incidence of so-called 'false positives'. Caspary & Field have developed a test which depends on the observation that lymphocytes from cancer patients when mixed with a basic protein commonly found in tumours, will release a factor which slows the electrophoretic mobility of added macrophages. The technique of cytopherometry which must be employed is fiddly and there has been some ambivalence in coming to terms with what might hold the seed of a potentially interesting phenomenon. The same considerations apply to the study of changes in fluorescence polarization induced by cancer basic protein. Identification of the cell type by surface markers is of increasing value for the diagnosis and treatment of childhood leukaemias such as non-T, non-B ALL (p. 115).

RELATION OF MHC TO THE COMPLEMENT SYSTEM

Genes controlling the levels of C3, C4, C2 and factor B are all located within the major histocompatibility complex. In addition, antisera to HLA-Bw4 and 6 (cf. legend, figure 9.7) block the formation of rosettes between human lymphocytes and C3d coated erythrocytes. C2 deficiency in man has been linked to the HLA-A10/Bw18 haplotype.

These genes therefore are concerned with C3 and the factors which react with it viz. the classical (C4,2) and the alternative pathway (factor B,C3b) enzymes which split C3, together with the binding site for C3d, and their clustering in this region is provocative. A function of the MHC relates to the interaction between cells in the immune response and it is tempting to consider that C3 related signals might be concerned in some of these intercellular events.

ASSOCIATION WITH DISEASE

An impressive body of data is accumulating which links specific HLA antigens with particular disease states in the human (table 9.2). Because of *linkage disequilibrium* (a state where closely linked genes on a chromosome tend to remain associated rather than undergo genetic randomization in a given population) which is often a feature of this region of the chromosome, the associations seen may be even more directly linked with a gene other than that coding for the HLA antigen in question. For example, in multiple sclerosis an association with the B7 allele was first established but when patients were typed for the D locus, a much stronger correlation with Dw2 emerged. The initial correlation with B7 resulted from linkage disequilibrium between B7 and Dw2. Carrying the argument a stage further, one cannot exclude the possibility of finding an even greater association with another closely linked gene.

TABLE 9.2. Association of HLA with disease

Disease	HLA	Estimated* relative risk
Ankylosing spondylitis	B27	81
Reiter's disease	B27	48
Psoriatic arthritis, Juvenile RA } when spine involved	B27	5·4
Acute anterior uveitis	B27	16·9
Psoriasis vulgaris	B13	4·3
Dermatitis herpetiformis	B8	4·3
Insulin dependent diabetes	B8	2.3
	Dw3	3.8
	Dw4	3·5
Addison's disease	B8	3·9
	Dw3	8·8
Thyrotoxicosis	B8	2·3
	Dw3	4·4
Myasthenia gravis	B8	4·4
	Dw3	2·3
Sjögren with Sicca syndrome	B8	3·2
Chronic active hepatitis	B8	2·9
	Dw3	6·8
Coeliac disease	B8	9·5
Rheumatoid arthritis	Dw4, DRw4	6·0
Behcet's disease	B5	4·6
Multiple sclerosis	B7	1·5
	Dw2	5·0
Subacute thyroiditis	Bw35	14
Ragweed hay fever	Haplotype linkage	
Hodgkin's disease	A1	1·4
	B5	1·6
	B8	1·3
	B18	1·9

No deviations from normal found in: rheumatoid arthritis; gout; non-insulin dependent diabetes; childhood asthma; leprosy; TB; *H.influenza* & infectious mononucleosis infection; ulcerative colitis & Crohn's; other liver disorders; sarcoidosis; SLE; rheumatic fever; essential hypertension; asbestosis; schizophrenia; pernicious anaemia; mammary carcinoma with respect to HLA-A and -B antigens. There is strong linkage disequilibrium between B7 and Dw2 and between B8 and Dw3.

Much of the data is taken from Ryder L.P. & Svejgaard A. (1976) *Associations between HLA and disease*. Published by the authors, State Univ. Hosp., Copenhagen.

* Increased chance of contracting the disease for individuals bearing the antigen relative to those lacking it.

Inevitably these findings call forth thoughts of immune response genes and, in the case of multiple sclerosis, it would imply that Dw2 individuals were poor T-cell responders to measles since defective cell-mediated immunity to this virus is to date the only major immunological abnormality recognized. However, the B7 allele also correlates positively with an increased incidence of paralytic polio and with relatively poor T-cell activity *in vitro* for heterologous target cells; perhaps the defect relates more to cellular interaction than to antigenic specificity. Somewhat more convincing evidence for an Ir gene is the clear *linkage* between IgE-mediated ragweed allergy and HLA haplotype within families but no *association* with particular A or B locus antigens, although D typing was not available in this study.

The association with HLA in ankylosing spondylitis is quite extraordinary; up to 95% of patients are of B27 phenotype as compared with around 5% in controls. The incidence of B27 is also markedly raised in other conditions when accompanied by sacro-iliitis, e.g. Reiter's disease, acute anterior uveitis, psoriasis and other forms of infective sacro-iliitis such as yersinia, gonococcal and salmonella arthritis. The very close association with B27 makes it unlikely that as good a correlation with any other gene will be found. The involvement of infective agents may provide a clue: does molecular similarity to B27 imply a tolerance to certain microbial antigens, or is there some more subtle interaction with microbial products? Reports by Ebringer and colleagues of a cross-reaction of B27 with *Klebsiella pneumoniae* and a higher faecal carriage rate for these organisms in patients with active disease are certainly provocative in this respect.

The B8-Dw3 axis is found with undue frequency in autoimmune diseases where cell surface antigens are prime targets. In Graves' disease and myasthenia gravis these have been identified as TSH and ACh receptors respectively and the question of some link between Dw3 and these receptors has been mooted. HLA antigens might also affect the susceptibility of a cell to viral attachment or infection, thereby influencing the development of autoimmunity to associated surface components.

Summary

Graft rejection is an immunological reaction: it shows specificity, the second set response is brisk, it is mediated by lymphocytes, and antibodies specific for the graft are formed. In each vertebrate species there is a major histocompatibility complex (MHC) which is responsible for provoking the most intense graft reactions. MHC antigens inherited from mother and father are codominantly expressed on the cell surface. The MHC in the mouse (H-2) is a complex region with two loci encoding major classical transplantation antigens, H-2K and H-2D each with many polymorphic specificities defined by the antibodies they so readily evoke. The molecules contain two peptides, one of H-2 specificity and the other β_2-microglobulin. Another major region, I, codes for lymphocyte activating determinants (Lad) which provoke a mixed lymphocyte reaction of proliferation and blast transformation when genetically dissimilar lymphocytes interact; this reaction stimulates the formation of helper T-cells required for the generation of cytotoxic T-cells directed against H-2D/K determinants (cf. T-B co-operation with carrier-hapten), the process being termed cell-mediated lympholysis. Lad (Ia) differences are responsible for the reaction of tolerated grafted lymphocytes against host antigens (g.v.h.). The genes in the whole MHC being closely linked tend to be inherited *en bloc* and are referred to as a haplotype. The MHC in man (HLA) consists of three loci (HLA-A, B & C) for classical transplantation antigens and one (HLA-D) for the major Lad. Individuals are typed by cytotoxic antisera and by the mixed lymphocyte reaction. Siblings have a 1 : 4 chance of identity with respect to MHC.

Grafts are rejected either by cytotoxic T-cells or by antibody inducing platelet aggregation or type II hypersensitivity reactions (e.g. antibody-dependent cell-mediated cytotoxicity). Rejection may be prevented by: (1) tissue matching including the D-locus, (2) anti-mitotic drugs (e.g. azathioprine), anti-inflammatory steroids and anti-lymphocyte globulin which produce general immunosuppression, (3) antigen-specific depression through tolerance induction or enhancement by deliberate immunization.

Cornea and cartilage grafts are avascular and comparatively well tolerated. Kidney grafting has been the most widespread although immunosuppression must normally be continuous. Bone marrow grafts for immunodeficiency and aplastic anaemia are accepted from matched siblings but it is difficult to avoid g.v.h. disease with allogeneic marrow.

The very high degree of polymorphism of the MHC may protect a species from molecular mimicry by parasites, maintain diversity of antigenic recognition and ensure heterozygosity ('hybrid vigour'). Differences between MHC of mother and fetus may be beneficial to the fetus but as a potential graft it must be protected against transplantation attack by the mother; suggested defence mechanisms are (i) lack of classical transplantation antigens on syncytiotrophoblast, (ii) mucopolysaccharide coat around trophoblast, and (iii) local production of immunosuppressant.

The MHC subserves recognition functions. The immune response (Ir) genes code for molecules (Ia) which in association with carrier determinants optimally regulate priming of T-cells by macrophage-processed antigen and interactions between T- and B-cells. Other MHC antigens are involved in the generation of cytotoxic T-cells in response to viral infection. Thus *the MHC would appear to be part of a system for signalling changes in 'self'* which enables the T-cells to make the appropriate immune response. Each cell in the body bears H-2D/K determinants so the cytotoxic T-cells use these to recognize a virally infected cell. The antigens of organisms such as TB, leishmania and toxoplasma which live within macrophages are processed to form an association with Ia on the macrophage surface which can stimulate 'delayed hypersensitivity' T-cells; these release factors enabling the macrophages to kill their intracellular parasites.

The immune surveillance theory of cancer postulates that changes in the surface of the neoplastic cell are recognized by the immune system and eliminated. However, although virally coded, idiotypic and oncofetal antigens may be detected on experimentally induced tumour cells together with components linked to cell division, the incidence of spontaneous cancers in immunosuppressed individuals is not generally higher than normal. Examples of immune responses to tumours in human cancer are known but attempts at control by immunization with tumour plus adjuvant have not been encouraging. Other strategies involve non-specific activation of macrophages and NK cells by adjuvants such as BCG, *C. parvum* and lecithin analogues. Oncofetal antigens may be useful in diagnosis (e.g. α-fetoprotein in primary hepatoma).

Genes controlling C3 and its complementary proteins map in the MHC. HLA specificities are often associated with particular diseases, e.g. HLA-B27 with ankylosing spondylitis, B8 with myasthenia gravis, Dw4 with rheumatoid arthritis and Dw2 with multiple sclerosis.

Further reading

Albert E. *et al.* (1978) Nomenclature for factors of the HLA system, 1977. *Bull. W.H.O.*, **56**, 461.

Billingham R. & Silvers W. (1971) *The Immunobiology of Transplantation.* Foundations of Immunology Series, Prentice-Hall, N. Jersey.

Bodmer W.F. (ed) (1978) The HLA System. *Brit. Med. Bull.*, **34** No. 3.

Castro J.E. (ed) (1978) *Immunological Aspects of Cancer.* M.T.P., Lancaster.

Dausset J. & Hors J. (1973) Statistics of 416 consecutive kidney transplants in the France-Transplant organization. *Transpl. Proc.*, **5**, 223.

Doherty P.C. & Zinkernagel R.M. (1975) A biological role for the major histocompatibility antigens. *Lancet*, **i**, 1406.

Festenstein H. & Demant P. (1978) *Immunogenetics of the major histocompatibility system.* Edward Arnold, London.

Fongerean M. & Dansset J. (eds) (1980) *Progress in Immunology* IV. Academic Press, London.

Kiesling R. & Haller O. (1978) Natural killer cells in mice. *Contemporary Topics in Immunobiology*, **8**, 171. Plenum, N. York.

Lance E.M., Medawar P.B. & Taub R.N. (1973) Antilymphocyte serum. *Adv. in Immunology*, **17**, 2.

Mitchison N.A. (1980) Protective immunity (to tumours) *in vivo.* In, *Clin. Aspects of Immunol.*, Peters K. & Lachmann P. (eds) 4th Ed. Blackwell Scientific Publications, Oxford.

Möller G. (ed) (1979) Natural killer cells. *Immunol. Rev.*, **44**.

Munro A. & Bright S. (1976) Products of the major histocompatibility complex and their relationship to the immune response. *Nature*, **264**, 145.

Rose N.R., Bigazzi P.E. & Warner N.L. (eds) (1978) *Genetic control of autoimmune disease.* Elsevier North-Holland Inc, New York.

Skinner M.D. & Schwartz R.S. (1972) Immunosuppressive Therapy. *N.Eng.J.Med.*, **287**, 221 and 281.

Smith R.T. & Landy M. (1975) *Immunobiology of the tumour–host relationship.* Academic Press, New York.

Zinkernagel R.M. & Doherty P.C. (1979) MHC-restricted cytotoxic T cells: studies on the biological role of polymorphic major transplantation antigens determining T-cell restriction—specificity, function and responsiveness. *Adv. Immunol.*, **27**, 51.

10 Autoimmunity

There are in the body appropriate mechanisms to prevent the recognition of 'self' components as antigens by the lymphoid system but, as with all machinery, there is always a chance that these mechanisms might break down, and the older the individual, the greater the chance of a breakdown. When this happens *autoantibodies* (i.e. antibodies capable of reacting with 'self' components) are produced. Grabar is of the opinion that autoantibodies have a biological function to act as 'transporting' agents for cellular breakdown products thereby aiding their disposal. While antibodies can act in this way, we are here concerned more with autoimmune phenomena which appear in relation to certain defined human diseases. Ideally we wish to apply the term 'autoimmune disease' to those cases where it can be shown that the autoimmune process contributes to the pathogenesis of the disease rather than situations where apparently harmless autoantibodies are formed following tissue damage, e.g. heart antibodies appearing after a myocardial infarction. Yet the role of autoimmunity in many disorders is still not clearly defined, and it is as a matter of convenience that we will refer to all maladies firmly associated with autoantibody formation as 'autoimmune diseases', except where it can be shown that the immunological phenomena are purely secondary findings.

The spectrum of autoimmune diseases

These disorders may be looked upon as forming a spectrum. At one end we have '*organ-specific diseases*' with organ-specific autoantibodies. Hashimoto's disease of the thyroid is an example: there is a specific lesion in the thyroid involving infiltration by mononuclear cells (lymphocytes, histiocytes and plasma cells), destruction of follicular cells and germinal centre formation, accompanied, as we showed originally, by the production of circulating antibodies with absolute specificity for certain thyroid constituents (Roitt, Doniach & Campbell).

TABLE 10.1. Spectrum of autoimmune diseases

Organ specific ←				→ Non-organ specific
Hashimoto's thyroiditis Primary myxoedema (bracketed together)	Goodpasture's syndrome	Autoimmune haemolytic anaemia	Primary biliary cirrhosis	Systemic lupus erythematosus (SLE)
Thyrotoxicosis	Myasthenia gravis	Idiopathic thrombocytopenic purpura	Active chronic hepatitis HB_S-ve	Discoid LE
Pernicious anaemia	Juvenile diabetes	Idiopathic leucopenia	Cryptogenic cirrhosis (some cases)	Dermatomyositis
Autoimmune atrophic gastritis	Pemphigus vulgaris		Ulcerative colitis	Scleroderma
Addison's disease	Pemphigoid		Sjögren's syndrome	Rheumatoid arthritis
Premature menopause (few cases)	Sympathetic ophthalmia			
Male infertility (few cases)	Phacogenic uveitis			
	(?? Multiple sclerosis ??)			

Moving towards the centre of the spectrum are those disorders where the lesion tends to be localized to a single organ but the antibodies are non-organ specific. A typical example would be primary biliary cirrhosis where the small bile ductule is the main target of inflammatory cell infiltration but the serum antibodies present—mainly mitochondrial—are not liver specific.

At the other end of the spectrum are the '*non-organ specific diseases*' exemplified by systemic lupus erythematosus (SLE) where both lesions and autoantibodies are not confined to any one organ. Pathological changes are widespread and are primarily lesions of connective tissue with fibrinoid necrosis. They are seen in the skin (the 'lupus' butterfly rash on the face is characteristic), kidney glomeruli, joints, serous membranes and blood vessels. In addition the formed elements of the blood are often affected. A bizarre collection of autoantibodies are found some of which react with the DNA and other nuclear constituents of all cells in the body.

An attempt to fit the major diseases considered to be associated with autoimmunity into this spectrum is shown in table 10.1.

Autoantibodies in human disease

At this stage in the discussion it may be of value to have a more precise account of the major autoantibodies detected in the different diseases to provide a framework for reference. Table 10.2 documents a list of these antibodies and the

TABLE 10.2. Autoantibodies in human disease
(IFT = Immunofluorescent test; CFT = complement fixation test)

Disease	Antigen	Detection of antibody
Hashimoto's thyroiditis, Primary myxoedema	Thyroglobulin	Precipitins; passive haemaggln.
	2nd Colloid Ag (CA2)	IFT on fixed thyroid
	Cytoplasmic microsomes	IFT on unfixed thyroid; passive haemaggln.
	Cell surface	IFT on viable thyroid cells; C′-mediated cytotoxicity
Thyrotoxicosis	Cell surface TSH receptors	Bioassay—stimulation of mouse thyroid *in vivo*; blocking combination TSH with receptors; stimulation adenyl cyclase
Pernicious anaemia[1]	Intrinsic factor	Neutralization; blocking combination with vit-B_{12}; binding to Int.Fact-B_{12} by copptn.
	Parietal cell microsomes	IFT on unfixed gastric mucosa
Addison's disease	Cytoplasm adrenal cells	IFT on unfixed adrenal cortex
Premature onset of menopause[2]	Cytoplasm steroid producing cells	IFT on adrenal and interstitial cells of ovary and testis
Male infertility (some)[3]	Spermatozoa	Sperm agglutination in ejaculate
Juvenile diabetes[4]	Cytoplasm of islet cells	IFT on unfixed human pancreas
	Cell surface	Leucocyte cytotoxicity
(Multiple Sclerosis)	Brain	Cytotoxic effects on cerebellar cultures by serum and lymphocytes (? secondary to disease)
Goodpasture's syndrome	Glomerular and lung basement membrane	Linear staining by IFT of kidney biopsy with fluorescent anti-IgG
Pemphigus vulgaris	Desmosomes between prickle cells in epidermis	IFT on skin
Pemphigoid	Basement membrane	IFT on skin
Phacogenic uveitis	Lens	Passive haemagglutination
Sympathetic ophthalmia	Uvea	(Delayed skin reaction to uveal extract)
Myasthenia gravis	Skeletal and heart muscle	IFT on skeletal muscle
	Acetyl choline receptor	Blocking or binding radioassay with α-bungarotoxin
Autoimmune haemolytic anaemia[5]	Erythrocytes	Coombs' antiglobulin test
Idiopathic thrombocytopenic purpura	Platelets	Shortened platelet survival *in vivo*

Table 10.2 (*contd.*)

Disease	Antigen	Detection of antibody
Primary biliary cirrhosis	Mitochondria (mainly)	IFT on mitochondria rich cells (e.g. distal tubules of kidney)
Active chronic hepatitis	Smooth muscle, nuclei	IFT (e.g. on gastric mucosa)
	Cell surface lipoprotein	Leucocyte cytotoxicity
Ulcerative colitis	Colon 'lipopoly-saccharide'	IFT; passive haemaggln. (cytotoxic action of lymphocytes on colon cells)
Sjögren's syndrome[6]	Ducts, mitochondria, nuclei, thyroid,	IFT
	IgG	Antiglobulin tests
Rheumatoid arthritis[7]	IgG	Antiglobulin tests: latex aggln., sheep red cell aggln. test (SCAT) & radioassay
	RANA[8]	IFT on EB-transformed cell line
	Collagen	Passive haemaggln.
Discoid lupus erythematosus } Dermatomyositis } Scleroderma[9] }	Nuclear	IFT
	IgG	Antiglobulin tests
Mixed connective tissue disease[10]	Extractable nuclear	IFT; countercurrent electro-phoresis
Systemic lupus erythematosus	DNA	Radioassay[11]; pptn; CFT
	Nucleoprotein	IFT; latex aggln. L.E. cells[12]
	Cytoplasmic sol.Ag	'Non-organ sp.CFT'
	Array of other Ag incl. formed elements of blood, clotting factors, IgG and Wasserman antigen	'Biological false positive' CFT

Notes:

1. Two major types of antibody to intrinsic factor are detected, viz. blocking and binding (figure 10.1). Binding antibody combines with preformed Int.Fact.—radioactive B_{12}($*B_{12}$) complex which can then be precipitated at 50 per cent ammonium sulphate (cf. Farr test—salt copptn., p. 144) and the radioactivity in the precipitate counted. Blocking antibody prevents binding of $*B_{12}$ to Int.Fact. and the uncombined $*B_{12}$ can then be adsorbed to charcoal and counted.

2. Antibodies occur in the minority of patients with associated Addison's disease.

3. Only small percentage show agglutinins. Spermatozoa may be agglutinated head to head, tail to tail or joined through their mid-piece. Seen also in small percentage of infertile women.

4. Most if not all juvenile (insulin dependent) diabetics have islet cell antibodies at some stage during the first year of onset. In contrast, islet cell antibodies in diabetic patients with an associated autoimmune polyendocrinopathy persist for many years.

5. The Coombs' test involves the demonstration of bound antibody on the washed red cell by agglutination with an antiglobulin. Erythrocyte autoantibodies, which bind well over the temperature range 0–37°C ('warm' Ab), are mostly IgG; approximately 60 per cent of cases are primary, the remainder being associated with other autoimmune disorders, e.g. SLE, ulcerative colitis. 'Cold' Ab, which react best over the

range 0–20°C, are mostly IgM and red cells coated with this Ab can often be agglutinated by anti-complement sera; approximately half are primary, the others being associated with *Mycoplasma pneumoniae* infection or generalized neoplastic disease of the lymphoreticular tissues.

6. Antibodies specifically reacting with the epithelium of salivary gland excretory ducts are demonstrable by immunofluorescence in up to half the cases.

7. The main antiglobulin factors react with the Fc portion of IgG which is usually adsorbed onto latex particles (human IgG) or present in an antigen–antibody complex (sheep red cells coated with subagglutinating dose of rabbit antibody). In the radioassay test, rabbit IgG is bound to a plastic tube, patient's serum added and the antiglobulin bound assessed by subsequent binding of labelled anti-human IgG or IgM (cf. p. 145).

8. The rheumatoid arthritis nuclear antigen (RANA) is revealed as speckled staining by IFT using cells transformed by EB virus; normal cells are negative.

9. In scleroderma (progressive systemic sclerosis) antinucleolar antibodies are frequently found.

10. This syndrome combines features of scleroderma, rheumatoid arthritis, SLE and dermatomyositis. The antigen is an extractable nuclear antigen which gives speckled fluorescence and RNase-sensitive precipitation by countercurrent electrophoresis.

11. Antibodies to single or double-stranded DNA are assayed by the Farr test (cf. p. 144) using labelled Ag, or by a DNA-coated tube test similar to the radioassay for antiglobulins (note 7 above).

12. When blood from an SLE patient is incubated at 37°C, some white cells are damaged and allow the entry of antibodies. Certain of the antibodies combining with the nuclear surface bind complement and attract polymorphs which strip away the cytoplasm and engulf the nucleus. The polymorph containing the engulfed homogenized nucleus is called an LE-cell (figure 10.3).

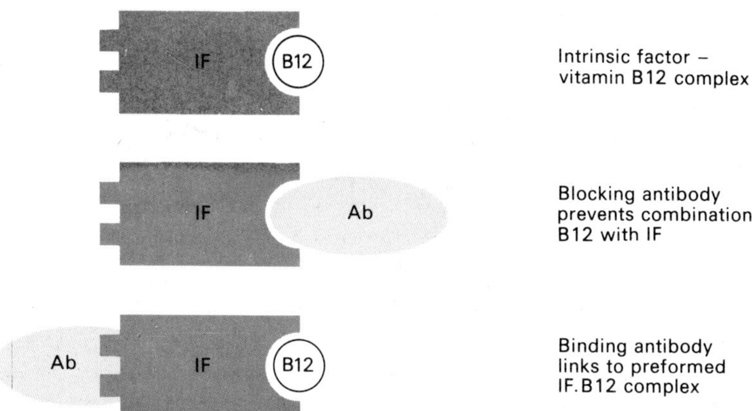

FIGURE 10.1. Intrinsic factor autoantibodies: sites of determinants for binding and blocking. (I. M. Roitt, D. Doniach & C. Shapland. *Lancet*, 1964, **2**, 469.)

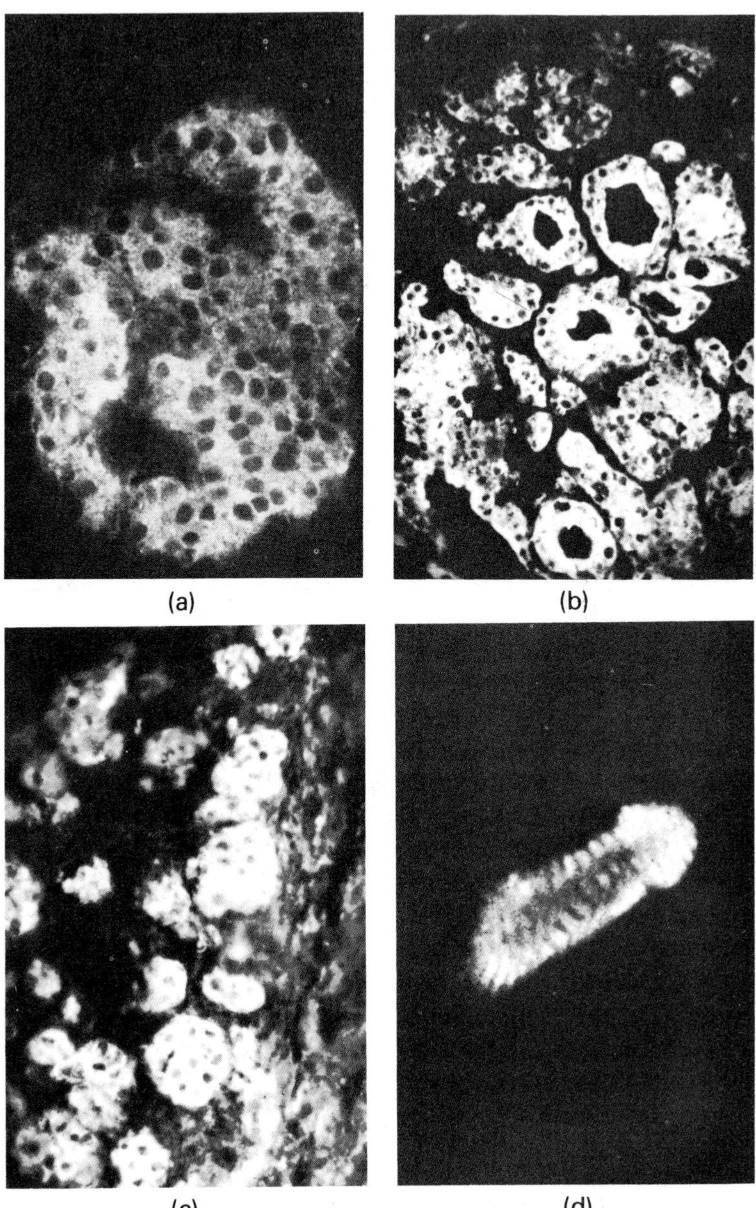

FIGURE 10.2. Autoantibodies demonstrable by indirect immunofluorescent test (section treated with patient's serum, washed, then stained with fluorescein-conjugate of anti-human Ig, cf. p. 149): (a) fluorescence of cells in the pancreatic islets of Langerhans after treatment with serum from insulin-dependent 'juvenile' diabetic; (b) thyroid microsomal antibodies staining cytoplasm of acinar cells; (c) serum of patient with Addison's disease staining cytoplasm of adrenal cells; (d) striated muscle antibodies in serum of patient with myasthenia gravis reacting with 'myoid' cell in human thymus; (e) fluorescence of distal tubular cells of the kidney after reaction with mitochondrial auto-

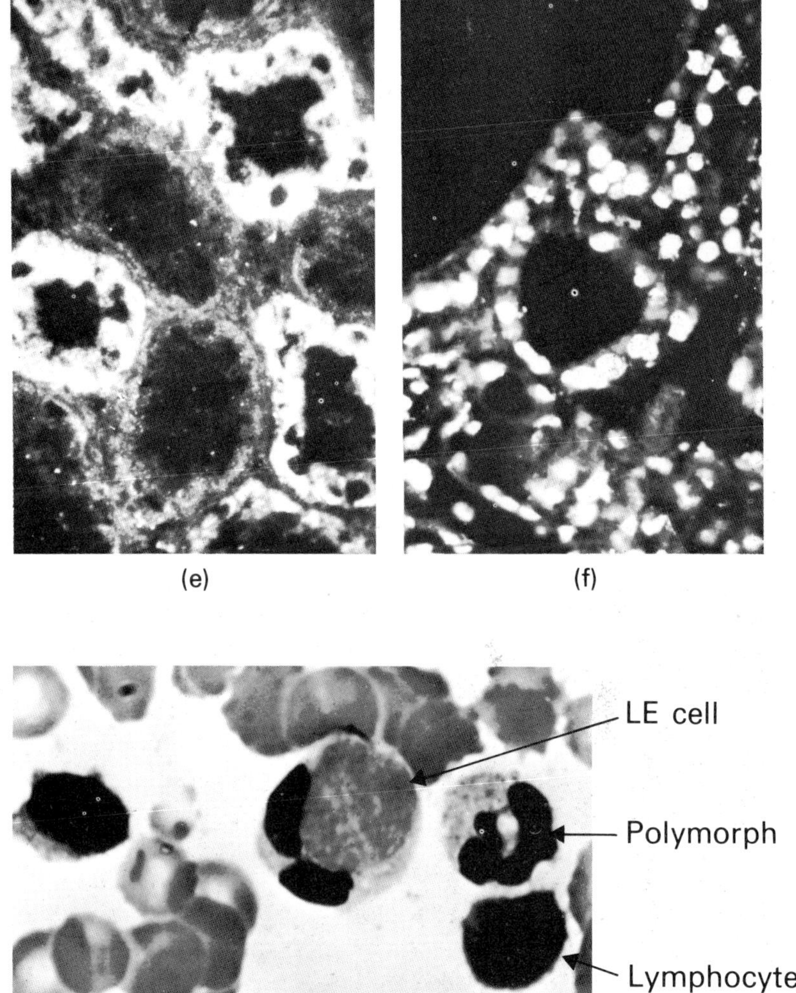

FIGURE 10.3. LE-cell in preparation from peripheral blood of SLE patient. The homogeneous nucleus lies within the polymorph which engulfed it by phagocytosis. Two normal polymorphs and two small lymphocytes are also present. (Photographed from material kindly provided by Prof. J.W. Stewart.)

---

antibodies; (f) diffuse nuclear staining obtained with nucleoprotein antibodies on a thyroid section. ((a) kindly provided by Dr. F. Bottazzo, (d) by Dr. T.E.W. Feltkamp, the others by courtesy of Dr. D. Doniach.)

methods employed in their detection. The notes following the table amplify specific points while some of the tests are illustrated in figures 10.1–10.3, 6.17 and 6.18.

Overlap of autoimmune disorders

There is a tendency for more than one autoimmune disorder to occur in the same individual and when this happens the association is often between diseases within the same region of the autoimmune spectrum (cf. table 10.1). Thus patients with autoimmune thyroiditis (Hashimoto's disease or primary myxoedema) have a much higher incidence of pernicious anaemia than would be expected in a random population matched for age and sex (10 per cent as against 0·2 per cent). Conversely both thyroiditis and thyrotoxicosis are diagnosed in pernicious anaemia patients with an unexpectedly high frequency. Other associations are seen between Addison's disease and autoimmune thyroid disease and in the rare cases of juveniles with pernicious anaemia and polyendocrinopathy which includes Addison's disease, hypoparathyroidism, diabetes and thyroiditis.

There is an even greater overlap in serological findings. 30 per cent of patients with autoimmune thyroid disease have concomitant parietal cell antibodies in their serum. Conversely, thyroid antibodies have been demonstrated in up to 50 per cent of pernicious anaemia patients. It should be stressed that these are not cross-reacting antibodies. The thyroid specific antibodies will not react with stomach and *vice versa*. When a serum reacts with both organs it means that two populations of antibodies are present, one with specificity for thyroid and the other for stomach.

At the non-organic-specific end of the spectrum, SLE is clinically associated with rheumatoid arthritis and several other diseases which are themselves uncommon: haemolytic anaemia, idiopathic leucopenia and thrombocytopenic purpura, dermatomyositis and Sjögren's syndrome. Antinuclear antibodies, non-organ-specific complement fixation reactions, and antiglobulin (rheumatoid) factors are a general feature of these disorders.

Sjögren's syndrome occupies an interesting position (table 10.3); aside from the clinical and serological features associated with non-organ-specific disease mentioned above, characteristics of an organ-specific disorder are evident. Antibodies reacting with salivary ducts are demonstrable

TABLE 10.3. Organ-specific and non-organ-specific serological interrelationships in human disease

Disease	% Positive reactions for antibodies to:				
	Thyroid*	Stomach*	Nuclei*	Non-organ-specific antigen**	IgG†
Hashimoto's thyroiditis	99·9	32	8	5	2
Pernicious anaemia	55	89	11	7	
Sjögren's syndrome	45	14	56	19	75
Rheumatoid arthritis	11	16	50	10	75
S.L.E.	2	2	99	66	35
Controls‡	0–15	0–16	0–19	0–10	2–5

* Immunofluorescence test ** CFT with kidney † Rheumatoid factor classical tests
‡ Incidence increases with age and females > males

and there is an abnormally high incidence of thyroid autoantibodies; histologically the affected lacrimal and salivary glands reveal changes of a similar nature to those seen in Hashimoto's disease, namely a replacement of the glandular elements by patchy lymphocytic and plasma cell granulomatous tissue. Associations between diseases at the two ends of the spectrum have been reported, but, as might be predicted from the serological data (table 10.3), they are not common.

There is still no entirely satisfactory explanation to account for the rare tendency to develop hypogammaglobulinaemia and the increased incidence of certain cancers occurring in autoimmune disease. Patients with organ specific disorders are slightly more prone to develop cancer in the affected organ whereas generalized lymphoreticular neoplasia shows up with uncommon frequency in non-organ-specific disease.

Genetic factors in autoimmune disease

Autoimmune phenomena tend to aggregate in certain families. For example, the first degree relatives (sibs, parents and children) of patients with Hashimoto's disease show a high incidence of thyroid autoantibodies and of overt and subclinical thyroiditis. Interestingly there is also an increased frequency of 'non-immunological' thyroid disorders, such as non-toxic nodular goitre. The proportion with autoantibodies is higher in those families where more than one member is clinically affected. Parallel studies have disclosed similar relationships in the families of pernicious anaemia patients in that gastric pariental cell antibodies are prevalent in the relatives who are wont to develop achlorhydria and atrophic gastritis. A somewhat unusual family is depicted in figure 10.4 which illustrates these features and reminds us of the thyroid–stomach link. Familial aggregation of mitochondrial antibodies has been observed, albeit to a lesser extent, in primary biliary cirrhosis. Turning to SLE, disturbances of immunoglobulin synthesis and a susceptibility to develop 'connective tissue diseases' have been reported but there are some conflicting accounts still not resolved.

These familial relationships could be ascribed to environmental factors such as an infective micro-organism, but there is evidence that one or more genetic components must be given serious consideration. In the first place, when thyrotoxicosis occurs in twins there is a greater concordance rate

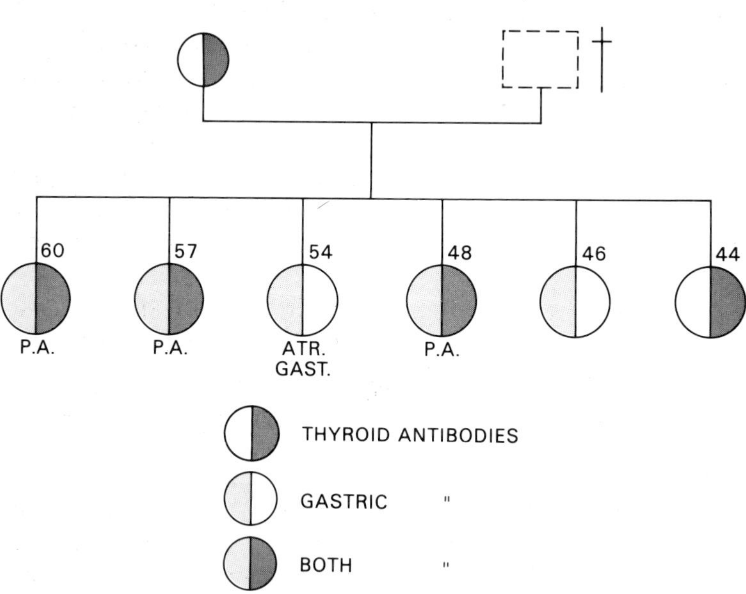

FIGURE 10.4. Familial aggregation of gastric autoimmunity. Six female siblings with their respective ages and autoantibodies are shown. Three had pernicious anaemia (PA) and another atrophic gastritis (Atr.gast.). The mother had myxoedema. (Courtesy Prof. D. Doniach.)

(i.e. both twins affected) in identical than in non-identical twins. Secondly, thyroid autoantibodies are more prevalent in individuals with ovarian dysgenesis having X-chromosome aberrations such as XO and particularly the isochromosome X abnormality. Furthermore, there are strong associations between several autoimmune diseases and particular HLA specificities, e.g. B8-Dw3 in Addison's disease and Dw4 in rheumatoid arthritis (Table 9.2, p. 288). Since only very restricted determinants on the autoantigenic molecules evoke autoantibodies (e.g. thyroglobulin of molecular weight 650,000, has a valency of 4), one is tempted to think in terms of Ir genes, it being precisely under such conditions that Ir genes can be recognized.

It is also intriguing to note that lines of animals have been bred which spontaneously develop autoimmune disease. In other words, the autoimmunity is genetically programmed. There is an obese line of chickens with autoimmune thyroiditis and the New Zealand Black (NZB) mouse with autoimmune haemolytic anaemia. The hybrid of NZB with another strain the New Zealand White (B × W hybrid) actually develops LE-cells, antinuclear antibodies and a fatal immune complex induced glomerulonephritis. Suitable intercross and backcross breeding of these mice has established that a *minimum* of three genes determines the expression of autoimmunity and that the production of both red cell and nuclear antibodies may be under separate genetic control, i.e. there may be different factors predisposing to autoimmunity on the one hand, and to the selection of antigen on the other. This view finds support in the genetic analysis of 'obese' chickens which has delineated an influence of the MHC, abnormalities in T-cell control and a defect in the thyroid gland.

The facts presented by human autoimmune disease also attest to multifactorial control. The overlaps in autoantibodies and disease discussed above point to a general tendency to develop autoimmunity in these individuals and further, the factors which predispose to organ-specific disease must be different from those in non-organ-specific disorders (as judged by the minimal overlap between them). There must be additional factors which are organ related in that the families of thyroiditis patients tend to have thyroid autoimmunity while relatives of patients with pernicious anaemia are prone to gastric autoimmunity.

Autoantibodies are demonstrable in comparatively low titre in the general population and the incidence of positive

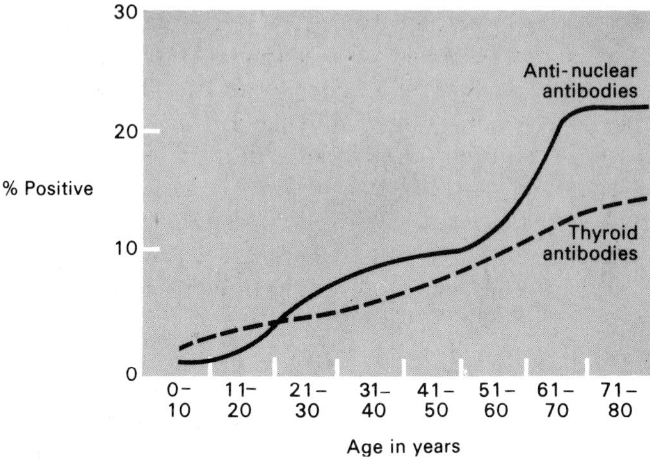

FIGURE 10.5. Incidence of autoantibodies in the general population. A serum was considered positive for thyroid antibodies if it reacted at a dilution of 1/10 in the tanned red cell test or neat in the immunofluorescent test and positive for antinuclear antibodies if it reacted at a dilution of 1/4 by immunofluorescence.

results increases steadily with age (figure 10.5) up to around 60–70 years. In the case of the thyroid and stomach at least, biopsy has indicated that the presence of antibody is almost invariably associated with minor thyroiditis or gastritis lesions (as the case may be), and it is of interest that post mortem examination has identified 10 per cent of middle-aged women with significant degrees of lymph-adenoid change in the thyroid similar in essence to that characteristic of Hashimoto's disease.

The point should also be made here that, in general, auto-antibodies and autoimmune diseases are found more frequently in women than in men.

Aetiology of autoimmune response

How do autoantibodies arise? Our earliest view, with respect to organ specific antibodies at least, was that the antigens were sequestered within the organ and through lack of contact with the lymphoreticular system failed to establish immunological tolerance. Any mishap which caused a release of the antigen would then provide an opportunity for auto-antibody formation. For a few body constituents this holds true and in the case of sperm, lens and heart for example, release of certain components directly into the circulation can provoke autoantibodies. But in general, the experience has been that injection of *unmodified* extracts of those tissues concerned in the organ-specific autoimmune disorders does not elicit antibody formation. Indeed detailed investigation of the thyroid autoantigen, thyroglobulin, has disclosed that it is not completely sequestered within the gland but gains access to the extracellular fluid around the follicles and leaves via the thyroid lymphatics (figure 10.6) reaching the serum in normal human subjects at concentrations of approximately 0·01–0·05 μg/ml.

Concentrations of this order produce 'low zone tolerance' in mice by affecting the T-lymphocytes, probably through suppressors. Extrapolating to man, we are presumably dealing with a situation in which T-cells are tolerant to thyroglobulin and B-cells are not. Indeed a small proportion of the B-cells in normal individuals bind human thyroglobulin through their surface Ig receptors. That these autoantigen binding cells are capable of autoantibody production is suggested by 'antigen suicide' experiments in which lymphocytes from

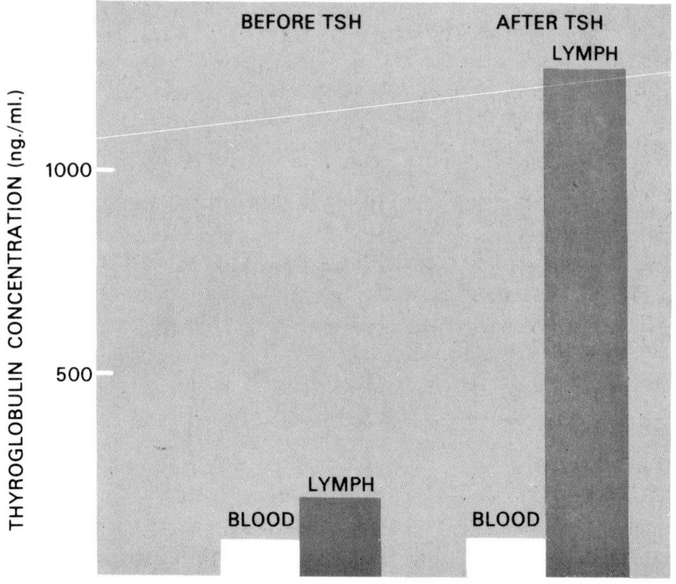

FIGURE 10.6. Thyroglobulin in the cervical lymph draining the thyroid in the rat. The concentration of thyroglobulin is increased after injection of pituitary thyroid stimulating hormone (TSH) suggesting that the release from thyroid follicles is linked to the physiological activity of the acinar cells (from Daniel P.N., Pratt O.E., Roitt I.M. & Torrigiani G., *Quart.J.exp.Physiol.* 1967, **52**, 184).

thyroglobulin-primed animals fail to make antibodies when challenged in a secondary host if they are allowed to bind thyroglobulin of very high specific radioactivity *in vitro* before transfer, the implication being that cells binding the 'hot' antigen through surface receptors are inactivated by irradiation.

Other molecules such as DNA and myelin basic protein are also bound by normal lymphocytes and it seems likely that B-cells reactive with a wide range of body constituents circulate normally. Other curious phenomena involving the generation of self-reactivity *in vitro* have been described, as for example the development of reactivity towards sertoli cells by spleen cells cultured with syngeneic testis. It is worth noting that anti-idiotypic responses are also essentially autoimmune in nature. The message then is that we are all sitting on a minefield of potentially self-reactive cells, but since autoimmune disease is more the exception than the rule, the body must have homeostatic mechanisms to prevent them being triggered under normal circumstances. We are now ready to examine ways in which these mechanisms may be circumvented to allow autoimmunity to develop.

PROVISION OF NEW CARRIER DETERMINANT

If, as discussed above, auto-reactive T-cells are rendered helpless through self-tolerance (cf. p. 109), then T-B collaboration to generate autoantibodies (reaction 1, figure 10.7) is not possible. Using this model, Allison and Weigle argued independently that provision of new carrier determinants to which no self-tolerance had been established would bypass this mechanism and lead to autoantibody production (reaction 2, figure 10.7).

(i) *Modification of the molecule*

A new carrier could arise through some modification to the molecule, for example, by defects in synthesis or by an abnormality in lysosomal breakdown yielding a split product exposing some new groupings. Experimentally it has been found that large proteolytic fragments of thyroglobulin are autoantigenic when injected alone but no evidence for such a mechanism has yet been uncovered in man; where antibodies to a split product such as the $F(ab')_2$ fragment of IgG have been detected, they have not reacted with the whole molecules.

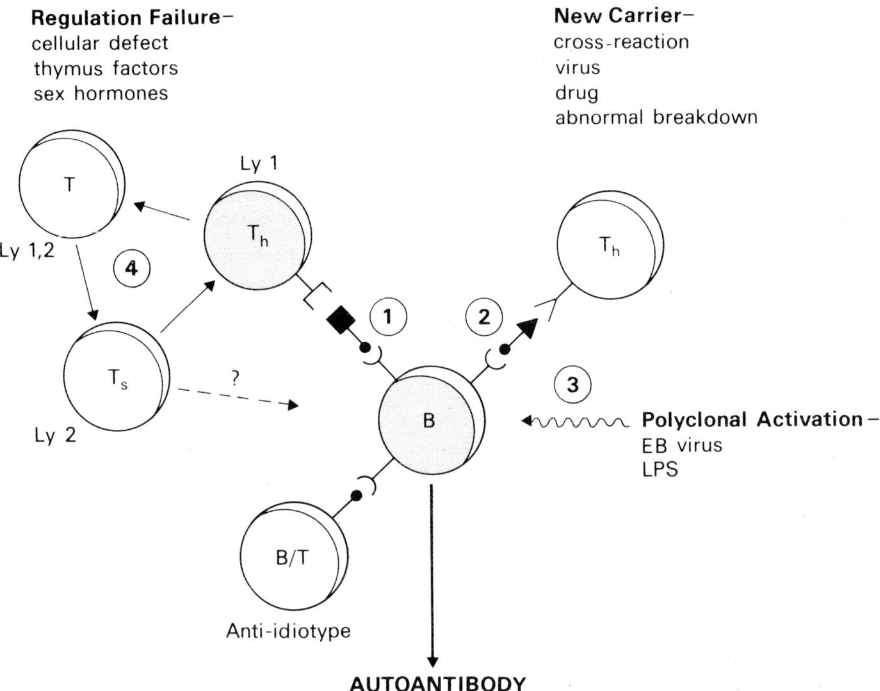

FIGURE 10.7. Mechanisms of autoantibody formation to non-sequestered body components. T-B co-operation in the response to an autoantigen (1) is normally held in check by immunoregulatory mechanisms (4). This may be circumvented by association of the autoantigen with a new carrier (2), by polyclonal activators (3) or by a failure in regulation (4). —● Autoantigenic determinant (hapten) recognized by B-cell, ■— autoantigenic determinant (carrier) recognized by T-cell, ◀— New carrier determinant. Shaded lymphocytes react with autoantigen. (After Drs. A. Cooke & P.M. Lydyard.)

Incorporation into Freund's complete adjuvant frequently endows these molecules with autoantigenic properties and as we shall see later this enables us to induce many autoallergic diseases in laboratory animals. It is conceivable that the physical constraints on the proteins at the water–oil interface of the emulsion provide the required alteration in configuration of the 'carrier portions' of the molecules.

Modification can also be achieved through combination with a drug. The autoimmune haemolytic anaemia associated with administration of α-methyl dopa might be attributable to modification of the red-cell surface in such a way as to provide a carrier for stimulating B-cells which recognize the Rhesus *e* antigen. This is normally regarded as a 'weak' antigen and would be less likely to induce B-cell tolerance than the 'stronger' antigens present on the erythrocyte.

Isoniazid may produce arthritis associated with nuclear antibodies and unlike most other cases of drug induced autoimmunity, synthesis of these antibodies is said to continue after cessation of drug therapy. A high proportion of patients on continued treatment with procainamide develop nuclear antibodies and 40% present with clinical signs of SLE. Myasthenia gravis and symptoms of pemphigus have been described in some patients on penicillamine. It is not clear in every case whether the drug provides carrier help through direct modification of the autoantigen or of some independent molecule concerned in associative recognition.

Associative recognition

This term applies to the phenomenon in which one membrane component may provide help for the immune response to another. In the context of autoimmunity, a new helper determinant may arise through drug modification as mentioned above, or through the insertion of viral antigen into the membrane of an infected cell. That this can promote a reaction to a pre-existing cell component is clear from the studies in which infection of a tumour with influenza virus elicted resistance to uninfected tumour cells. The appearance of cold agglutinins often with blood group I specificity after *Mycoplasma pneumonia* infection could have a similar explanation.

Cross-reactions

Many examples are known in which potential autoantigenic determinants are present on an exogenous cross-reacting antigen which provides the new carrier to provoke autoantibody formation. Post rabies vaccine encephalitis is thought to result from an autoimmune reaction to brain initiated by heterologous brain tissue in the vaccine (cf. experimental allergic encephalomyelitis below). Some micro-organisms carry determinants which cross-react with the human and this may prove to be an important way of inducing autoimmunity. In rheumatic fever antibodies produced to the streptococcus also react with heart, and the sera of 50% of children with the disease who develop Sydenham's chorea give neuronal immunofluorescent staining which can be absorbed out with streptococcal membranes. Colon antibodies present in ulcerative colitis have been found to cross-react with *Escherichia coli* 014. There is also some evidence for the view that antigens common to *Trypanosoma cruzi* and cardiac muscle provoke some of the immunopathological lesions seen in Chagas' disease.

POLYCLONAL ACTIVATION

Microbes often display adjuvant properties through their possession of polyclonal lymphocyte activators such as bacterial endotoxins which may act by providing the second (non-specific) inductive signal for B-cell stimulation (p. 75), so bypassing the need for specific T-cell help. This can occur by direct interaction with the B-lymphocyte or indirectly through stimulating the secretion of non-specific factors from T-cells or macrophages. A good example is the thymus-dependent production of autoantibodies by injection of mice with thyroglobulin and endotoxin (LPS). The variety of autoantibodies detected in cases with infectious mononucleosis must surely be attributable to the polyclonal activation of B-cells by EB virus. They are seen also in lepromatous leprosy where the abundance of mycobacteria reproduces some of the features of Freund's adjuvant. However, unlike the usual situation in human autoimmune disease, these autoantibodies tend to be IgM and, in addition, do not persist when the microbial components are cleared from the body. Curiously, lymphocytes from mice with spontaneous autoimmunity (e.g. NZB) produce abnormally large amounts of IgM when cultured *in vitro* as if they were under polyclonal activation.

FAILURE OF IMMUNE REGULATION

Body constituents circulating in high concentration are thought to induce tolerance through clonal abortion, whereas unresponsiveness to other molecules present at low levels is probably controlled through some form of T-suppression (p. 109 and figure 10.7). If this regulation mechanism were to fail, then autoreactive lymphocytes would be triggered. In accord with this view, manipulations which reduce T-suppressors encourage the development of autoantibodies. Irradiated mice reconstituted with spleen cells deprived of Ly2 positive T-cells produce antibodies to thyroglobulin, nuclei and lymphocytes. When rats were thymectomized at a few weeks of age and given divided doses of X-rays, they developed thyroglobulin autoantibodies and thyroiditis. Neonatal thymectomy which greatly depletes the T-suppressor population, induces or exacerbates spontaneous autoimmune states in susceptible animals—autoimmune haemolytic anaemia in NZB mice and thyroiditis in Obese strain chickens and Buffalo rats. Coombs' positivity (i.e. the state in which circulating red cells are coated with antibody) can be transferred with the spleen cells of a Coombs' positive NZB to a young negative mouse of the same strain, but the continued production of red cell antibodies is short-lived unless the recipient's T-cells are first depleted by pre-treatment with anti-lymphocyte serum. Other changes seen with age in the NZB are an increasing resistance to the induction of tolerance to soluble proteins and a sudden fall in the plasma concentration of thymic peptide (FTS; p. 112) before the onset of disease (note: FTS is said to inhibit the autoreactive response of spleen cells to syngeneic fibroblasts in culture). Thus, there is a widely held view that one defect in the NZB is a progressive loss of T-suppressors with age and it is relevant that Ly1,2 cells which are needed for the induction of suppressors are low in diseased mice. Defects are possible at various control points in the regulatory mechanism: for example another mutant mouse strain with a spontaneous SLE-like syndrome, the MRL/l, has ample numbers of effective Ly1,2 cells but Ly1 helpers are resistant to their suppressor action.

Less is known of regulatory circuits in man although there is increasing evidence that non-specific T suppressor function in SLE may be poorly regulated. B-lymphocytes from patients with active disease secrete larger amounts of Ig when cultured *in vitro* than normal B-cells. Concanavalin A-induced non-specific suppressors are reduced or absent and T_G cells which suppress pokeweed mitogen-stimulated lymphocytes (p. 102) are low, the defect being greater the more active the disease. The thymic factor FTS is also depressed in these patients.

The origins of such defects are obscure. They might be the consequence of some subtle viral infection of the lymphoid system; the shedding of tremendous amounts of a C type oncornavirus from NZB T-cell lines may be of relevance to this. Or one may be dealing with some ageing process affecting the thymus or the lymphoid stem cells. Sex hormones may also contribute to the increased frequency of autoimmunity in females. Thus, oopherectomy and testosterone treatment alleviate the disease in female (NZB $\times$ NZW)F1 hybrids.

These considerations apply in general to non-specific suppressor mechanisms, yet the different autoimmune states are usually associated with specific autoantigens. If idiotype network interactions are involved in these T-cell control circuits, this could provide one explanation for antigen-specific defects. Furthermore, anti-idiotype may provide a persistent *stimulus* to autoantibody production even when the circumstances initiating synthesis are only temporary (e.g. virus infection).

Pathogenic mechanisms in autoimmune disease

We have mentioned that despite certain exceptions as, for instance, myocardial infarction or damage to the testis, traumatic release of organ constituents does not in general elicit antibody formation. Destruction of thyroid tissue by therapeutic doses of radio-iodine does not initiate thyroid autoimmunity nor does damage to the liver in alcoholic cirrhosis result in the synthesis of mitochondrial antibodies, to give but two examples. We should now look at the evidence which bears directly on the issue of whether autoimmunity, however it arises, plays a *primary* pathogenic role in the production of tissue lesions in the group of diseases labelled as 'autoimmune'.

EFFECTS OF HUMORAL ANTIBODY

Blood

The erythrocyte antibodies play a role in the destruction of red cells in autoimmune haemolytic anaemia. Normal red cells coated with autoantibody eluted from Coombs' positive erythrocytes have a shortened half-life after reinjection into the normal subject. Normal red cells also have a shortened survival when infused into patients with haemolytic anaemia, but only if they possess the antigens against which the patient's autoantibodies are directed showing that the destructive process must be linked to the autoimmune response. Platelet antibodies are apparently responsible for idiopathic thrombocytopenic purpura (ITP). IgG from a patient's serum when given to a normal individual causes a depression of platelet counts and the active principle can be absorbed out with platelets. The transient neonatal thrombocytopenia which may be seen in infants of mothers with ITP is explicable in terms of transplacental passage of IgG antibodies to the child.

Some children with immunodeficiency associated with very low white cell counts have a serum lymphocytotoxic factor which requires complement for its activity. Lymphopenia occurring in patients with SLE and rheumatoid arthritis may also be a direct result of antibody since non-agglutinating antibodies coating the white cells have been reported.

Thyroid

Cytotoxic antibodies. The serum of patients with Hashimoto's disease is cytotoxic for human thyroid cells growing in monolayer culture after dispersal by trypsin. This is a typical complement-mediated antibody reaction directed against cell surface antigens but it is still difficult to assess the extent to which this can operate *in vivo.* In the first place, simple fragments of thyroid gland grow out well in medium containing cytotoxic antibody and complement, and secondly, there is no evidence that infants born to Hashimoto mothers have defective thyroid function despite the presence of the antibody in their serum. Perhaps thyroid damage only occurs when there is collaboration with other factors such as immune complex deposition, ADCC or mechanisms mediated by sensitized T-cell effectors.

Thyroid stimulating antibodies. Under certain circumstances antibodies to the surface of a cell may stimulate rather than destroy (cf. type V sensitivity; chapter 8). This would seem to be the case in thyrotoxicosis (Graves' or Basedow's disease). There has long been indirect evidence suggesting a link between autoimmune processes and this disease: thyroid antibodies are detectable in up to 85 per cent of thyrotoxic patients and histologically the majority of the glands removed at operation show varying degrees of thyroiditis and local antibody formation in addition to the characteristic acinar cell hyperplasia (figure 10.8); thyrotoxicosis is found with undue frequency in the families of Hashimoto patients; there is an association with gastric autoimmunity in that 30 per cent have gastric antibodies and up to 10 per cent pernicious anaemia. The direct link came with the discovery by Adams and Purves of thyroid stimulating activity in the serum of thyrotoxic patients. Using a new bioassay they found that the serum caused a stimulation of the thyroid

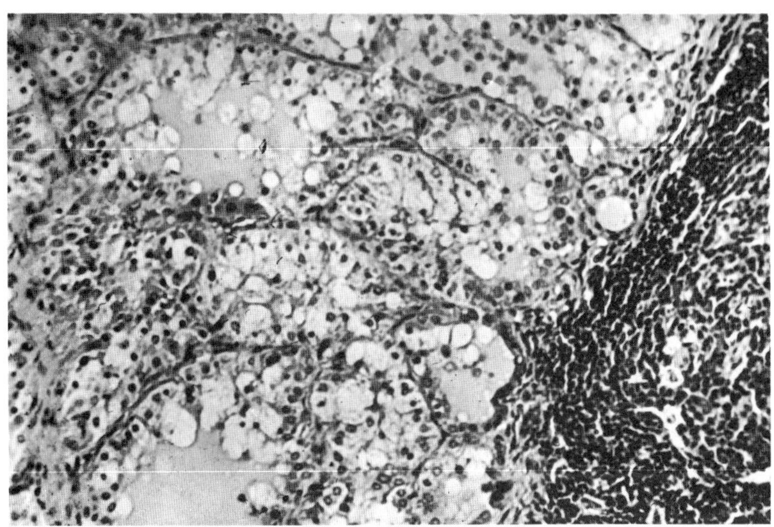

FIGURE 10.8. Lymphoid follicle adjacent to hyperactive thyroid cells in gland taken from patient with thyrotoxicosis.

gland of the recipient animal which was considerably prolonged relative to the time course of action of the physiological thyroid stimulating hormone (TSH) from the pituitary; it was ultimately shown that this was due to the presence of thyroid stimulating antibodies (TSAb). These antibodies can block the binding of TSH to thyroid membranes and seems to act in the same manner as TSH, probably by stimulating the identical receptors (cf. figure 8.17). Both operate through the adenyl cyclase system as indicated by the potentiating effect of theophylline, and both produce similar changes in ultrastructural morphology in the thyroid cell, but it is one of Nature's 'passive transfer experiments' which links TSAb most directly with the pathogenesis of Graves' disease. When TSAb from a thyrotoxic mother crosses the placenta it is associated with the production of neonatal hyperthyroidism, which resolves after a few weeks as the maternal IgG is catabolized.

There is a good correlation between the titre of TSAb and the severity of hyperthyroidism, because TSAb act independently of the pituitary–thyroid axis, and iodine uptake by the gland is unaffected by administration of thyroxine or tri-iodothyronine, whereas normally this would cause feedback inhibition and suppression of uptake; this forms the basis of an important diagnostic test for thyrotoxicosis.

There is reason to believe that enlargement of the thyroid

in this disorder is due to the action of growth-promoting antibodies which directly stimulate cell division as distinct from metabolic hyperactivity.

Intrinsic factor

Autoantibodies to this product of gastric mucosal secretion were first demonstrated in pernicious anaemia patients by oral administration of intrinsic factor, vitamin B_{12} and the serum from a patient with this disease. The serum was found to prevent intrinsic factor from mediating the absorption of B_{12} into the body, and further studies showed the active principle to be an antibody. Circulating antibody does not seem to be capable of neutralizing the physiological activity of intrinsic factor; a patient immunized parenterally with hog intrinsic factor in complete Freund's adjuvant had high serum antibody levels and good cell-mediated skin responses but still absorbed B_{12} well when fed with hog intrinsic factor. These data imply that the antibodies have to be present within the lumen of the gastrointestinal tract to be biologically effective, and indeed they can be identified in the gastric juice of these patients, synthesized by plasma cells in the gastritic lesion.

Sperm

In some infertile males, agglutinating antibodies cause aggregation of the spermatozoa and interfere with their penetration into the cervical mucus.

Glomerular basement membrane (gbm)

With immunological kidney disease the experimental models preceded the finding of parallel lesions in the human. Injection of cross-reacting heterologous gbm preparations in complete Freund's adjuvant produces glomerulonephritis in sheep and other experimental animals. Antibodies to gbm can be picked up by immunofluorescent staining of biopsies from nephritic animals with anti-IgG. The antibodies are largely if not completely absorbed out by the kidney *in vivo* but they appear in the serum on nephrectomy and can passively transfer the disease to another animal of the same species.

An entirely analogous situation occurs in man in certain cases of glomerulonephritis, particularly those associated with lung haemorrhage (Goodpasture's syndrome). Kidney biopsy from the patient shows *linear* deposition of IgG and C3 along the basement membrane of the glomerular capillaries (figure 8.12a). After nephrectomy, gbm antibodies can be detected in the serum. Dixon and his colleagues eluted the gbm antibody from a diseased kidney and injected it into a squirrel monkey. The antibody rapidly fixed to the gbm of the recipient animal and produced a fatal nephritis (figure 10.9). It is hard to escape the conclusion that the lesion in the human was the direct result of attack on the gbm by these complement-fixing antibodies. The lung changes in Goodpasture's syndrome may be attributable to cross-reaction with some of the gbm antibodies.

Muscle

The transient muscle weakness seen in babies born to mothers with myasthenia gravis calls to mind neonatal

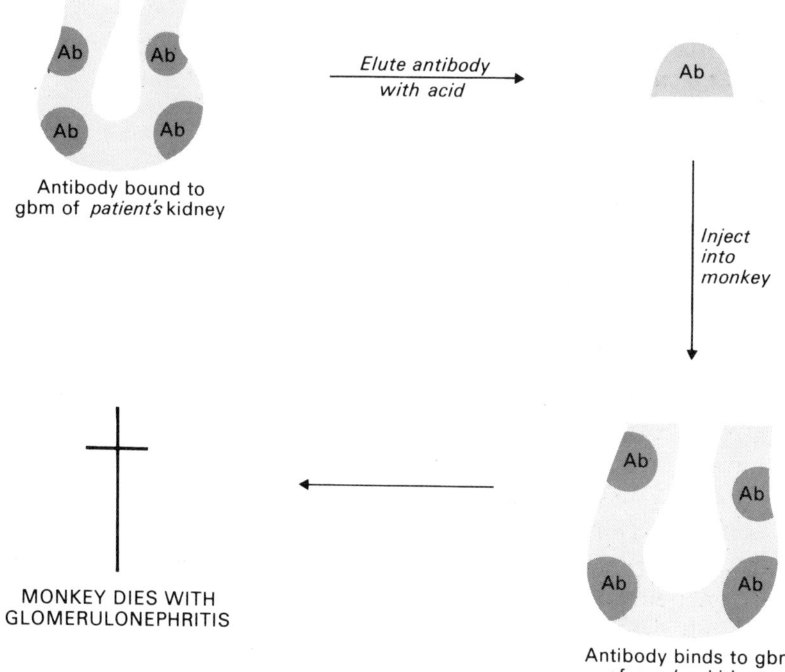

FIGURE 10.9. Passive transfer of glomerulonephritis to a squirrel monkey by injection of antiglomerular basement membrane (anti-gbm) antibodies isolated by acid elution from the kidney of a patient with Goodpasture's syndrome (after Lerner R.A., Glassock R.J. & Dixon F.J., *J.exp.Med.* 1967, **126**, 989).

thrombocytopaenia and hyperthyroidism and would certainly be compatible with the transplacental passage of an IgG capable of inhibiting neuromuscular transmission. Strong support for this view is afforded by the consistent finding of antibodies to muscle acetyl choline receptors in myasthenics and the depletion of these receptors within the motor end plates.

Table 10.4 summarizes these direct pathogenic effects of humoral autoantibodies.

EFFECTS OF COMPLEXES

Systemic lupus erythematosus (SLE)

Where autoantibodies are formed against soluble components to which they have continual access, complexes may be formed which can give rise to lesions similar to those occurring in serum sickness (cf. 237). In SLE, complexes of DNA and other nuclear antigens, and possibly

TABLE 10.4. Direct pathogenic effects of humoral antibodies

Disease	Autoantigen	Lesion
Autoimmune haemolytic anaemia	Red cell	Erythrocyte destruction
Lymphopenia (some cases)	Lymphocyte	Lymphocyte destruction
Idiopathic thrombocytopenic purpura	Platelet	Platelet destruction
Male infertility (some cases)	Sperm	Agglutination of spermatozoa
Pernicious anaemia	Intrinsic factor	Neutralization of ability to mediate B_{12} absorption
Hashimoto's disease	Thyroid surface antigen	Cytotoxic effect on thyroid cells in culture
Thyrotoxicosis	TSH receptors	Stimulation of thyroid cells
Goodpasture's syndrome	Glomerular basement membrane	Complement mediated damage to basement membrane
Myasthenia gravis	Acetyl choline receptor	Blocking and destruction of receptors
Acanthosis nigricans (type B) & ataxia telangiectasia with insulin resistance	Insulin receptor	Blocking of receptors

C-type viral components, together with immunoglobulin and complement can be detected by immunofluorescent staining of kidney biopsies from patients with evidence of renal dysfunction. The staining pattern with a fluorescent anti-IgG or anti-C3 is punctate or 'lumpy-bumpy' as some would describe it (figure 8.12b) in marked contrast with the linear pattern caused by the gbm antibodies in Goodpasture's syndrome (figure 8.12a; p. 231). The complexes grow in size to become large aggregates visible in the electron microscope as amorphous humps on the epithelial side of the glomerular basement membrane. During the active phase of the disease, serum complement levels fall as components are affected by immune aggregates in the kidney and circulation. Attempts to detect autoantigens in the circulating complexes have not been conspicuously successful; immunoglobulins and complement components make up the usual tally of constituents which can be identified. Although in a way negative evidence, this is consistent with the possibility that anti-idiotype perpetuates an autoimmune state once it is initiated (i.e. acts as a surrogate autoantigen) and generates circulating idiotype–anti-idiotype complexes.

Immunofluorescent studies on skin biopsies from patients with the related disease discoid lupus erythematosus also reveal the presence of immune complexes.

Rheumatoid arthritis

A strong case can be made for the fairly straightforward proposition that an autoimmune response to the Fc portion of IgG gives rise to complexes which are ultimately responsible for the pathological changes characteristic of the rheumatoid joint. Virtually all patients with rheumatoid arthritis have demonstrable antibodies to IgG—the so-called rheumatoid or anti-globulin factors. The majority have IgM antiglobulins which react in the classical latex and sheep cell agglutination tests (table 10.2; note 7) and both they and the 'sero-negative' patients who fail to react in these tests can be shown to have elevated levels of IgG antiglobulins detectable by tube absorption techniques (cf. p. 145) (figure 10.10). Sensitization to self IgG is therefore an almost universal feature of the disease.

The synovium typically is very heavily infiltrated with mononuclear cells often aggregated in the form of lymphoid follicles; there are many plasma cells and it has been estimated that the synthesis of IgG can be as high as that

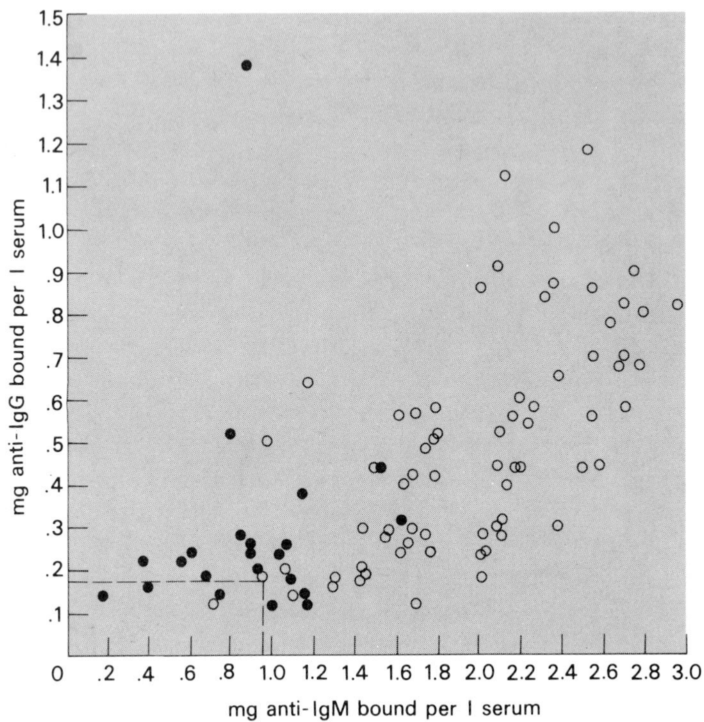

FIGURE 10.10. IgM and IgG antiglobulins determined by tube radioassay in patients with seropositive (○) and seronegative (●) rheumatoid arthritis. The dotted lines indicate the 95% confidence limits (mean + 2 S.D.) of the normal group. (From Nineham L., Hay F.C. & Roitt I.M. *J. clin. Path.* 1976, **29**, 1121.)

of a stimulated lymph node. If IgG is the main antigen responsible for evoking this response, most of the plasma cells should be synthesizing antiglobulins, yet only a minority (say 10–20%) bind fluoresceinated IgG, either in the form of heat-aggregated material or immune complexes (rheumatoid factor is a low affinity antibody and good binding is only seen when multivalent IgG is used as antigen). However, we must take into account a strange and unique feature of IgG antiglobulins; because they are both antigen and antibody at the same time, they are capable of self-association (figure 10.11b) and this hides the majority of free antiglobulin valencies. Cleverly realizing that destruction of the Fc regions by pepsin would liberate these hidden binding sites (figure 10.11c), Munthe & Natvig observed that as many as 40–70% of the plasma cells in the synovium displayed an anti-IgG specificity following treatment with this enzyme.

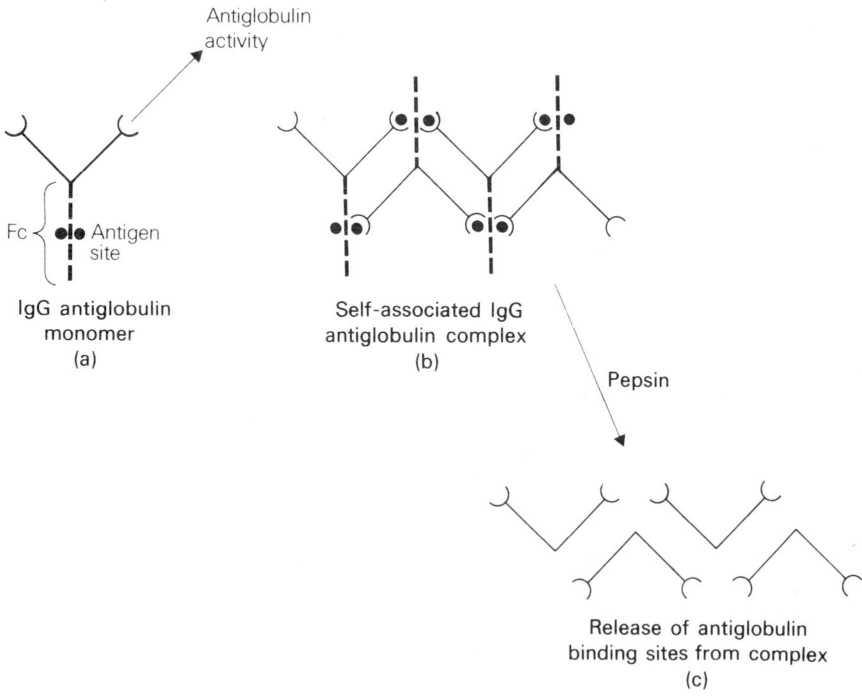

FIGURE 10.11. Self-associated complexes of IgG antiglobulins and the exposure of 'hidden' binding sites by pepsin. Such complexes in the joint may be stabilized by IgM antiglobulin and C1q which have polyvalent binding sites for IgG.

IgG aggregates, presumably products of these plasma cells, can be regularly detected in the synovial tissues and fluid. Analysis shows them to consist almost exclusively of immunoglobulins and complement while a major proportion of the IgG is present as self-associated antiglobulin as shown by binding to an Fcγ immunosorbent after treatment with pepsin. The complexes can mediate cartilage breakdown through different pathways (figure 10.12). In the joint space itself they initiate an Arthus reaction leading to an influx of polymorphs with which they react to release lysosomal enzymes. These include neutral proteinases and collagenase which can damage the articular cartilage by breaking down proteoglycans and collagen fibrils. More damage results if the complexes are adherent to the cartilage since the polymorph binds but is unable to internalize them ('frustrated phagocytosis'); as a result the lysosomal hydrolases are released extracellularly into the space between the cell and

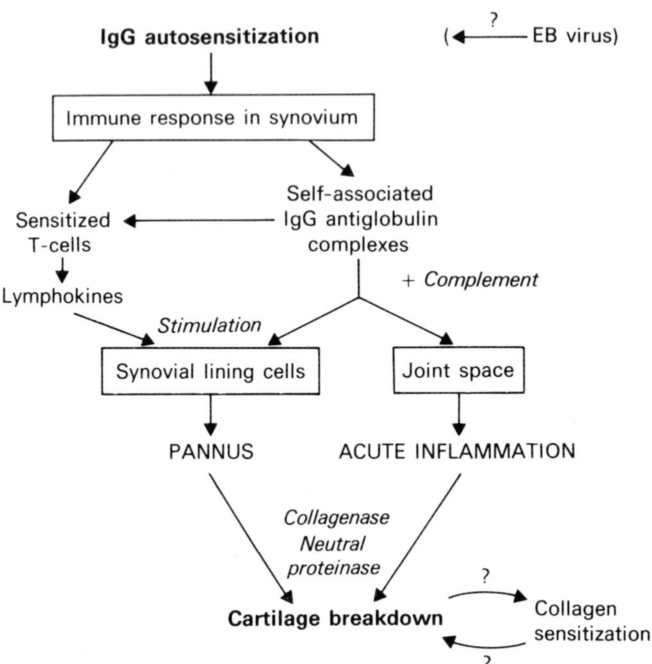

FIGURE 10.12. Hypothetical scheme showing how initial autosensitization to IgG can lead to the pathogenetic changes characteristic of rheumatoid arthritis.

the cartilage where they are protected from enzyme inhibitors such as α_2-macroglobulin.

The aggregates may also stimulate the macrophage-like cells of the synovial lining, either directly through their surface receptors or indirectly through the release of lymphokines from sensitized T-cells. The activated synovial cells grow out as a malignant pannus (cover) over the cartilage and at the margin of this advancing granulation tissue, breakdown can be seen, almost certainly as a result of enzyme release. Activated macrophages also secrete plasminogen activator and the plasmin formed as a consequence activates a latent collagenase produced by synovial cells. Sensitization to partially degraded collagen may occur and this could lead secondarily to amplification of the lesion. Prostaglandin E_2, another product of the stimulated macrophage, can bring about bone resorption which is a further complication of severe disease. Subcutaneous nodules are granulomata possibly formed through local production of insolubilized self-associating antiglobulins.

The rheumatological pulse has quickened perceptibly

with the recent discovery that a high proportion of patients with rheumatoid arthritis have circulating antibodies to a nuclear antigen present in EB virus transformed but absent from normal lymphocytes. Whether this betokens a primary aetiological role for EB virus infection or whether this is a phenomenon secondary to the disease will, one expects, be decided by investigation of patients with very early disease.

CELLULAR HYPERSENSITIVITY

The inflammatory infiltrate in organ specific autoimmune disease is usually essentially mononuclear in character and, although not an infallible guide, this has been taken as an expression of cell-mediated hypersensitivity. Direct evidence is still thin. At the time of writing, skin reactions to autoantigens have proved difficult to assess and *in vitro* leucocyte inhibition tests have not been unequivocally accepted although for example in autoimmune thyroiditis and thyrotoxicosis there is a consistent finding of inhibition of leucocyte migration by thyroid microsomes. The killing of colon cells in culture by lymphocytes from patients with ulcerative colitis is encouraging and it has been reported that long-term culture of thyroid target cells with Hashimoto leucocytes leads to significant failure in the metabolic handling of iodine. Firm evidence for a direct participation of T-lymphocytes in any of these reactions has yet to be provided. There is more inclination to think in terms of K-cell killing, either by pre-armed cells or of targets coated with antibody secreted into the cultures by the effector cell population. Thus the destruction of isolated liver cells by leucocytes from patients with HB_S-negative active chronic hepatitis can be blocked by antigen (hepatic lipoprotein) or by aggregated normal IgG (which would bind to K-cell Fc receptors), but is not affected by removal of T-cells.

Indirect evidence for a destructive role of the inflammatory cells comes from the observation that high doses of steroids may restore gastric function in certain patients with pernicious anaemia. In one such case studied, biopsy after intensive treatment with prednisone showed a diminution in the cellular infiltrate and new formation of parietal and chief cells in the gastric mucosa; acid and intrinsic factor were now produced after histamine stimulation and the ability to absorb vitamin B_{12} assessed by the Schilling test was restored to near normal values. The most likely explanation is that attack by the inflammatory cells and attempts to regenerate by mucosal cells were more or less in balance in the atrophic mucosa. Elimination of inflammatory cells by the prednisone allowed the regeneration of gastric mucosal cells to become evident.

Our views on the pathogenesis of pernicious anaemia may be stated as follows. Autoimmune attack based on the parietal cell antigen gives rise to an atrophic gastritis which in many cases settles down to a dynamic equilibrium where the rate of destruction roughly balances the rate of regeneration; the loss of capacity to make intrinsic factor is evident in tests showing defective B_{12} absorption but sufficient vitamin is absorbed to keep the body in balance. These patients often have parietal cell antibodies and go on for 15 years or so without developing megaloblastic anaemia. However, if they should produce antibodies to intrinsic factor in the lumen of the gastrointestinal tract, these will neutralize the small amount of intrinsic factor still available and the body will move into negative balance for B_{12}. The symptoms of B_{12} deficiency will then appear some considerable time later as the liver stores become exhausted (figure 10.13).

The nature of the cellular attack in organ-specific disorders is still not resolved but it is not improbable that cell-mediated hypersensitivity, direct antibody cytotoxicity and inflammatory reactions due to immune complexes may operate alone or in concert.

EXPERIMENTAL MODELS OF AUTOIMMUNE DISEASE

If autoimmune processes are pathogenic in human diseases we would expect that the production of autoimmunity should lead to comparable lesions in experimental animals.

Experimental autoallergic disease

When animals are injected with extracts of certain organs emulsified in oil containing killed tubercle bacilli (i.e. in complete Freund's adjuvant), autoantibodies and destructive inflammatory lesions specific to the organ used for immunization result. Thus, Rose and Witebsky found that rabbits receiving rabbit thyroglobulin in Freund's adjuvant developed antibodies to thyroglobulin and thyroiditis involving invasion of the gland by mononuclear cells of lymphocytic and histiocytic types with destruction of the normal follicular

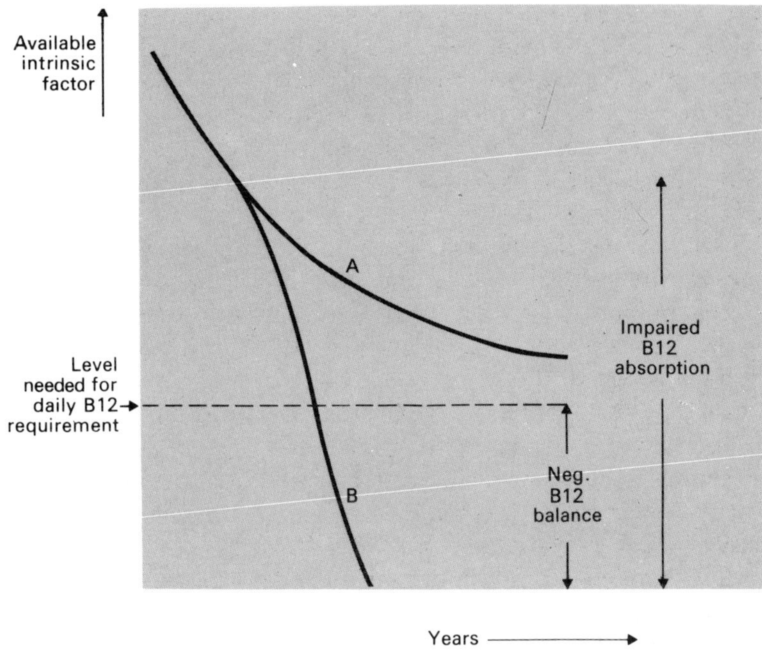

FIGURE 10.13. Pathogenesis of pernicious anaemia. Group A: Patients with long standing atrophic gastritis having parietal cell but no intrinsic factor antibodies. Group B: Pernicious anaemia patients with intrinsic factor antibodies superimposed upon the atrophic gastritis. (After Doniach D. & Roitt I.M., *Seminars in Hematology* 1964, **1**, 313.)

architecture. Histologically there are many points of similarity between this experimental autoallergic lesion and human autoimmune thyroiditis as seen in Hashimoto's disease and primary myxoedema (figure 10.14).

In some of the earliest work in this field it was shown that injection of central nervous tissue produced encephalomyelitis and paralysis in monkeys and guinea-pigs; the parallel with post rabies vaccine encephalitis is clear since the vaccine contains brain extracts, and optimistic comparisons with multiple sclerosis have been made. Similarly lesions can be induced in the adrenal (cf. Addisonian idiopathic adrenal atrophy), the testis (? model for granulomatous orchitis) and stomach (cf. atrophic gastritis of pernicious anaemia). Heterologous glomeruli stimulate the formation of glomerular basement membrane autoantibodies which localize in the kidney of the host to cause severe glomerulonephritis (Steblay model) resembling closely that seen in Goodpasture's syndrome.

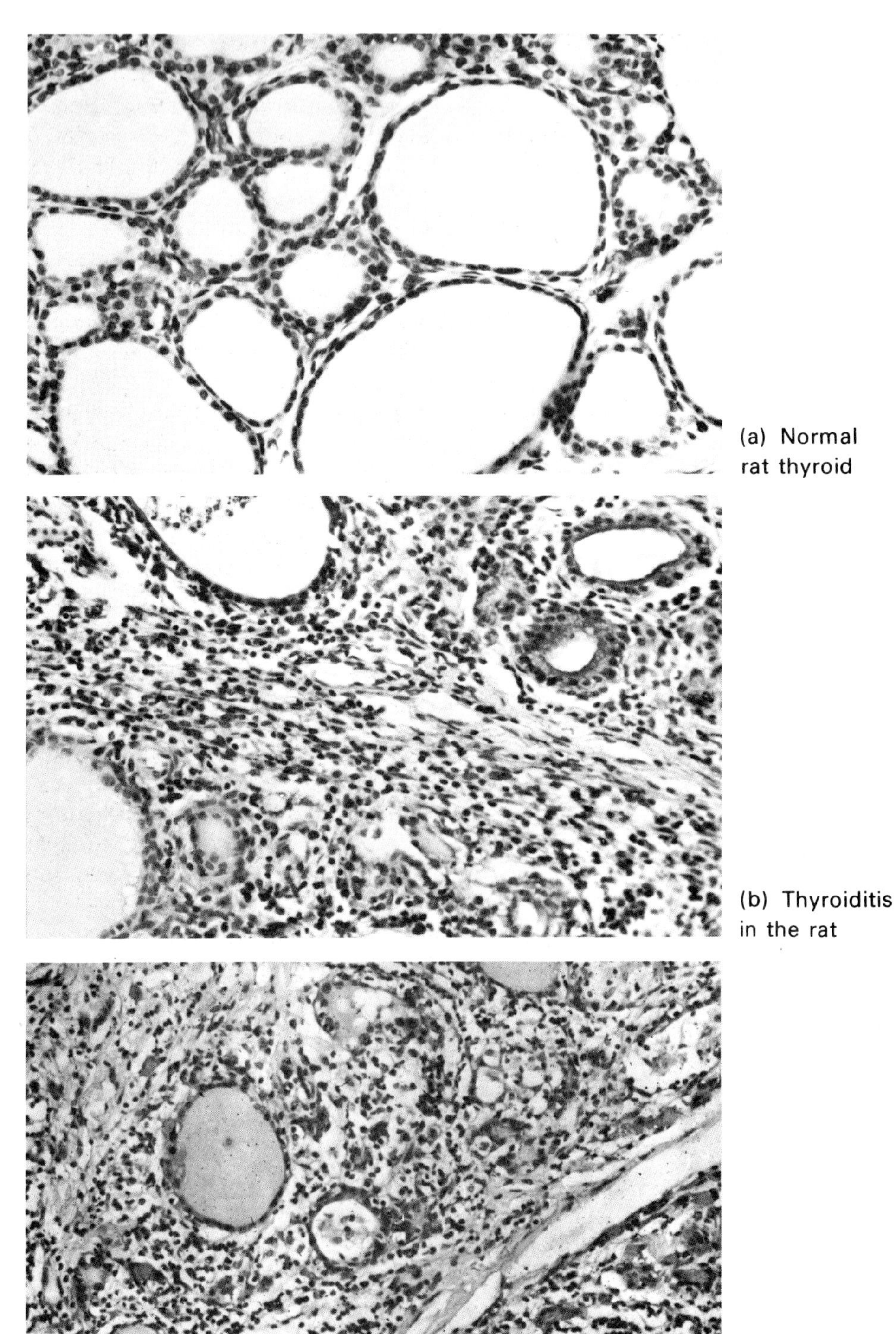
(a) Normal rat thyroid

(b) Thyroiditis in the rat

(c) Hashimoto disease

The experimental disease can usually be transmitted to syngeneic animals by lymphoid cells from immunized donors and occasionally by serum. In the case of experimental autoallergic orchitis, a synergism between cell-mediated hypersensitivity and antibody was recognized in the transfer studied.

Abnormalities of neuromuscular conduction resembling those seen in myasthenia gravis together with muscle autoantibodies can be evoked in guinea-pigs by muscle or thymus in Freund's adjuvant. Because these neuromuscular changes were *not* observed when the same experiments were carried out in thymectomized adults even though similar antibodies were formed, Goldberg put forward the view, independently supported by histological observations, that the fundamental lesion in myasthenia is an autoimmune reaction with the thymus as a target releasing a soluble factor which acts as an inhibitor of neuromuscular conduction. These results will have to be reconciled with the finding of functionally inhibitory antibodies to acetyl choline receptors in the human disease, and the production of an experimental myasthenic syndrome in rabbits by immunization with purified receptor from the electric eel.

The pre-eminent ability of Freund's complete adjuvant to enhance the production of experimental autoallergic disease may depend upon several factors acting concomitantly: modification of antigen, stimulation of T-helpers and (more controversially) disruption of normal T-suppressor feedback. Although the precise nature of the events leading to tissue damage have yet to be resolved, it is abundantly clear that the deliberate provocation of an autoallergic state can produce lesions which closely mimic those seen in human organ specific autoimmune disease and add weight to the notion that the immunological events are directly concerned in the pathogenesis of these disorders.

Spontaneous autoimmune disease

The message from animal models in which autoimmune disease develops spontaneously is the same. Neonatal bur-

---

FIGURE 10.14. Similarity of lesions in Hashimoto's disease of the human and experimental autoallergic thyroiditis produced by injection of rats with homologous thyroid in complete Freund's adjuvant. Other features of Hashimoto's disease such as the eosinophilic metaplasia of acinar cells (Askenazy cells) and local lymphoid follicles are not seen in this experimental model although the latter occur in the spontaneous thyroiditis of Obese strain chickens.

sectomy largely prevents the appearance of thyroglobulin antibodies and thyroiditis in Obese strain chickens, so pointing to a primary involvement of thyroid antibodies in the tissue lesions. Immunological control is also implicated by the exacerbation of disease caused by neonatal thymectomy.

The now famous strain of mouse, the New Zealand Black (NZB), consistently develops an autoimmune haemolytic anaemia with positive Coombs' tests (agglutination of antibody coated erythrocytes by an antiglobulin serum). As discussed earlier, the disease can be provoked in young unaffected NZB's by transfer of spleen cells from a Coombs' positive donor suggesting that it is the production of red cell antibodies which leads to shortened erythrocyte survival and consequent anaemia. A high proportion of these mice, and especially their hybrids with the partially related New Zealand White (B × W F1), have circulating antinuclear antibodies, may give a positive LE-cell test (cf. SLE p. 299) and have an immune complex induced glomerulonephritis. Several other mutant mouse strains which have SLE-like symptoms are also positive for anti-DNA and die with type III hypersensitivity kidney lesions.

Diagnostic value of autoantibody tests

Serum autoantibodies frequently provide valuable diagnostic markers. The most useful routine test is screening of the serum by immunofluorescence on a frozen section prepared from a composite block of unfixed human thyroid and stomach, and rat kidney and liver. This is supplemented by agglutination tests for rheumatoid factors and for thyroglobulin, thyroid microsome and red cell antibodies and by radioassay for antibodies to intrinsic factor, DNA and IgG (see table 10.2). The salient information is summarized in table 10.5.

The tests will also prove of value in screening for people at risk, e.g. relatives of patients with autoimmune disease, thyroiditis patients (for gastric autoimmunity and *vice versa*) and ultimately the general population.

Treatment of autoimmune disorders

The majority of approaches to treatment, not unnaturally, involve manipulation of immunological responses (figure 10.15). However, in many organ-specific diseases, metabolic control is usually sufficient, e.g. thyroxine replacement in

TABLE 10.5. Autoantibody tests and diagnosis

Disease	Antibody	Comment
Hashimoto's thyroiditis	Thyroid	Distinction from colloid goitre, thyroid cancer and subacute thyroiditis Thyroidectomy usually unnecessary in Hashimoto goitre
Primary myxoedema	Thyroid	Tests +ve in 99 per cent of cases. If suspected hypothyroidism assess 'thyroid reserve' by TRH stimulation test
Thyrotoxicosis	Thyroid	High titres of cytoplasmic Ab indicate active thyroiditis and tendency to post-operative myxoedema: anti-thyroid drugs treatment of choice although HLA-B8 patients have high chance of relapse
Pernicious anaemia	Stomach	Help in diagnosis of latent P.A., in differential diagnosis of non-auto-immune megaloblastic anaemia and in suspected subacute combined degeneration of the cord
Idiopathic adrenal atrophy	Adrenal	Distinction from tuberculous form
Myasthenia gravis	Muscle	When positive suggests associated thymoma (more likely if HLA-B12)
	ACh receptor	Positive in > 80%
Pemphigus vulgaris and pemphigoid	Skin	Different fluorescent patterns in the two diseases
Autoimmune haemolytic anaemia	Erythrocyte (Coombs' test)	Distinction from other forms of anaemia
Sjögren's syndrome	Salivary duct cells	
Primary biliary cirrhosis (PBC)	Mitochondrial	Distinction from other forms of obstructive jaundice where test rarely +ve Recognize subgroup within cryptogenic cirrhosis related to PBC with +ve mitochondrial Ab
Active chronic hepatitis	Smooth muscle anti-nuclear and 20 per cent mitochondrial	Smooth muscle Ab distinguish from SLE
Rheumatoid arthritis	Antiglobulin, e.g. SCAT and latex fixation	High titre indicative of bad prognosis
SLE	High titre antinuclear, DNA;LE-cells	DNA antibodies present in active phase Ab to double-stranded DNA characteristic
Scleroderma	Nucleolar	
Other 'collagenoses'	Nuclear	

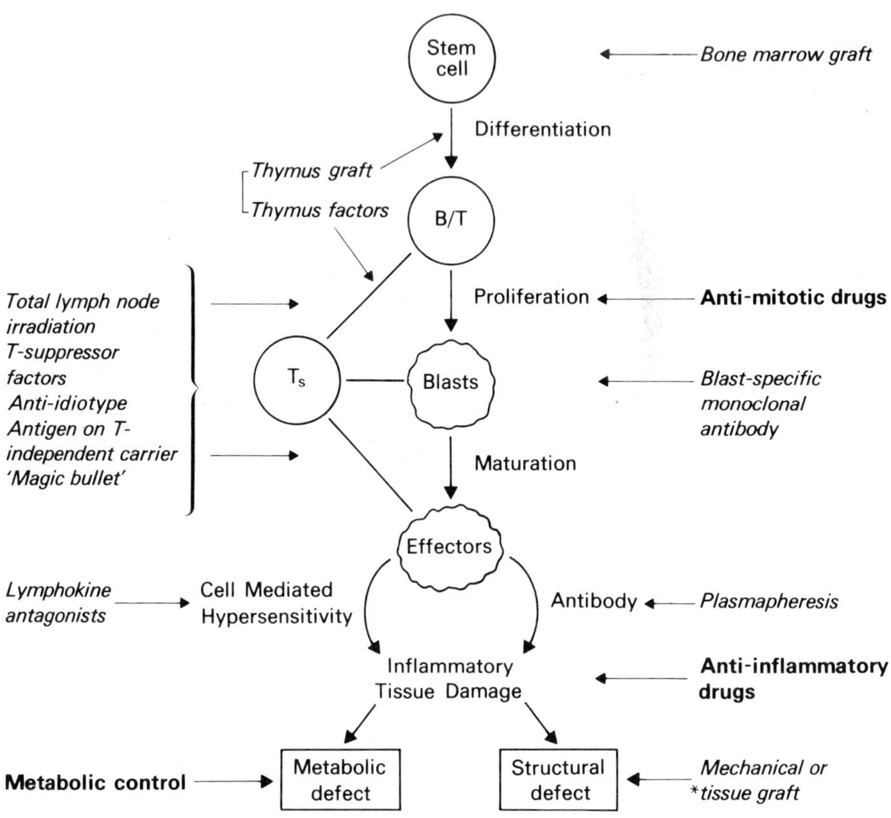

FIGURE 10.15. The treatment of autoimmune disease. Current conventional treatments are in bold type; some feasible approaches are given in italics. (*In the case of a live graft, the immunosuppressive therapy used may protect the tissue from the autoimmune damage which affected the organ being replaced.)

primary myoedema, insulin in juvenile diabetes, vitamin B12 in pernicious anaemia, anti-thyroid drugs for Graves' disease and so forth. Anticholinesterase drugs are commonly used for long-term therapy in myasthenia gravis. Thymectomy is of benefit in most cases and it is conceivable that the gland contains ACh receptors in a particularly antigenic form.

Patients with severe myasthenic symptoms respond well to high doses of steroids and the same is true for serious cases of other autoimmune disorders such as SLE and immune complex nephritis where the drug helps to suppress the inflammatory lesions.

In rheumatoid arthritis, apart from steroids, anti-inflammatory drugs such as salicylates, indomethacin, phenylbutazone and newer preparations such as fenoprofen and ibuprofen are widely used. Penicillamine, gold salts and antimalarials such as chloroquine all find an important place in therapy but their mode of action is unknown.

Therapeutic blocking of other mediators directly concerned in immunological tissue damage will be feasible if lymphokine and complement antagonists become available. Plasma exchange to lower the rate of immune complex deposition in SLE provides only temporary benefit although it may be of value in life-threatening cases of arteritis. Successful results have been obtained in Goodpasture's syndrome when the treatment has been applied in combination with anti-mitotic drugs, the rationale being an increased tendency for antigen reactive cells to divide as the negative feedback effect of IgG is lowered following removal of plasma proteins.

Cyclosporin A which preferentially hits dividing lymphocytes (p. 271) should similarly discriminate against the antigen-sensitive cells responding during autoimmune disease, but a pilot study in SLE has not been encouraging. If these cells carry a characteristic blast specific antigen, they should be vulnerable to attack by an appropriate anti-lymphocyte globulin. Several groups are trying to evolve a strategy based upon the 'magic bullet' (for some, the immunologists' 'holy grail'), the essence of which is to fashion different types of cytotoxic weaponry by coupling bacterial toxins or lots of radioactivity onto the antigen which selectively homes onto the lymphocytes bearing specific surface receptors.

While awaiting more selective therapy, conventional non-specific anti-mitotic agents such as azathioprine, cyclophosphamide and methotrexate have been used effectively in SLE, chronic active hepatitis and autoimmune haemolytic anaemia for example. It should one day be practical to correct any relevant defects in stem cells or in thymus processing by bone marrow or thymus grafting or perhaps, in the latter case, by thymic hormones.

We have already discussed the possible role of thymic factors in maintaining T-suppressor control of autoimmunity and one anticipates some interesting advances as the purified materials become available. Hybridoma technology or even gene cloning should ultimately provide the clinician with antigen-specific suppressor factors. The powerful immunosuppressive action of anti-idiotype antibodies has led to much rumination on the feasibility of controlling autoantibody production by provoking appropriate interactions within the immune network (cf. p. 102). Another potentially valuable approach for the future involves 'switching off' primed B-cells by presenting hapten linked to a thymus-independent carrier like the copolymer of D-glutamic and D-lysine (D-GL) or isologous IgG particularly when given with high cortisone doses. This has certainly worked well in NZB hybrid mice where anti-DNA levels have been reduced using nucleosides as the haptens: we shall have to see whether man and mouse really are that different.

Summary: comparison of organ-specific and non-organ-specific diseases

Organ-specific (e.g. Thyroiditis, Gastritis, Adrenalitis)	Non-organ specific (e.g. Systemic Lupus Erythematosus)
Differences	
1. Antigens only available to lymphoid system in low concentration	Antigens accessible at higher concentrations
2. Antibodies and lesions organ-specific	Antibodies and lesions non-organ-specific
3. Clinical and serologic overlap—thyroiditis, gastritis and adrenalitis	Overlap SLE, rheumatoid arthritis, and other connective tissue disorders
4. Familial tendency to organ-specific autoimmunity	Familial connective tissue disease ? Abnormalities in immunoglobulin synthesis in relatives
5. Lymphoid invasion, parenchymal destruction by ? $\pm$ cell mediated hypersensitivity ? $\pm$ antibodies	Lesions due to deposition antigen–antibody complexes
6. Therapy aimed at controlling metabolic deficit	Therapy aimed at inhibiting inflammation and antibody synthesis
7. Tendency to cancer in organ	Tendency to lymphoreticular neoplasia
8. Antigens evoke organ-specific antibodies in normal animals with complete Freund's adjuvant.	No antibodies produced in animals with comparable stimulation
9. Experimental lesions produced with antigen in Freund adjuvant	Diseases and autoantibodies arise spontaneously in certain animals (e.g. NZB mice and hybrids and some dogs) or after injection of parental lymphoid tissue into F1 hybrids

Similarities
1. Circulating autoantibodies react with normal body constituents
2. Patients often have increased immunoglobulins in serum
3. Antibodies may appear in each of the main immunoglobulin classes
4. Greater incidence in women
5. Disease process not always progressive; exacerbations and remissions
6. Association with HLA
7. Spontaneous diseases in animals genetically programmed
8. Autoantibody tests of diagnostic value

Further reading

Allison A.C. (1971) Unresponsiveness to self antigens. *Lancet*, **ii**, 1401.

Brent L. & Holborow E.J. (eds) (1974) *Progress in Immunology*. North Holland, Amsterdam.

Cooke A. & Lydyard P.M. (1980) The role of T cells in autoimmune diseases. In *Pathology, Research & Practice* **1**, 70. G. Fischer Verlag, Stuttgart.

Doniach D. & Bottazzo G.F. (1977) Autoimmunity and the endocrine pancreas. *Pathobiology Annual*, Iochim H.L. (ed.). Appleton–Century–Crofts, New York.

Fudenberg H.H., Stites D.P., Caldwell J.L. & Wells J.V. (1978) *Basic and clinical immunology*. 2nd ed. Lange Medical Publications, Los Altos, California.

Gell P.G.H., Coombs R.R.A. & Lachmann P. (eds.) (1975) *Clinical Aspects of Immunology*, 3rd ed. Blackwell Scientific Publications, Oxford

Glynn L.E. & Holborow E.J. (1964) *Autoimmunity and Disease*. Blackwell Scientific Publications, Oxford

Johnson P.M. & Faulk W.P. (1976) Rheumatoid factor: its nature, specificity and production in rheumatoid arthritis. *Clin.Immunol.Immunopath.*, **6**, 414.

Maini R.N. (1977) *Immunology of the rheumatic diseases*. Arnold, London.

Marchalonis J.J. & Cohen N. (eds) (1980) *Self/non-self discrimination*. Contemp. Topics in Immunobiol, Vol. 9. Plenum Press, New York.

Miescher P.A. *et al.* (1978) Menarini Symposium on *Organ Specific Autoimmunity*. Schwabe & Co., Basle.

Miescher P.A. & Muller-Eberhard H.J. (eds) (1976) *Textbook of Immunopathology*, 2nd ed. Grune & Stratton, New York.

Roitt I.M. & Doniach D. (1967) Delayed hypersensitivity in autoimmune disease. *Brit. med. Bull.* **23**, 66.

Rose N.R., Bigazzi P.E. & Warner N.L. (eds) (1978) *Genetic Control of autoimmune disease*. Elsevier/North Holland, New York.

Samter M. (ed) (1971) *Immunological Diseases*. Little Brown, New York

Talal N. (ed) (1977) *Autoimmunity*. Academic Press, New York.

Turk J.L. (1978) *Immunology in Clinical Medicine*, 3rd ed. Heinemann, London.

World Health Organization Technical Report Series (1973) No. 496, *Clinical Immunology*.

Appendix

TABLE 1. Recommended schedule for active routine immunization of normal individuals in the United Kingdom[1]

Age	Vaccine	Interval	Notes
During the first year of life	Dip/tet/pert and oral polio vaccine (first dose)		The earliest age at which the first dose should be given is three months, but a better general immunological response can be expected if the first dose is delayed to six months of age
	Dip/tet/pert and oral polio vaccine (second dose)	Preferably after an interval of six to eight weeks	
	Dip/tet/pert and oral polio vaccine (third dose)	Preferably after an interval of four to six months	
During the second year of life	Measles vaccine	After an interval of not less than three weeks	Although measles vaccination can be given in the second year of life, delay until three years of age or more will reduce the risk of occasional severe reactions to the vaccine which occur mainly in children under the age of three years
At five years of age or school entry	Dip/tet and oral polio vaccine or dip/tet/polio vaccine		These may be given, if desired, at three years of age to children entering nursery schools, attending day nurseries or living in children's homes.
Between 10 and 13 years of age	BCG vaccine		
All girls aged 11 to 13 years	Rubella vaccine	There should be an interval of not less than three weeks between BCG and rubella vaccination	All girls of this age should be offered rubella vaccine whether or not there is a past history of an attack of rubella
At 15 to 19 years of age or on leaving school	Polio vaccine (oral or inactivated) and tetanus toxoid		

[1] Data from *Immunisation Against Infectious Diseases* (1972), DHSS, London. (Reproduced from 'Immunisation', G. Dick, Update Books with permission of author and publishers.)

TABLE 2. Recommended schedule for active routine immunization of normal individuals in the USA[1]

Age	Vaccine	Notes
2 months	Dip/tet/pert and oral polio vaccine	Suitable for breast-fed as well as bottle-fed babies
4 months	Dip/tet/pert and oral polio vaccine	
6 months	Dip/tet/pert and oral polio vaccine	
1 year	Measles, rubella, mumps, tuberculin test	May be given at 1 year as combined measles–rubella or measles–mumps–rubella vaccines Measles vaccine may be given at 6 months in places where measles frequent in first year of life. In such circumstances a repeat dose should be given at 1 year. Frequency of repeated tuberculin tests depends on risk of exposure and prevalence of tuberculosis. Initial test should be at time of, or preceding, measles immunization
1½ years	Dip/tet/pert and oral polio vaccine	
4 to 6 years	Dip/tet/pert and oral polio vaccine	
14 to 16 years	Tet	And every 10 years thereafter

[1] Data from *Report of the Committee on Infectious Diseases* (1974), 17th edition, American Academy of Pediatrics, Evanston, Illinois. (Reproduced from 'Immunisation' by G. Dick, Update Books with permission of author and publisher.)

Index